TREATING SOMATIC SYMPTOMS
IN CHILDREN AND ADOLESCENTS

The Guilford Child and Adolescent Practitioner Series

Editors: **John Piacentini** *and* **John T. Walkup**

This series offers effective, innovative intervention strategies for today's child and adolescent practitioners. Focusing on persistent clinical challenges that cut across diagnoses and often come up in practice, books in the series present evidence-based tools for conceptualizing and addressing clients' individualized needs. These concise volumes provide what is missing from many evaluation and treatment manuals: the nuts-and-bolts techniques required for everyday clinical work. Each accessible guidebook includes a treasure trove of suggested interventions, complete with case examples, practical tips, sample dialogues, and practitioner-friendly resources, such as reproducible handouts and forms.

Teen Suicide Risk:
A Practitioner Guide to Screening, Assessment, and Management
Cheryl A. King, Cynthia Ewell Foster, and Kelly M. Rogalski

Psychological Interventions for Children with Sensory Dysregulation
Ruth Goldfinger Golomb and Suzanne Mouton-Odum

Treating Somatic Symptoms in Children and Adolescents
Sara E. Williams and Nicole E. Zahka

Treating Somatic Symptoms in Children and Adolescents

SARA E. WILLIAMS
NICOLE E. ZAHKA

Series Editors' Note by
John Piacentini and John T. Walkup

THE GUILFORD PRESS
New York   London

The authors have checked with sources believed to be reliable in their efforts to provide information that is
complete and generally in accord with the standards of practice that are accepted at the time of publication.
However, in view of the possibility of human error or changes in behavioral, mental health, or medical sciences,
neither the authors, nor the editor and publisher, nor any other party who has been involved in the preparation or
publication of this work warrants that the information contained herein is in every respect accurate or complete,
and they are not responsible for any errors or omissions or the results obtained from the use of such information.
Readers are encouraged to confirm the information contained in this book with other sources.

Library of Congress Cataloging-in-Publication Data

Names: Williams, Sara Elizabeth, 1976– author. | Zahka, Nicole E., author.
Title: Treating somatic symptoms in children and adolescents / Sara E. Williams and Nicole E.
    Zahka.
Other titles: The Guilford child and adolescent practitioner series.
Description: New York, NY : The Guilford Press, 2017. | Series: The Guilford child and
    adolescent practitioner series | Includes bibliographical references and index.
Identifiers: LCCN 2016049135 | ISBN 9781462529520 (hardcover : alk. paper)
Subjects: | MESH: Somatoform Disorders—therapy | Cognitive Therapy |
    Signs and Symptoms | Child | Adolescent
Classification: LCC RC552.S66 | NLM WM 170 | DDC 616.85/24—dc23
LC record available at *https://lccn.loc.gov/2016049135*

Illustrations by Scott Stoll.

About the Authors

Sara E. Williams, PhD, is a pediatric psychologist at Cincinnati Children's Hospital Medical Center, where she is Clinical Director of the Functional Independence Restoration (FIRST) program for inpatient pediatric chronic pain rehabilitation. She is also Associate Professor of Pediatrics at the University of Cincinnati College of Medicine. Dr. Williams specializes in assessing, treating, and researching pediatric chronic pain conditions.

Nicole E. Zahka, PhD, is a pediatric psychologist at Cincinnati Children's Hospital Medical Center. Her practice includes children and adolescents with chronic medical conditions and anxiety disorders, with a specialty in assessment and treatment of conversion and functional movement disorders, as well as syncope and gastrointestinal disorders.

Series Editors' Note

In The Guilford Child and Adolescent Practitioner Series, our goal is to provide practitioners with a library of relatively short, practical, theory-driven books focused on common clinical problems and key intervention techniques. The books in this series differ from existing treatment manuals in that they do not focus on specific disorders such as obsessive–compulsive disorder (OCD), major depression, or attention-deficit/hyperactivity disorder (ADHD), but rather on clinical issues that cut across specific disorders or fall between the so-called diagnostic "cracks." These clinical challenges—including the treatment of sleep and somatic problems, sensory intolerance, unwanted habits, and adolescent noncompliance, among others—are common in children and adolescents in therapy and can confound clinicians, many of whom have not encountered them in training or in their clinical work.

By offering clearly and coherently organized titles that provide relentlessly practical, step-by-step guidance, we hope to help busy practitioners select and implement the assessment and intervention strategies best suited to their needs. Common to each of these titles is an emphasis on the functional understanding of the antecedents (e.g., triggers) and consequent factors that serve to elicit and maintain the presenting problem. This theoretical framework provides a clear conceptual link between the target psychopathology and specific assessment and treatment techniques. Ample case examples illustrate case conceptualization and treatment selection and implementation. The technical aspects of the intervention are explained through clinical illustrations, sample dialogue, and handouts, forms, and other practitioner-friendly material.

Each book in the series provides relevant information about the topic problem, including a description of how the behavior begins and is maintained, and how the problem may manifest and change over development and across different settings and contexts. The theoretical models underlying the problem behavior and intervention strategies are presented along with existing research support for these strategies. Guidelines for recognizing and addressing challenges that may arise during treatment are also detailed. Finally, given the common occurrence of the target behaviors covered in this series with other clinical problems, strategies for integrating the selected treatment into a more comprehensive treatment plan are provided.

In this book, Sara Williams and Nicole Zahka describe the evaluation and treatment of children and adolescents with somatic symptoms, a challenging situation in which kids experience real, physical symptoms without known medical cause or easy explanation. As defined in this volume, somatic symptoms lasting for several months or more and leading to significant impairment are common in youth with medical and psychological disorders and can be highly perplexing, not only for the children and their families, but also for the medical and therapeutic communities with whom these individuals come into contact. As a result, affected youth can endure numerous costly and invasive medical procedures that fail to yield causal information or relief. Not surprisingly, high levels of frustration, distress, and disability are common.

Drs. Williams and Zahka, both expert pediatric psychologists with considerable experience working with children and adolescents suffering from somatic symptoms and with their families, present a comprehensive biopsychosocial model for evaluating and treating this often vexing problem. They expertly describe how the therapist can bridge the gap between the medical and psychological aspects of the child's experience and teach the child and family the connection between physical symptoms and underlying psychosocial stressors. Once the child and family have developed a reasonable understanding of these connections, cognitive-behavioral therapy is used to teach children how to respond to their stressors in a more adaptive way. Of critical importance, the authors also provide clear guidelines for therapists to use in navigating the larger treatment context, including step-by-step instruction in effective strategies for collaborating with other family members, schools, and health care professionals necessary to ensure generalizable and durable treatment outcomes.

Highly detailed case material and sample treatment plans provide therapists with the hands-on clinical material that is rarely available in treatment manuals. If you need expert guidance in dealing with puzzling presentations of complex symptom patterns, this is the right book for you. We are very familiar with the work of these authors and know their treatment approach to be very helpful in improving the lives of children and adolescents with somatic symptoms and those of their families. We trust the highly valuable information in this book will be extremely useful to you in your practice.

JOHN PIACENTINI, PHD
JOHN T. WALKUP, MD

Preface

It is Tuesday night, and Johnny feels sick. "Mom! I don't feel good," he groans. "I'm hot, my throat is scratchy, and my stomach hurts."

"Well, let's get you to bed and see how you feel in the morning," says his mom, feeling his head.

And so begins a usual interaction between a parent and a child that occurs when a child does not feel well. Often, the child wakes up in the morning having forgotten all about the previous day's complaint. Sometimes, however, even a good night's sleep is not enough to get back on track. When kids like Johnny wake up in the morning still feeling poorly, another chain of events takes place: children do not get out of bed and parents become worried. Maybe Mom remembers a note sent home from school warning of strep throat, so she stays home from work to take Johnny to the doctor. In straightforward medical encounters, children and families are in luck. They get a knowing look from the physician and complete a medical test right there in the office. A follow-up phone call later that afternoon confirms the suspicion—strep throat indeed—and a prescription is written along with a reminder not to share snacks with classmates. After five doses of medicine, a couple of days on the couch, and too many bowls of ice cream to mention, Johnny is back in action. He returns to school, his mom goes back to work, and life goes on.

This is the situation that medicine is made for and excels at in the modern scientific world. When a child's symptom complaints are clearly linked to organic processes, such as infections or bone breaks, the health problem is readily identified through routine testing and a diagnosis is confirmed. Closely on the heels of that smooth transaction follows a treatment plan, usually consisting of a medicine and instructions for rest. The collective expectations of the medical encounter are met; a disease is identified, medicines are prescribed to cure it, rest makes any lingering symptoms vanish, and everyone moves on. Modern medicine is truly a miracle.

But what about when it doesn't work this way? When children like Johnny go to the physician with the same complaints and complete the same tests, but this time the tests all come back negative? Everyone hopes the symptoms are just due to a bad cold or a lingering flu and will go away on their own, but they do not. They persist for weeks, then months. Follow-up tests are completed and those come back negative, too. So do the ones by the specialists. There is no infection, no injury or damage, nothing to explain the symptoms. Eventually, children and families are told that there is just no medical reason for these symptoms, never mind a treatment plan. With no answers and a sick child who is missing out on life as a result of these mysterious problems, suddenly modern medicine feels more like a nightmare than a dream.

This is the world of somatic symptoms: the presence of real, physical symptoms without easy explanation.

Imagine the frustration, confusion, and worry that children and families experience in these situations. Instead of heading home with a condition to search and a pill to swallow, the outcome of the visit to the doctor is quite *un*expected. In the place of a clear medical explanation for what the problem *is,* there is a lot of discussion about what the problem is *not*. Inevitably, an exasperated medical provider makes the dreaded statement that perhaps the child's symptoms are "all in his head," which is neither true nor helpful. There is no clear treatment plan or prescription to fill at the pharmacy. And with all of this confusion and uncertainty, there is definitely no indication of what to do tomorrow when that child wakes up with the same symptoms, which, quite likely, will be worse in the morning. The world of somatic symptoms is difficult to navigate for children and families, as well as the medical and therapeutic community. When these children and families show up in a mental health provider's office, it is important to have an understanding of their experience with these challenges and to share with them that, finally, there is something to offer as a way of coping with—and overcoming—somatic symptoms.

In the following chapters, we present a summary of what somatic symptoms are, who has them, where they come from, and how to understand them within a biopsychosocial framework. Throughout the book, the term "somatic symptoms" is used to represent a wide array of physical symptom descriptions, categories, and diagnoses that are common among children and adolescents. No matter what we call them, where they come from, or whether they rise to the level of a psychological disorder, somatic symptoms are best understood from a biopsychosocial approach and respond to the treatment described in this book. In-depth coverage of how to conduct effective assessment, education, and intervention for somatic symptoms will be provided. Finally, the importance of the larger treatment context, including how to collaborate with families, schools, and health care colleagues, will be reviewed. The goal of each of these aspects of treatment is to take the understanding of these conditions and apply the very best strategies for children to cope with symptoms and improve function (see Figure P.1).

We wrote this book as a resource to help mental health providers understand and treat children with somatic symptoms. This is the book we wish we had when we were training as pediatric psychologists, working in settings that ranged from outpatient mental health clinics to inpatient children's hospitals. If you are just starting out in your therapeutic work with children, this book will teach you the basics of assessment, education, and treatment for children with somatic symptoms. If you are experienced in treating children with anxiety and depression using a cognitive-behavioral approach, this book will allow you to integrate your existing tools within a somatic symptoms treatment framework and apply them to children with this presentation. A referral for conversion disorder may strike fear in the heart of even the most seasoned

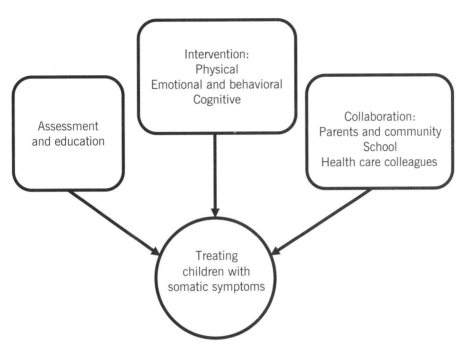

FIGURE P.1. Scope of the book.

mental health provider. With this book, we hope to reduce that fear and demystify the treatment of somatic symptom presentations. For all readers, this book provides a solid, evidence-based foundation and conceptual framework, and practical advice for effectively treating children and adolescents with somatic symptoms.

Throughout the book, there are many case examples as well as tips and tricks for working with children and families in this patient population, taken from our combined years of practice. We teach you how to explain these concepts in real terms to children and provide a framework within which to incorporate this information into your practice, but our true goal is for you to add your own familiar language and style to make it yours. All case material in this book is either composite or thoroughly disguised in order to protect privacy.

The materials presented in this book are designed to be practical and user friendly. There is a table of contents for the worksheets in the Appendix that can be used as a guide for treatment delivery, as the worksheets are presented in the order in which treatment is delivered. The treatment approach described in this book is applicable for young school-age children (6 and older) through older adolescents (18 years). For consistency's sake, the term "children" is used throughout the book, but the strategies are appropriate and effective for *both* children and adolescents. When applicable, different considerations are noted for younger children versus adolescents. Similarly, the term "parent" is used throughout this book, but families can be made up of many different people, and it is appropriate to think of any caregiver when "parent" strategies are discussed. Overall, through these materials, we hope that mental health providers take away a broader understanding of somatic symptoms and enhance their ability and confidence to treat children with these presentations.

Although the role of psychological intervention and the application of cognitive-behavioral therapy (CBT) to the treatment of children with somatic symptoms are the focus of this book, the importance of interdisciplinary treatment when it comes to working with this patient population cannot be overemphasized. Truly, CBT for children with somatic symptoms is most successful when done in collaboration with health care colleagues. As stated in upcoming chapters, understanding the biological role of symptoms is a core component of delivering effective treatment, and working with health care colleagues, including physicians, psychiatrists, nurses, physical therapists, and others, is essential to supporting children's success in physical areas in which they are struggling. In fact, a mental health provider should engage in treatment of a child with somatic symptoms *only* if the child has undergone medical consultation for his or her symptoms or is in the active care of a physician. While this book focuses on delivering outpatient care, this treatment can also be effectively implemented in other settings, such as medical or psychiatric inpatient or day treatment, where the content and order of intervention would remain the same but the frequency of sessions and ability to collaborate closely with team members would increase. Finally, children with somatic symptoms struggle in the social realms of their lives, and collaborating with families, friends, and teachers is also part of the process. When working with children, the larger context should always be kept in mind.

We are grateful to so many people for their influence in our personal and professional lives that has led us to complete this work. First, we thank our families for their love, editing, and general life expertise. We are indebted to the mentors with whom we have worked throughout our training and careers, who helped us find and grow our own passion for working with children with somatic symptoms and their families. We recognize how fortunate we are to work with a truly outstanding group of psychology and medical colleagues whom we learn from every day. And finally, we would like to acknowledge the children and families with whom we work, who are truly the source of inspiration for this book. We are grateful for their willingness to work with us, for the trust they showed by taking that first step toward wellness, and for teaching us about courage and perseverance. It is our sincere hope that more children and families are able to regain their lives through the treatment described in this book.

Contents

PART IV. COLLABORATION

Understanding Somatic Symptoms

INTRODUCTION

The first part of the book provides an overview of somatic symptoms in terms of definition, theory, and conceptualization. Essentially, this section gives mental health providers a good understanding of what somatic symptoms are, where they come from, and how to think about them. This foundation will allow effective engagement in the treatment approach outlined in upcoming chapters. Overall, the goal of Part I is to understand the nature of somatic symptoms prior to engaging with the sections on assessment, education, intervention, and collaboration that follow.

The role of cognitive-behavioral therapy (CBT) in the treatment of children with somatic symptoms is described in Chapter 1. Even for mental health providers who have experience working with children from a CBT perspective, the potential benefit or role of CBT for children with somatic symptoms may not be easy to see if one is not experienced in working within this patient population. However, CBT has something to offer to children with somatic symptoms in terms of managing distress and improving function, which is the ultimate goal of treatment. A theoretical review of the interplay between cognition, emotion, and behavior as applied to stress and coping provides the framework for understanding the application and efficacy of this treatment approach.

In Chapter 2, somatic symptoms are defined and presented in a historical context from both psychological and medical perspectives, including a review of the four major somatic symptom categories: neurological, cardiac, pain, and gastrointestinal. Somatic symptoms are real physical symptoms, sometimes with and sometimes without easy medical explanation, that impair function and quality of life and are associated with psychological distress and high levels of health care utilization. Demographic characteristics are reviewed, as well as the research on the nature of somatic symptoms. Although limited, empirical research suggests that the development and maintenance of somatic symptoms is multifaceted. In addition to what somatic symptoms are, information is presented on what somatic symptoms are *not,* with specific discussion of their distinction from factitious disorders and the role of unintentional secondary gain.

Finally, Chapter 3 discusses the application of the biopsychosocial model to somatic symptoms, which is grounded in the idea that somatic symptoms reflect an intersection of biological, psychological, and social factors. The theoretical foundation of biopsychosocial assessment and education is also presented, including explanations of the role of the autonomic nervous system, anticipatory anxiety, and gate control theory of pain. The chapter also provides clinical descriptions of these theories that can be used for education and intervention.

CHAPTER 1

Treating Children
with Somatic Symptoms

This chapter provides a basic introduction to somatic symptoms and the role of CBT in the treatment of children with this symptom presentation.

WHAT ARE SOMATIC SYMPTOMS?

Somatic symptoms are persistent physical health complaints that may or may not be associated with an identified medical or psychological condition, such as abdominal pain associated with irritable bowel syndrome, heart palpitations associated with panic disorder, or gait imbalance associated with no known reason. The majority of the literature on somatic symptoms in children focuses on symptoms that are medically unexplained or functional in nature, meaning they are symptoms in the absence of known disease (Stone, Carson, & Sharpe, 2005). This definition of somatic symptoms is fitting for most children who present for psychological intervention with these types of concerns and is the primary focus of this book, although, as stated in the preface, this treatment approach is also relevant for children with medically explained somatic symptoms.

Somatic symptoms are quite common, observed in nearly every area of pediatric specialty care, such as unexplained heart palpitations in cardiology and functional abdominal pain in gastroenterology (Campo & Fritsch, 1994). Other common somatic symptoms include dizziness, headache, fatigue, muscle weakness, nausea, or a combination of any of the above. Within the existing health care system, many children with somatic symptoms undergo multiple, costly medical procedures to rule out disease and return for multiple follow-up medical visits in continued pursuit of the cause of the symptoms (Belmaker, Espinoza, & Pogrund, 1985; Kaplan, Ganiats, & Frosch, 2004). However, many times, despite all of the tests and interventions, children and families do not find a diagnosis or symptom relief from a solely medical approach.

Children with persistent somatic symptoms experience high levels of disability and distress (e.g., Campo & Fritsch, 1994). Moreover, those who experience somatic

3

symptoms as children report higher levels of pain, disability, and health care utilization as adults compared to those without a childhood history of somatic symptoms
(Walker, Garber, Van Slyke, & Greene, 1995). Such current correlates and long-term
outcomes underscore the negative impact of somatic symptoms on children's lives,
adding to the importance of improving the understanding and treatment of children
with these conditions.

The traditional biomedical model of symptoms and disease does not explain
somatic symptoms, nor provide treatment guidance (Engel, 1977). Fortunately, a
paradigm shift has taken place in medicine toward the adoption of a biopsychosocial
model of symptoms and disease that better accounts for somatic symptoms (Drossman, 1998). Very simply put, this model acknowledges that regardless of etiology,
somatic symptoms are real *and* they are influenced by a child's emotional and behavioral responses, as well as the context in which children live. Health care providers'
difficulty with providing explanation and treatment for somatic symptoms has been
associated with frustration for children and families (Walker, Katon, Keegan, Gardner, & Sullivan, 1997a). Understanding and treating somatic symptoms from a biopsychosocial framework with an interdisciplinary team (e.g., physician, mental health
provider, and physical therapist) has the potential to improve the clinical encounter
and thereby enhance health outcomes for children with somatic symptoms. This is
what we seek to do in this book—provide information on psychological assessment,
education, and treatment for somatic symptoms that mental health providers can use
to significantly improve the lives of children with these conditions.

Somatic Symptoms Are Real

Somatic symptoms are true physical complaints, produced by and experienced in
the body; however, their distinguishing feature is that they are not dangerous in the
sense that they are not signs of identifiable damage or illness. As will be discussed in
detail in Chapters 2 and 3, somatic symptoms are often the result of false signaling
and maladaptive patterns in the nervous system. This is what makes somatic symptoms unique. Typically, physical symptoms signal disease or bodily distress and are
good indicators of when our body needs attention. We are biologically predisposed
to attend to these alarms that alert us to danger and allow us to either prevent further
damage or conduct further investigation to promote healing. They are the body's best
communication tools for surviving and staying a healthy course in life. It makes sense
that a person would take note when they arise and, in the best-case scenario, solve the
problem that is causing the symptom. Then symptoms usually go away, as their job is
done and restored health is on its way.

The problem with somatic symptoms is that they *are not* signaling imminent
danger, and in this sense, they are like a false signal. Unfortunately, because of this,
there is often no quick solution that will turn off the signal and as a result, symptoms
do not easily go away. Instead, they get attention, as the body is trained to do, and
over time this can create significant problems both in terms of feeling quite ill, and
of becoming significantly disabled by the symptoms. For example, as anyone knows
who has heard the pinging of a smoke detector in the middle of an otherwise quiet
night, sometimes even the best alarm systems get it wrong. But we jump every time

because we are trained to do it, and over time that response creates problems of its own. Such is the case for somatic symptoms, like a series of drills without any smoke or fire.

Ping, Ping, Ping

To get an even better sense of the somatic symptom experience, imagine for a minute what it would be like to have a false signal wreaking havoc in *your own life*. Most people have had the experience of hearing the noise of a pinging smoke detector in their home and are trained to pay attention to this type of signal—missing the cue that a fire is happening in your home would have negative consequences, after all. Because these types of situations always seem to happen at 3:00 A.M., imagine that you are sound asleep and are woken up by that very sound: Ping! Ping! Ping! Most likely, you dutifully get out of bed to investigate. Right away, you are relieved to see that there are no flames. Phew! But you still have a problem, because while you know the signal is false in the sense that it is not alerting you to danger, it is still ringing, and that is going to make it very hard to get back to sleep. You quickly think of the next obvious solution—it must be a low battery. You locate a spare, fumble with the smoke detector cover, and make the replacement. You hop back into bed, but no sooner than your head hits the pillow, you hear it again, Ping! Ping! Ping! Oh dear—you sit back up.

What could be going on? There is no fire (you check again just to be sure) and you just put in a brand-new battery. The signal is very real and bothersome, yet it is also completely unhelpful. You decide that this situation must be complicated, certainly more than you can handle at 3:00 A.M., and defer further investigation until the morning. You insert a pair of earplugs, gather up as many pillows as you can find to cover your head, and get back to bed, telling yourself that while this sound is incredibly annoying, it does not mean that you are in danger. It is a tough night. Turns out, it is really hard to ignore a signal to which you are trained to attend.

In the morning, you have an extra cup of coffee and declare your determination that this is a problem you can solve. You do a quick review: the most likely causes of this sound—either a fire or a low battery—have to do with the smoke detector itself, and you have ruled both of those out. You realize that you have to think outside the box—this is hard, you did not sleep so well—so you consult with a particularly handy friend who is also better rested than you. Together you realize that there is a third plausible, yet less obvious, solution: perhaps the problem is not at the source, maybe it is *systemic*, such as a glitch in the wiring or home alarm system. Now you are getting somewhere. You realize this must be why your previous solutions did not work; although it *seemed* like the problem was at the location of the signal—the smoke alarm itself—it must be bigger than that. With a call to the specialists—in this case, the electrician and the home alarm company—you have a technician visit your house later that day, the faulty wiring is identified, the system is reset, and you hear the best sound you have ever heard in your life: silence. You did it! The solution was not obvious, but it was there. You just had to look in a different place.

Now, take this example one step further. It is a fanciful extension, but a very real one when it comes to the experience of somatic symptoms. Imagine that it did not occur to you that the cause of your pinging smoke detector was systemic, and you remained convinced it was a problem at the source of the ringing, which despite all your attempts could not be turned off. What would life be like living with this noise? No matter how many times you reassure yourself that there is no fire, the fact that the alarm keeps ringing begins to create problems of its own. Your sleep becomes disrupted, for one. The accumulated sleep deprivation makes it difficult to function well at work. Pretty soon, even when you are out of the house, all you can think about is that terrible sound. It is hard to tell anymore if the signal is "real" or just a very vivid recollection. Your stress level climbs and you develop the world's shortest fuse. Think of the time and effort you would spend trying to figure out why this was happening and attempting to fix it. You might enlist all of the "right" help from handymen, neighbors, or anyone who was willing to listen to your struggles; but, alas, imagine that none of these folks looked at the bigger picture either, and thus their efforts to fix the problem were also to no avail. Ping, ping, ping. Your friends and family may question your sanity at some point—they might even have the audacity to suggest that you are just making this sound up or that you've engineered this whole situation as a desperate cry for attention. Imagine how frustrating *that* would be! As if you would ever *choose* to torture yourself in this manner!

Take a moment to really imagine this situation, however extreme it may seem. Imagine how stuck you would feel and how exhausted you would become. For children with somatic symptoms who have an alarm ringing all the time that they haven't been able to turn off, these are *exactly* the types of challenges they face on a daily basis. For some children and families, they haven't yet figured out that there might be a systemic reason for the problem (and more important, a systemic solution), while others may understand that it is systemic but still be having a hard time resetting the system. Just like pinging smoke detectors, somatic symptoms also have a solution; it is just not the obvious one and because of that, initially at least, it may be harder to implement.

Diagnoses and Disorders

When somatic symptoms persist, become severely distressing, and impact function, they rise to the level of being considered as a disorder. Somatic symptom diagnoses go by many different names, which adds to the confusion of understanding, explaining, and treating children with these problems. A few examples of somatic symptom conditions are the more historical term "somatoform disorder," any kind of functional disorder or syndrome, conversion disorder, and also medically unexplained physical symptoms, or MUPS. The term "functional" is often used interchangeably with "somatic" to describe these kinds of symptoms, which refer to physiological systems in the body that are not working or functioning well together. Disorders of function are different from "organic" disorders, which are more traditionally thought to come from disease or injury. Despite the disagreement in nomenclature, all of these terms and phrases refer to symptoms that are real and distressing, stem from a larger problem usually rooted in the nervous system, and are difficult to treat solely in a medical setting. For the purposes of this book, the term "somatic symptoms" is used to broadly refer to symptoms without disease across a wide variety of body systems.

The medical and psychological diagnoses that are used for children presenting with somatic symptoms are described in detail in Chapter 2.

It is also important to note that when the term "somatic symptom" is used in this book, it does not refer to an intermittent stomachache or headache that keeps a child out of school for a day or two. Somatic symptom diagnoses are reserved for children who have more than just transient experiences and impairment. In children, impairment is measured by how much symptoms interfere with or prevent engagement in typical or developmentally appropriate activities. This can include school absence, receiving poorer-than-usual grades, mobility impairment (e.g., in walking, running, climbing stairs), difficulty engaging in gym or sports, lack of engagement with friends or extracurricular activities, or inability to complete activities of daily living (e.g., feeding, dressing, bathing).

Medical Evaluation and Treatment

Because somatic symptoms present as physical problems, most children initially seek treatment in a medical setting. To the physician, these patients present like any other patient and his or her family, having a physical problem and seeking a medical solution. Patients and families similarly expect a "routine" medical encounter in which they will receive a medical diagnosis and treatment plan. However, when these expectations are not met, as is often the case for somatic symptoms, children and their families, and sometimes even health care providers, become quite frustrated. As mentioned above, using a biopsychosocial assessment and treatment approach is advantageous for all of the child's providers, as well as patients and families. Engaging in this approach provides a diagnosis (e.g., "I know what you have, and it is called 'functional abdominal pain'"), explains the symptoms from a physical standpoint to validate the role of biological factors, and opens the door to discussing psychosocial factors that may be contributing to and maintaining the somatic symptoms. The biopsychosocial model is reviewed in detail in Chapter 3.

Unfortunately, some children and families still may be resistant to this multidisciplinary, biopsychosocial approach based on their expectation that treatment for *any* physical symptom should be a more traditional medical solution, such as undergoing surgery or another procedure or being prescribed a medication. They may also expect a more passive treatment recommendation, which is a common expectation for medical treatment, meaning that they would expect to be given something (e.g., medication) and then rest while waiting for it to work. However, this is far from the message that families hear from their providers when given the diagnosis of a somatic symptom condition. They may receive an explanation of somatic symptoms from a biological standpoint, but they are now asked to consider the psychosocial aspects that contribute to the illness, which may represent an entirely new way of thinking for them. Moreover, a passive treatment approach is rarely effective for any condition, as it ignores the activity requirements that are part of the recovery from a physical condition, especially a somatic one; however, families do not expect to hear this. The greatest treatment success will be realized by providers from all disciplines who encourage families to see that their children *themselves* need to have the primary role in improving their overall health and well-being.

THE ROLE OF PSYCHOLOGICAL INTERVENTION

Eventually, at some point in their search for answers, these children and families show up in the office of a mental health provider—a psychologist, social worker, counselor, or therapist—if not for help managing the stress that may have been suggested as a root cause of these unexplained symptoms, then certainly for the stress that has been created by having something so mysterious that no medicine can even fix it. In more traditional medical models, somatic symptom diagnoses are those of *exclusion* ("The test is negative, so it is *not* this or that . . .") versus diagnoses of *inclusion* ("The test is positive, so it *is* this!"), so children and families have usually been through a lot of tests with few conclusions, deepening their sense of frustration and confusion. When a family arrives in a mental health provider's office, they may share experiences such as "Our doctor said there must be psychological problems causing these symptoms because they cannot find anything else," or "We were told to come see you but really we think more medical tests need to be done," or "We are at our wits' end and literally have no idea what else do to." Children and families are looking for someone, anyone, to help. As part of a team of health care colleagues, the mental health provider plays a central and prominent role in treatment.

Understanding the Journey

When working with children with somatic symptoms and their families, it is safe to assume they have been on a frustrating and sometimes long journey, filled with confusing messages. Mental health providers are charged with the responsibility of communicating to children and families that just because medical intervention did not work or is not straightforward, this does not mean that symptoms are "all in their heads." It is not mind versus body, but mind *and* body, and by understanding these connections instead of fighting against them, children and families can learn very effective ways to manage and overcome somatic symptoms.

First, the mental health provider, like the child and family, needs to recognize that this is not a typical referral. Many times, children with somatic symptoms did not begin their journey toward wellness by intending to seek out mental health treatment. These are children who initially presented in a health care setting with suspected medical problems but through a series of twists and turns end up with a referral to a mental health provider. For example, just as an anxious child expects to seek treatment from a mental health provider, a child with somatic symptoms expects to receive treatment from a health care provider. This is why some children and families have a difficult time coming to terms with a mental health referral.

And, as much as children with somatic symptoms and their families might be surprised to see a mental health provider, mental health providers might be surprised to know that *children with somatic symptoms are already in the office*. They are the same children who presented for treatment of anxiety but, by the way, have terrible daily stomachaches. They just might not think to mention it, because they are there for treatment of worries, and stomachaches get reported to the primary care provider, after all. Mental health providers might be surprised by how often current patients report stomachaches or headaches during the course of a week.

Both for the children who never expect to meet a mental health provider and for the ones who are already receiving treatment, coping skills can be offered for somatic symptoms. Children with somatic symptoms are not unlike the children already seen in mental health practices for treatment of anxiety or behavioral issues. Some children who present with mental health concerns may be more aware, vocal about, or demonstrative of their anxiety or mood challenges compared to children who present with somatic complaints, who may have more pronounced physical symptoms, difficulty labeling their feelings, or feelings of stigma surrounding mental health. However, there are many more similarities than differences between these populations.

The Search for "Truth"

Sometimes when patients are referred to a mental health provider and the medical provider has not been able to determine a solely organic source for the symptoms, a suggestion is made that the child must have experienced a significant stress or trauma that caused the symptoms, and the mental health referral is made with the idea that the hidden "true" cause will be uncovered. This is yet *another* frustrating experience for families, who often understand their child is stressed by this whole experience but are adamant that nothing significant happened that started off the chain of events. There is not support in the literature for the supposition of a significant stressor preceding somatic symptom presentation. If a stressor does happen around the time that symptoms begin, it usually happens in combination with a physical process, and an association forms between the stressor and the symptoms. It is important to consider that a stressor can be something as "little" as returning to school after missing a big test due to an episode of food poisoning, or the additive effects of childhood stressors rather than one big event. Additionally, a stressor does not have to be emotional: it can be pushing the body through a physical challenge on a hot day without enough fluids. Sometimes, just being a kid with confusing health problems is stressful enough to cause disability. Rarely is there one stressor underlying the symptom presentation. The question of whether a stressor has "caused" somatic symptoms comes up almost immediately upon meeting children with somatic symptoms, which can be related to unhelpful feelings of guilt or shame on the part of the child and family. As a mental health provider, be aware of this question, as children and families have often not been validated in their prior experiences and this is an assurance that can be swiftly provided. This is one way that a mental health provider brings relief and understanding to children with somatic symptoms.

The Role of the Mental Health Provider

Like parents and medical providers, mental health providers are often stymied by the problems these children present. If children do not have a straightforward diagnosis of anxiety or depression along with their symptoms, it can be hard to know what treatment, if any, will benefit them. It could be argued that the unique place a mental health provider occupies in children's treatment—a bridge between the medical and psychological worlds—offers an *advantage* in understanding how to effectively provide treatment and have a real, lasting impact on children and families.

The mental health provider in this role is part educator and part therapist, a partner to the child and family in communicating their experience to school and the community, as well as a partner to medical providers in improving treatment of children's symptoms. It requires patient practice in the art and science of giving enough explanation to help children and families better understand and move forward from symptoms without feeling overwhelmed. Most times, the role is an exceedingly positive one that provides hope and a real solution, while teaching children to become more resilient copers. A mental health provider is a firm but empathic listener and teacher who enables children to realize achievements in their lives that they believed to be unattainable and empowers parents and schools to set limits they felt were impossible to impose on a struggling child—limits that are exactly what are needed to get the child back on track. Overall, a mental health provider gives much-needed understanding, support, and guidance to children with somatic symptoms and their families, all of which can be done through the application of treatment skills that are likely already familiar.

COGNITIVE–BEHAVIORAL THERAPY

When children and families arrive in a mental health provider's office, not only have they been on a difficult journey in terms of understanding somatic symptoms, they have heard confusing messages about why they have been referred or what therapy will entail. When children are asked why they are seeing a therapist, they might say, "Well, my doctor told me I needed to learn some coping skills." And when asked to clarify, they say, "I don't know, but my doctor felt pretty convinced you would help me!" At best, children have the good impression that a mental health provider is a helper. At worst, they have preconceived notions regarding what a mental health provider does or what psychological therapy entails and as a result may be fearful or uncertain of what is about to occur. Either way, education about *how* psychological intervention is applied to somatic symptoms is given in order to provide children and families with a clear understanding of what they will do in treatment. Understanding somatic symptoms through the biopsychosocial model allows providers to see the connection between physical symptoms and psychosocial stressors, and cognitive-behavioral therapy (CBT) provides the tools to teach children how to respond to these stressors in a more adaptive way. To begin the discussion of how to treat children with somatic symptoms, we review the theoretical basis and application of CBT (Beck, Rush, Shaw, & Emery, 1979), the best evidence-based psychological intervention for children in this patient population.

The Theory of Stress and Coping

The Lazarus and Folkman (1984) model of stress and coping offers a theoretical framework for understanding cognitive, emotional, and behavioral responses to stress that provides the foundation for the therapeutic work of CBT as applied to somatic symptoms. In this model, stress is conceptualized as "a relationship between the person and the environment that is appraised as taxing or exceeding resources and endangering well-being" (Lazarus & Folkman, 1984, p. 21). By this definition, a situation is not *inherently* stressful or benign; stress results only when the individual *thinks* of the encounter as threatening. Thoughts then influence feelings and actions, and together this pattern determines an individual's experience, which then provides feedback to the person to remember for the next time (e.g., "That fire alarm *did* mean there was a fire, and next time I better respond to it even faster!"). In this way, a person's thought process is the starting point from which emotions and actions follow, which can lead to either maladaptive or adaptive results. These are the connections that are addressed in the application of CBT for somatic symptoms.

To understand how the theory of stress and coping applies to children with somatic symptoms, consider the relationship of the cognitive, emotional, and behavioral factors involved in the symptom experience. As posited by Lazarus and Folkman (1984), any negative response or reaction that a person experiences in a stressful situation—such as unpleasant affect or maladaptive changes in behavior—is a *consequence* of negative thinking. In traditional CBT models, this is usually the result of what are considered to be "automatic" negative beliefs, cognitive distortions, or possible misinterpretations of a situation (Beck et al., 1979). Applied to children with somatic symptoms, the initial stressor could be conceptualized as the experience of the somatic symptoms themselves. Whether the child was calm and coped positively (adaptive outcome) or became anxious and coped negatively (maladaptive outcome) would be determined by the child's thoughts about where that symptom came from (e.g., "I'm just tired" or "What if I have cancer?") and what it meant to his or her current state of being (e.g., normal and transient vs. threatening and dangerous).

As previously mentioned, a unique feature of somatic symptoms is that they are real, but not dangerous in terms of alerting us to acute bodily harm. However, the mind is set up to think of *any* symptom as dangerous, in which case it is easy to see the effect of a corresponding negative emotional and action pattern. Alternatively, an initial stressor could be conceptualized as a child taking a test in school, and a negative thought pattern about the situation could promote a feeling of worry or fear that would fuel somatic symptoms and result in a poor outcome on the test for the child. In this way, the model of stress and coping allows for somatic symptoms to be conceptualized as the stressor itself or as an effect of other stressors that children encounter in their daily lives.

Cognitive Triad

In applying this theory of stress and coping to CBT, the points of intervention can be found and used to identify unhelpful patterns and change them. Thoughts, feelings, and actions are interrelated, as illustrated in the cognitive triad (Figure 1.1). CBT works from the concept that there are two points on the triangle that can be directly changed: thoughts and actions (Beck et al., 1979). Feelings are not something that can be directly changed, as it is not the common experience that an emotional or physical state can be changed without thinking or doing something differently. Because negative thoughts lead to unpleasant affect and maladaptive behaviors, changing *thoughts* should result in more neutral or even positive feelings and behaviors. Additionally, *doing* something different is another way to influence the thinking

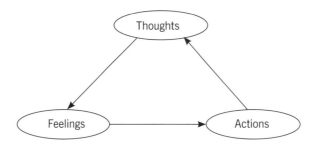

FIGURE 1.1. The CBT model.

and feeling pattern in a positive way. When providing CBT to children with somatic symptoms, both of these points are important during intervention; the motto "Just do it" would certainly apply here, and additionally, "Just think it." Examining thoughts and changing behavior are the goals of CBT for somatic symptoms, to turn maladaptive stress and coping responses into more adaptive patterns that improve children's function.

Automatic Negative Thoughts

In cognitive theory, it is considered part of the normal human experience to have what are termed *automatic* negative thoughts, as these are designed to protect a person by alerting them to danger (Beck et al., 1979). However, in cases where acute danger is *not* present, automatic negative thoughts may lead people down an unnecessarily anxious, symptom-amplifying, and avoidant path. This is where CBT comes in as an effective treatment for somatic symptoms: CBT teaches people become aware of inaccurate or automatic negative thinking patterns and change them so that they will have more balanced feelings—both physical and emotional—and action patterns.

The fact that many negative thoughts are automatic and a common human experience is not pathological in and of itself; this becomes problematic only when these thought patterns significantly increase negative feelings and impair function and, in the case of somatic symptoms, perpetuate symptoms and reinforce negative thinking as if to say, "See! I told you something bad would happen and it did." These problems with automatic negative thinking are addressed through CBT by learning to view challenging situations in a more balanced, realistic fashion and responding more effectively, which improves physical and emotional functioning. Cognitive strategies for intervention are reviewed in Chapter 8.

Function

In addition to changing their thinking patterns, children need to develop new actions and behaviors in response to symptoms in an effort to improve their function. Research has shown that function improves before symptoms, as demonstrated with chronic pain (Lynch-Jordan et al., 2014). During the course of treatment, fluctuation of symptoms is to be expected. Rather than immediate symptom resolution, there is typically a slow, but not necessarily linear, improvement of symptoms over time as function increases. There may be ups and downs in symptoms along the way, sometimes with acute flares around times when children are reengaging in normal activities such as school, sports, or family events. Children may continue to have symptoms into the future, although they are typically less intense and disabling. Children and families need to be reassured that this is the natural course of recovery and not an indication that CBT is the wrong treatment for them; much as anxiety increases at first when children face their fears in treatment, symptoms often rise when children are first asked to increase their function.

Of course, increasing function is the hardest thing to do in the face of intense, persistent symptoms, and this is where the strategies that children learn through CBT are critical. Part of what helps them achieve increased function is teaching them new behavioral responses, such as doing an activity *anyway* even if symptoms are present, as well as engaging in regular daily schedules, taking care of their bodies, learning relaxation, and addressing unhelpful thinking patterns. Children must understand that these strategies will improve their symptom experience because of the connections of thoughts, feelings, and actions, which is why education is crucial to their buy-in of this approach (Chapters 3 and 5).

Logistics and Efficacy

There are several core features of CBT that also hold in its application to children with somatic symptoms. First, CBT is time limited. A course of CBT for children with somatic symptoms is typically eight to 16 weekly to every-other-week sessions, depending on the level of disability and comorbid psychological problems. Second, CBT is a structured intervention. It follows a typical course of treatment, which is outlined in this book, in addition to being structured within each session, with time for check-ins, homework review, skills training, and homework assignments. Third, the skills taught in session are practiced as "homework"; the point of children learning coping skills is so they can use them out in the world. CBT is an evidence-based treatment for children with somatic symptoms (Garralda, 1999). Reviews of CBT for chronic pain conditions (including abdominal pain and headache) and other somatic symptoms have demonstrated good efficacy of these interventions for improving symptoms and function in children with lasting effects (e.g., Eccleston, Palermo, Williams, Lewandowski, & Morley, 2009; Hofmann, Asnaani, Vonk, Sawyer, & Fang, 2012). Similarly, CBT has been found to decrease somatic complaints in children with anxiety (Kendall & Pimental, 2003). Mechanistically, one way that CBT works is through targeting factors that maintain symptoms (e.g., avoidance), which leads to symptom reduction (Deary, Chalder, & Sharpe, 2007). Overall, research supports that CBT is beneficial for *all* children with physical symptoms, regardless of origin (Creed, 2009).

In describing CBT to children and families, first communicate that this treatment is evidence based. The analogy of putting tools in your toolbox and learning how to use them to build a better daily experience works well here. A benefit of engaging in CBT interventions is that not only can children acquire tools to improve their ability to cope with somatic symptoms, but the tools also provide them with coping skills for their lives. Many parents have shared that they, too, want to learn and use these tools with their children. That can be a wonderful way for parents to support their children in learning new skills, as well as to positively manage their own stress that comes along with taking care of a child with somatic symptoms.

Overall, providing CBT to children with somatic symptoms is an evidence-based, active approach to get children and families back on track in their lives, which improves children's symptoms. The goal of CBT is to teach children about symptoms, help them reframe their thinking, and provide them with behavioral strategies they can apply to reduce symptoms and associated impairment. *In other words, children learn that if they feel a way that they do not want to feel, physically or emotionally, they can change their thoughts and actions through the skills they develop in treatment to improve their feelings.* Addressing children's barriers to function, whether biological, psychological, or social, and tailoring coping strategies to particular situations results in improved function, and therefore improvement in symptoms over time. This is the foundation on which treatment for children with somatic symptoms is built.

ADDITIONAL TREATMENT CONSIDERATIONS

Finally, there are three considerations that are essential to keep in mind in the application of CBT for children with somatic symptoms, including factors related to referrals, the child's and family's role in treatment, and differential diagnosis.

Referrals

There are a few standard referral scenarios for children arriving in a mental health provider's office with somatic symptoms. The first scenario is that of a child with a long history of medical visits and treatments that may (or may not) have been successful in reducing symptoms or improving function in the short term but have not worked in the long term. In this case, the referral for mental health support is the proverbial "end of the line," when the medical team has run out of options and it may have been suggested that symptoms are being driven by something other than a medical condition. This is the "it's all in your head" referral, and these children sometimes have the most intractable and tough-to-treat symptoms. At this point in their journey, families range from being willing to try anything, and therefore being very open to CBT, to feeling like they have not been heard by the medical teams and are suspicious that everyone has given up. If it is the former, the mental health provider is in good shape. If it is the latter, emphasize that regardless of the cause of the symptoms, children and families are experiencing great distress, and there is no harm in helping them cope with the symptoms and the factors that relate to them, whatever they may be.

The second scenario is when the child is referred *before* there has been significant loss of functioning or impairment. This is a great referral, because it usually indicates that the referring provider is also assessing the child from a biopsychosocial standpoint, which facilitates multidisciplinary treatment from the start. In addition, when it is early on, the symptoms usually have not become too impairing and functioning has not become too limited, so children require less unraveling of maladaptive patterns and return to functioning more quickly. Children and families in this position are quite open to understanding the symptoms as stemming from biopsychosocial factors, and as a result they engage well in treatment.

The third referral possibility is the surprising one mentioned earlier, when a mental health provider shifts his or her thinking into the biopsychosocial model and recognizes the presence of somatic symptoms in children who are in treatment already. In this scenario, these treatment strategies may be blended into existing work. As long as the understanding of somatic symptoms is incorporated *before* introducing children to the strategies for coping with them, there is no bad time to weave this information into established treatment.

Active Role

Send the message that both children and their families will take an active role in CBT treatment. They will be *participants* in this care, not recipients of it. Communication between the mental health provider and the family provides the education on what to do, but it is the child (with the family's support) who is the most important person to make the changes that will result in eventual treatment success. In this regard, CBT is not something that one receives, which may represent a different expectation than children and families have regarding treatment for what they at least initially believed to be a medical problem, and they may have a hard time buying into mental health treatment as a result. In the worst-case scenario, a family may feel that psychological intervention doesn't "count" as doing anything or that it is somehow less valid than a medical approach. It is understandable that anyone who is sick or who is caring for a sick child would want nothing more than an easy fix that could make it all better. However, more and more in medicine, this passive approach is recognized as not providing benefit in the long run. These days, even patients who have undergone major surgery are discharged from the hospital the same day because it has been found that movement and getting back to a normal routine actually improve treatment outcomes. Similarly, patients with arthritis are encouraged to exercise because movement is a protective factor for long-term disease management. Regardless, this can be a difficult message for children and families to hear when children are sick and do not feel like doing anything and parents cannot bring themselves to push them.

As a provider in this situation, it can be similarly difficult to sit with families as they struggle with this fundamental shift in how they view treatment, and to hear statements like "no one is doing anything to help" or be told that despite improvements in therapy, "no doctor has been able to understand this." In the face of these challenges, the provider must continue to promote the child's role in his or her own care and view that as the biggest benefit to treatment. That way, the child is the one who gets the credit for the improvements that are made, which is the best way to increase the child's confidence, and the confidence of the family as well. When asked who is responsible for his or her success in treatment, a child should be able to say

"Me!" The knowledge that a young person can effect such great change in his or her own life is a powerful message to convey.

Differential Diagnosis

For the mental health provider, consider the importance of distinguishing somatic symptom presentations from other psychological problems. As mentioned earlier in this chapter, when meeting a child with somatic symptoms it is most important *not* to assume that he or she has had a significant trauma or stressor or that major psychopathology has led to somatic symptoms. That being said, some children may have had traumatic experiences (connected to their symptoms or not) or exhibit psychological comorbidities, which become evident through the assessment and treatment process. If larger psychological challenges than the somatic symptom difficulty are present, our approach is to treat the somatic symptoms first from the CBT perspective that we describe because it is still a biopsychosocial process and the additional psychological factors are likely affecting symptoms too. Once a child in this situation has gained some traction in treatment and demonstrates improvement in function, which is the goal of treatment, the child then would likely benefit from more intensive psychological and/or psychiatric treatment to address the comorbid psychological issues. Engaging in additional treatment for significant and possibly more impairing mental health challenges is often necessary to make further gains or lasting change in somatic symptom presentations.

Alternatively, children and families may present who have been acutely aware of additional psychological issues but have not pursued psychological treatment because they and/or their medical providers were so focused on the somatic symptoms. This is an understandable situation: How can families effectively engage children in psychological treatment for trauma or anxiety when a child may not be able to walk or to sit through a session because of somatic symptoms? Sometimes psychiatric facilities or programs will not accept children for treatment until they are physically functional and medically stable, which children may not be when they are struggling with somatic symptoms. From both of these standpoints, sometimes the physical symptoms do seem more pressing, and therefore there is good reason to address those challenges first. Still, relay to families the need to get intervention for other psychological symptoms as soon as possible so as not to dismiss the importance of those additional challenges.

It is also beneficial to help families understand the necessity of additional intervention for other psychological concerns, because if they engage in just the treatment for somatic symptoms, it is very likely that their children will not fully return to normal functioning in their lives because of the barriers posed by the other psychological factors. For example, if a child is able to work through chronic headaches in treatment but then is stymied in the return to school because of overwhelming social phobia, the intervention will not be successful. This book should be used to address the treatment of somatic symptoms—other psychological concerns need further treatment using evidence-based modalities (e.g., treatment for anxiety, trauma-focused CBT, dialectical behavior therapy, mindfulness-based CBT). For the population that is the focus of this work, treating somatic symptoms with the CBT approaches described in this book is enough most of the time.

GOING FORWARD

Engaging in CBT with children with somatic symptoms and their families can be a challenging, yet extremely rewarding experience. Families we have worked with have emphasized how much they valued having mental health providers treat their children "like people" and meet children where they were in terms of talking about symptoms. Other families have shared that they initially thought psychological treatment would be scary, or worse, ineffective, and they were pleasantly surprised at how easy it was to engage in the conversation and how helpful the suggestions were. One family put it quite simply in saying, "You were the only helpful doctor." Children have gone from using wheelchairs to running races, from failing in high school to attending college, and from feeling anxious about their symptoms to confidently managing them. Overall, it is a privilege to be part of a child's and family's journey from impairment and confusion to function and confidence.

CHAPTER SUMMARY AND TAKE-AWAY POINTS

- Somatic symptoms are real, physical experiences that are influenced by a combination of biological, psychological, and social factors.
- Children and families often have been through a confusing and frustrating medical journey to arrive at a diagnosis of somatic symptoms. Understanding their unique presenting concerns will help the therapist engage them in a psychological approach to symptom management.
- CBT is an evidence-based approach to treating children with somatic symptoms. Teaching children the connection between thoughts, feelings, and actions provides the foundation for learning coping skills to improve function, which is the primary target for improving children's overall symptom experience.

CHAPTER 2

Describing Somatic Symptoms

In this chapter, somatic symptoms are defined, including a review of the four major somatic symptom categories as well as historical and current terminology from a medical and psychological standpoint. Finally, we review what is known and unknown about the development and associations of somatic symptoms.

DEFINITION

In defining somatic symptoms, the concepts of symptoms and disease must first be distinguished. "Symptoms are the patient's subjective experience of changes in his or her body, whereas disease is objectively observable abnormalities in the body" (Sharpe & Carson, 2001, p. 926). Symptoms comprise the *feeling* of physical phenomena whereas disease represents *evidence* explaining the underlying reason for the symptoms (Eisenberg, 1977). In the case of acute illness, symptoms are the feelings of fatigue, nausea, and fever, and disease is the infection. From this viewpoint, symptoms and disease are *separate constructs*. While they can happen together, they also can happen apart, making it possible for disease to occur in the absence of symptoms and for symptoms to occur in the absence of disease. Symptoms without disease, or somatic symptoms, are the primary focus of this book. Even symptoms without disease are still biological in nature and are no less *real* in their presentation.

Medical Terminologies

Broadly speaking, there are four major categories of somatic symptoms, divided by body system/medical specialty: neurological, cardiac, pain, and gastrointestinal. The various medical diagnoses associated with each somatic symptom category are listed below, along with a brief description of the symptoms, testing options, and recommended treatment. Note that a unique aspect of being a mental health provider who treats children with somatic symptoms is the need to be fluent in both medical and psychological languages. For mental health providers with less experience in the medical world, these descriptions may seem technical and the terminologies unfamiliar. If this is the case, spend a little extra time on this information, as it is critical that both the medical *and* psychological sides of children's experience with these symptoms are understood and can be easily discussed. The more familiarity a mental health provider has with somatic symptoms, the more confidence is instilled in children and families as they embark on treatment.

That being said, when working with health care colleagues, you will find variability in terminology and diagnostic approach between children or even within the same child, which usually reflects a different focus and training between providers. It is good to remember that a mental health provider *does not need to be a medical expert* in the underlying biomechanics of these presentations or bear the responsibility of coming up with the one true diagnosis for symptoms. No matter what the symptoms are called, there is always a role for CBT to help children manage and cope with symptoms to improve function. Staying focused on those larger goals avoids the confusion that can result from the variety of terminologies used for symptom descriptions.

Neurological Symptoms

Neurological symptoms present as conversion disorder, functional neurological symptom disorder, psychogenic nonepileptic seizures (PNES), nonepileptic seizures, pseudoseizures, functional movement disorder, functional gait disorder, functional gait imbalance, psychogenic movements, spells, numbness, tingling, paresthesia, and psychogenic blindness. The descriptions and diagnoses in the neurological symptoms category are largely consistent with a fundamental diagnosis of conversion disorder. They represent different presentations of a deficit of motor movement or sensation that are not due to an underlying organic neurological disease process (e.g., brain tumor, multiple sclerosis, epilepsy, meningitis). Assessment includes examination of motor and sensory symptoms, looking for neurological signs that are present and those that are conspicuously absent, including laterality, inconsistency in presentation (e.g., gait normal in room vs. abnormal in hallway), weakness, sensory disturbance, speed of gait, triggers, changes in center of gravity, speech, and visual/auditory function (Stone et al., 2005).

In specialty care, children see neurologists, and diagnostic tests are those of *exclusion*, meaning that a *lack* of test results supports a functional diagnosis after organic disease is ruled out. These include electroencephalogram (EEG), video EEG, and magnetic resonance imaging (MRI) of the brain. Treatment includes referral to psychiatrists, psychologists, and/or physical therapists. If children are significantly impaired (e.g., cannot walk or care for themselves), they may be referred to an inpatient rehabilitation program, although this occurs less frequently.

Cardiac Symptoms

Cardiac symptoms present as neurocardiogenic syncope, neurally mediated syncope, vasovagal syncope, vasodepressor syncope, neurally mediated hypotension, syncope, passing out, fainting, psychogenic syncope, presyncope, dizziness, shortness of breath, noncardiac chest pain, dysautonomia, postural orthostatic tachycardia syndrome (POTS), and orthostatic intolerance. Somatic symptoms that are cardiac in nature include feelings of heart rate change, dizziness, or fainting. Neurocardiogenic syncope, also called vasovagal or vasodepressor syncope, is the most common cardiac somatic symptom (Strieper, Auld, Hulse, & Campbell, 1994). This is a condition where, in response to a stressor (e.g., pain, emotion, sight of blood), there is an abrupt release of epinephrine, which causes rapid heart rate (tachycardia), followed by a rapid slowing of the heart rate (bradycardia) that drops blood pressure, limiting oxygenated blood flow to the brain and causing fainting (syncope) or dizziness (presyncope), either of which can be associated with blurry vision, weakness, sweating, or nausea. Psychogenic syncope, the presence of symptoms without accompanying heart rate or blood pressure change, may occur without a triggering event or in unexpected circumstances (e.g., lying down; Grubb et al., 1992). POTS is another type of cardiac symptom related to dysregulation of the autonomic nervous system. It is associated with sustained increase in heart rate upon standing, which is usually the more unpleasant symptom rather than accompanying dizziness (Raj, 2013; Grubb & Karabin, 2008). POTS is more common in people with connective tissue disorders (e.g., Ehlers-Danlos syndrome, joint hypermobility; Keller & Robertson, 2006).

In the diagnosis of cardiac symptoms, children typically see cardiologists. Testing may include an electrocardiogram (EKG) to rule out problems with electrical activity in the heart, an exercise or stress test to examine heart function, or a tilt-table test, which uses a mechanical table that slowly moves children from a prone to a standing position for 30 minutes or until symptoms are produced (e.g., fainting, dizziness, nausea, low heart rate, hypotension; Strieper et al., 1994). Treatment includes symptom management (e.g., sitting down), counterpressure movements to increase blood return to the heart (e.g., tensing lower leg muscles, flexing/crossing arms and legs; van Dijk et al., 2006), improving overall conditioning (aerobic and strength exercises), healthy habit improvement (increasing hydration and improving sleep), as well as medications such as midodrine, a vasoconstrictor that raises the blood pressure, or fludrocortisone, a mineralocortoid that promotes fluid retention.

Pain Symptoms

Pain symptoms present as amplified musculoskeletal pain syndrome (AMPS), chronic widespread pain, fibromyalgia, complex regional pain syndrome (CRPS), reflexive sympathetic dystrophy (RSD), chronic migraine, chronic headache, any type of functional pain disorder, any type of chronic pain syndrome, and primary pain disorder. A chronic pain syndrome is characterized by recurrent or chronic pain that has persisted for 3 or more months in the absence of identifiable organic disease or that lasts longer than what would be expected from an organic cause (Merskey & Bogduk, 1994). Chronic pain syndromes are understood to be disorders of the nervous system in which the brain regards a part of the body as acutely damaged when it is not. It is also understood through processes of central sensitization and pain amplification, in which pain signals become magnified, sometimes for unknown reasons, or persist instead of quiet down after an initial insult, such as an acute injury that has healed. The pain is real, it's just not happening for a protective reason. Some physicians have suggested adoption of the term "primary pain disorder" to account for chronic pain syndromes to make the terminology less confusing and to better explain the primary role of the nervous system in chronic pain as opposed to identifying the disorder by body location (Schechter, 2014).

Tests for chronic pain syndromes also are tests of exclusion, in which injury or disease is ruled out (e.g., X-ray, MRI, blood test). Many children initially see rheumatologists for systemic concerns, neurologists for headache, or orthopedists for musculoskeletal concerns. Children are either treated by those providers or referred to multidisciplinary pain centers with anesthesiologists, psychologists, and physical therapists who specialize in chronic pain management. Treatment includes medication (typically *not* narcotic or opiate pain medicines, but rather medications in the antiseizure or antidepressant category, such as gabapentin or amitriptyline that address nervous system dysfunction), physical therapy, and CBT/biofeedback.

Gastrointestinal Symptoms

Gastrointestinal (GI) symptoms present as functional gastrointestinal disorders (FGIDs), disorders of brain–gut interaction, functional abdominal pain (FAP), functional bowel disorder (FBD), irritable bowel syndrome (IBS), gastroparesis, belly pain, rumination, functional nausea, functional vomiting, and abdominal migraine. These somatic symptoms all share the hallmark feature of persistent or recurring GI symptoms—such as vomiting, nausea, abdominal pain, bloating, diarrhea, or constipation—resulting from abnormal GI *functioning* rather than a structural or disease-based abnormality. Somatic GI symptoms are well researched, with positive, symptom-based criteria for FGIDs known as the Rome Criteria, understood to stem from a central mechanism of disordered brain–gut interaction (Drossman, 2016). Children typically see pediatricians or gastroenterologists for these concerns. In addition to the positive Rome Criteria signs, tests of GI symptoms are also tests of exclusion (e.g., colonoscopy, stool test). Treatment includes pharmacological management to address symptoms hydration and good nutrition intake to support proper digestive function, and referral for CBT/biofeedback to help children cope with symptoms and improve function.

Having gone through the four major somatic symptom categories, it is probably easy to see from where some of the confusion regarding what to call somatic symptoms stems. No wonder children and families are confused about these diagnoses—the array of medical terminology describing somatic symptoms is astounding. For these reasons, to eliminate confusion and streamline communication, we recommend picking a single terminology for the symptoms that children are experiencing, which can be as simple as asking the child and family what they usually call it, and use that consistently throughout treatment.

Psychological Terminologies

From a psychological standpoint, there are several diagnoses that can apply to children with somatic symptoms. Many somatic symptoms can be accounted for within a larger psychological diagnosis, such as depression, anxiety, or adjustment disorder, if the symptoms occur in the presence of other concerns. The fifth edition of the

Diagnostic and Statistical Manual of Mental Disorders (DSM-5) has a specific category, called "Somatic Symptom and Related Disorders," that includes diagnoses with prominent physical complaints, associated psychological distress, and impaired function (American Psychiatric Association, 2013). There are seven diagnoses in this category: somatic symptom disorder, illness anxiety disorder, conversion disorder (functional neurological symptom disorder), psychological factors affecting other medical conditions, factitious disorder, other specified somatic symptom and related disorder, and unspecified somatic symptom and related disorder. Common features of these disorders include prominent physical symptoms together with abnormal concern about them, impairment in daily life, and persistence of the symptoms for between 3 and 6 months, depending on the disorder. It is important to note that a chief feature of somatic symptom disorder is that the associated psychological distress and impairment is *excessive*; children would *not* qualify for this diagnosis based on the presence of symptoms and normative concern alone. To illustrate this difference, a large population study of Swedish youth found that while 22.7% of adolescents reported at least one persistent somatic symptom, only 10.5% of the population—fewer than half of those experiencing symptoms—met criteria for a somatic symptom disorder (van Geelen, Rydelius, & Hagquist, 2015).

There was a significant revision to the "Somatic Symptom and Related Disorders" category in DSM-5 to emphasize the importance of making a positive diagnosis based on the *presence* of symptoms and distress rather than basing the diagnosis on the absence of medical explanation (American Psychiatric Association, 2013). Changes from previous editions of the DSM also included shifting away from the term "somatoform disorder," which placed more emphasis on mental illness, to "somatic symptom disorders," which places more emphasis on a biopsychosocial presentation. Previous diagnostic criteria for somatoform disorders focused on the prominence of symptoms being "medically unexplained," with more attention placed on the mental health contribution to the symptom presentation. As the medical and psychological community has recognized that there are limits to how reliably one can determine that a symptom is truly medically unexplained, a more balanced approach has been struck between the role of physical *and* psychosocial factors contributing to these presentations in DSM-5; as such, somatic symptom disorders can accompany medically explained or unexplained symptoms. Additionally, grounding a diagnosis on the *absence* of something reinforced the biomedical approach (mind vs. body), while basing it on the *presence* of something is consistent with a biopsychosocial approach (mind *and* body). This is a critical difference that aids in the understanding of somatic symptoms that we review in more detail in the next chapter.

While this biopsychosocial language facilitates a better understanding of somatic symptoms from a mind–body perspective, the biomedical terminologies that make a stronger distinction between medical and psychological causes for symptoms are still used in the medical world, and you will still encounter them when seeing children in this population. The medical community uses the *International Statistical Classification of Diseases and Related Health Problems* (ICD), a diagnostic manual, and the current 10th revision still includes somatoform disorder and other "psychogenic" conditions as diagnoses for somatic symptom disorders (World Health Organization, 2015). Future revisions of the ICD are expected to align more with DSM-5 conceptualizations. From our base of operation as psychologists, our use of terminologies for somatic symptoms reflects the terminology in DSM-5, with corresponding diagnoses assigned based on those criteria. For a mental health provider working in a medical setting, health and behavior codes can be used for the corresponding medical diagnosis as an alternative to using a DSM-5 diagnosis.

Both medical and psychological terminologies for somatic symptoms have changed and will continue to change over time, mirroring the evolution of our understanding of these symptom presentations and the corresponding changes in diagnostic criteria. Many times, terminologies are used interchangeably; it is beneficial to be familiar with historical *and* current terms to provide the best possible understanding of these disorders and communicate it effectively to providers, children, and families. There is a remarkable amount of discussion in the somatic symptoms world regarding the labeling of these symptoms, including whether they should be diagnosed in a medical or psychological context, and the threshold at which they move from being a physical symptom that causes appropriate psychological concern to one with a highly distressing level of psychological concern. Although it can be very easy to get caught up or lost and confused in what diagnosis to use for these symptoms, remember this: regardless of the label, somatic symptoms cause impairment in children's lives, and the treatment described in this book will help them understand their symptoms and improve their function.

SOMATIC SYMPTOMS IN THE POPULATION

Somatic symptoms are quite common in children, prevalent in both primary and specialty medical care settings and observed in nearly every body system (Campo & Fritsch, 1994; Stone et al., 2005). The most common somatic symptoms include headache, fatigue, dizziness, aching muscles, limb pain, nausea, abdominal pain, and neurological symptoms (e.g., changes in eyesight, balance, sensation, or gait; Beck, 2008; Campo, 2012; Fritz, Fritsch, & Hagino, 1997). A review of patient records indicated that 38% of pediatric and adult patients seeking care at an internal medicine clinic presented with a primary somatic symptom complaint; after further examination and testing, 85% of those cases had no identifiable disease that accounted for symptoms (Kroenke & Mangelsdorff, 1989). In other words, about one-third of patients seen in that outpatient care environment had somatic symptoms. In pediatric specialty care, the percentage of children who present with somatic symptoms ranges from 15 to 90%, depending on the area (Carson et al., 2000). For example, pediatric patients with FGIDs account for up to 50% of gastroenterology clinic referrals, syncope and unexplained chest pain account for 90% of cardiology referrals, and chronic widespread pain accounts for up to 40% of referrals to rheumatology (Anthony & Schanberg, 2005; Rouster, Karpinski, Silver, Monagas, & Hyman, 2016; Stone et al., 2005; Tunaoglu et al., 1995). Although the initial focus may be on one body system, the presence of one somatic symptom usually predicts more, with headache and abdominal pain representing the most common combination (Campo, 2012).

Studies of children with somatic symptoms have confirmed that these problems are rarely found to be associated with identifiable disease later (Kroenke &

Mangelsdorff, 1989). In fact, a review of the pediatric literature reported that fewer than 10% of children initially presenting with somatic symptoms were later found to have disease that could have accounted for those symptoms (Campo & Fritsch, 1994). From these studies, we can conclude that somatic symptom presentations are prevalent and do not mean that we are simply "missing something" from a medical standpoint.

Organic Overlap

There can also be overlap between organic disorders and somatic symptoms. Children who have an organic disease can later develop somatic symptoms, or conditions can be comorbid and present at the same time, for example, comorbid nonepileptic and epileptic seizures, postviral dysautonomia, an orthopedic injury that heals but evolves into AMPS, or inflammatory bowel disease and comorbid IBS. Studies have found that there may be a central nervous system explanation for these overlapping conditions. For example, among patients with inflammatory bowel disease in remission, abnormal brain activity was identified in patients who also had abdominal pain but not in patients without pain, showing that pain can be present in the absence of active disease (Bao et al., 2016). A possible mechanism for this is autonomic nervous system activation, which happens when the body fights off disease and eventually heals but forgets to turn off, and somatic symptoms result. These connections will be discussed in more detail in Chapter 3. As diagnostic technology improves, more overlap between somatic symptoms and organic disease is discovered (Drossman, 2016).

When organic disease and somatic symptoms overlap, it can be an exquisitely difficult situation clinically because it leads children and families to believe that there is something organically wrong—there was before, after all—and it can be particularly challenging to explain somatic symptoms under these circumstances. For example, consider the case of a child who had a brain tumor that presented as headache and gait disorder. After the tumor was removed, he had residual headaches in the area of tumor removal, making it difficult for him and his family to attribute the pain to anything other than tumor regrowth, despite multiple clear scans. Close collaboration with his oncology team was critical in terms of assuring all parties in moving forward with a CBT approach that focused on functional improvement and coping with pain.

Demographics

Both children and adolescents experience somatic symptoms. While younger children (ages 3–5) can have somatic symptoms, they are more common among school-age children, ages 6–18. Girls are more likely to have somatic symptoms than boys, although this may differ based on age; there is a more equal gender presentation during childhood, with increasing frequency of girls presenting with symptoms during adolescence (Campo, 2012). The onset of puberty may play a role in the development of somatic symptoms, such that mood and behavior interact with physiological factors (e.g., hormones), all of which are changing during this point in development (Susman, Dorn, & Schiefelbein, 2003). There are a host of social factors that likely contribute to gender differences in symptom presentation as children get older. Research has shown that somatic symptoms can carry over into adulthood. For example, children with functional abdominal pain were more likely as adults to have other chronic pain problems (Walker, Dengler-Crish, Rippel, & Bruehl, 2010), somatic symptoms (Dengler-Crish, Horst, & Walker, 2011), and anxiety (Shelby et al., 2013), compared to children who did not have a history of abdominal pain.

For somatic symptoms to be considered as rising to the level of a clinical problem, *significant impairment* from these symptoms must also be present. If children have these symptoms at a low intensity or frequency and/or cope with them well, the symptoms are not considered clinically impairing and no diagnosis—medical or psychological—is made. However, children who experience symptoms with more frequency, intensity, and/or are coping poorly in terms of exhibiting emotional distress and functional impairment are considered to have a clinically significant problem worthy of diagnosis. For some somatic symptoms diagnoses, there is a time consideration. Recurrent or chronic pain symptoms have to exist for 3 months or longer to be classified as a chronic pain condition. Other somatic symptoms, such as functional neurological disorders, require symptoms to be present for 6 or more months to meet diagnostic criteria.

Impairment

Children with somatic symptoms experience high levels of disability and psychological distress (Campo & Fritsch, 1994). Functionally, somatic symptoms are associated with physical impairment, social difficulties, and activity limitations that can range from minimal to moderate, such as missing a few days of school or sitting out a sports practice or two, to severe, such as no longer attending school, dropping out of sports and social activities, and using an assistive device to get around (e.g., crutches, wheelchair).

Children with somatic symptoms can have more impairment from symptoms than children with organic disorders. A study of children with inflammatory bowel disease, a serious organic gastrointestinal disorder, found that they were *less* disabled by their symptoms than children with functional abdominal pain (Walker, Garber, & Greene, 1993). A possible reason for this is that children with an organic diagnosis received corresponding medical treatment that more effectively managed their symptoms compared to children with somatic symptoms, or that the organic medical problems were less chronic than somatic symptoms once treatment was received, or that the diagnosis was less uncertain and therefore less worrisome once identified.

In terms of psychological distress, somatic symptoms can occur on their own or in addition to common mental health disorders of childhood and adolescence (Campo, 2012). The most frequent co-occurring diagnoses are anxiety and depressive disorders, or subclinical presentations of these symptoms; however, children with somatic symptoms rarely have other psychiatric conditions (Campo, 2012). Some research has indicated a higher rate of learning disorders specifically in children with nonepileptic seizures (Sawchuk & Bucchalter, 2015). Assessment and treatment of comorbid psychological concerns are crucial for successful outcomes. For instance, if a child has abdominal pain and also has generalized anxiety disorder, the child's physiological arousal and distress may be too great for him to benefit from CBT alone, and a referral to a psychiatrist prior to or during treatment would likely result in a better treatment outcome. Similarly, a child with untreated ADHD may have difficulty engaging in relaxation strategies due to attentional dysregulation and may not gain as much benefit if those symptoms remain untreated. For all children, the goal of treatment is to manage symptoms and return to function, while also accounting for the degree to which psychological factors impact impairment and referring for or providing intervention for those additional concerns as needed.

Health Care Utilization

It is common for children with somatic symptoms to undergo multiple, costly medical procedures to rule out disease and return for multiple follow-up medical visits in continued pursuit of the cause of the symptoms (Kaplan, Ganiats, & Frosch, 2004). This pattern of increased health care utilization has economic importance in terms of the cost of health care as well as the effect of the lost educational time for children and productivity at work for parents (Levant, 2005; Kaplan et al., 2004).

Research within specific somatic symptom populations has examined the effects of psychological treatment on health care utilization patterns. For instance, children with nonepileptic seizures frequently undergo many medical and diagnostic procedures, which can delay referral to effective therapies such as psychological intervention (LaFrance, Reuber, & Goldstein, 2013). In Sawchuck and Bucchalter's (2015) retrospective review of nonepileptic seizures in children, they found that there was a *sevenfold* decrease in emergency room visits after initial psychology intake, and partial to full remission of symptoms in children who received psychological care in their model. Teaching children how to improve their ability to manage symptoms and reduce impairment has the potential to reduce overall health care costs to the system and to the families; this is the role of CBT.

Treatment Setting

As noted in the first chapter, the strategies outlined in this book are geared toward delivery in an outpatient treatment setting. The assumption is that the children are able to effectively learn the treatment strategies in this setting and apply them in their daily lives (i.e., symptoms are not so impairing as to affect the child's ability to attend sessions or learn skills). However, some children struggle to gain benefit within those parameters and require a higher level of care. Determining the treatment setting requires clinical judgment, taking into account assessment of functioning, duration of symptoms, and impairment level. If a child has daily headaches that are distressing but do not impair school attendance or participation in activities, this child would be appropriately served in outpatient care. Another child with daily headaches that cause significant mood changes, prevent school attendance, and persist despite medical, psychological, and other intervention may require a more intensive approach, either through more frequent outpatient sessions or referral to a partial day treatment, or inpatient psychiatric or pain rehabilitation program. The strategies in this book are applicable to treatment in any of those settings; the difference is the structure the higher levels of care provide to the child to better facilitate learning or application of the treatment strategies to improve function and symptom coping that is often necessary when impairment is severe.

So far we have covered the basics of somatic symptoms: they are biological in nature, not due to an acute or identified disease process, can occur on their own or with other medical or mental health diagnoses, and go by many different names. Somatic symptoms present in primary and specialty care with great frequency in every body system, occur most frequently in school-age children, and during adolescence, more often in girls than boys. They are associated with significant impairment and high levels of health care utilization. While they may be effectively treated in outpatient settings, children with more significant levels of impairment might require a higher level of care. After understanding what somatic symptoms are, next up is why they develop.

THEORY AND RESEARCH

Several theoretical explanations have been offered for the nature and development of somatic symptoms through a small but growing body of research. Biologically, one possibility is that an underlying disease *is* present that is not detectable with current medical techniques (Aronowitz, 2001). Additionally, individual differences in physiology, stress reactivity, attention, and sensitization to symptoms may account for onset and maintenance of somatic symptoms (Mayer, Naliboff, Chang, & Coutinho, 2001; Tache, Martinez, Million, & Rivier, 1999). Psychologically, there is a strong association between somatic symptoms and internalizing disorders that, in combination with the experience of physical symptoms, may overwhelm coping efforts (Walker, Smith, Garber, & Van Slyke, 1997b). Environmental and behavioral factors that children experience in their interaction with others, reinforcement, and secondary gain also contribute to symptom presentations (Walker & Zeman, 1992). In sum, the somatic symptoms that children experience are likely the result of a combination of all of these factors.

It is important to note that there are also cross-cultural differences in the presentation and understanding of somatic symptoms. Reviews of research in this area have concluded that there are some patterns of somatic and mental health symptoms that can be thought of as universal signs of distress, particularly for physical symptoms associated with depressive disorders (Bagayogo, Interian, & Escobar 2013). The way in which these symptoms are reported, identified, discussed, understood, accepted, and treated varies across cultures due to a host of sociocultural factors (Escobar & Gureje, 2007).

While there is not enough research to make concrete claims about the exact set of factors that combine to put children at risk for developing somatic symptoms, applying these theoretical bases to clinical presentations in children with somatic symptoms, the following general patterns can be described; they are hypersensitive to bodily signals (biological), have a difficult time identifying or coping with emotion (psychological), and experience modeling of symptoms or secondary gain/reinforcement of disability (social). Each of these factors is addressed in detail to more fully understand the influence of each one.

Biological Factors

A number of theories have been proposed with regard to biological factors involved in the development of somatic symptoms, including preexisting disease (Rangel, Garralda, Levin, & Roberts, 2000), automatic responses in pain perception and autonomic nervous system reactivity including arousal and hypervigilance (McGrath, 1995), and the relation of stress reactivity to internalizing disorders (Boyce et al., 2001). Theoretically, the role of "stress" has been studied in a variety of ways in terms of the biological effects of this process on the body and the strong role it plays in the development of somatic symptoms. Stress can be defined as "an event or experience that expends the resources of an individual" (Blount et al., 2008), which can be physical or emotional in nature. Stress is associated with poor biological outcomes, including immune function (Kiecolt-Glaser, McGuire, Robles, & Glaser, 2002) and psychosocial function (Kanner, Feldman, Weinberger, & Ford, 1987). Stress can be associated with objectively distressing events (e.g., acute threat) or subjective ones (e.g., perceived threat; Blount et al., 2008). It is common for somatic symptoms to be present after a physical illness or injury as well as after an emotionally stressful event (Garralda, 1999). Research has demonstrated that in predisposed individuals, stressors activate *and* change the reactivity of the nervous system, both central and autonomic, such that individuals may develop somatic symptoms that are retriggered or exacerbated in reaction to subsequent stressors (Mayer et al., 2001). We now consider the evidence for the biological and stress factors related to different somatic symptom presentations.

There is a long history of research in the field of conversion disorder on the relation of biological factors to somatic symptoms. Prior to the 20th century, conversion symptoms were thought to arise in context of threatening situations that resulted in an intense emotional experience that was then translated or "converted" into a physical expression of symptoms (Kozlowska, Scher, & Williams, 2011). Initially, it was not well understood how and why strong emotions produced conversion symptoms, or why some people were more susceptible to developing them than others. During the 21st century, advances in technology made it possible to use neuroimaging techniques, which advanced research in this and many other medical science fields. This allowed scientists in the fields of neurobiology and information processing to investigate conversion symptoms from new perspectives, including study of the role of sensorimotor, cognitive, emotional, and motor processes (Black, Seritan, Taber, & Hurley, 2004; Vuilleumier, 2005).

While research has not determined that any one of these processes alone results in conversion symptoms, interconnections *between* these processes likely contribute to conversion disorder presentations. For instance, research has shown that distressing feelings can result in neurological activity that changes sensorimotor processes (Kozlowska et al., 2011). Clinically, this explains how a stressful situation could trigger a process of neurological activation that results in symptoms such as gait impairment. Cognitively, children with conversion symptoms have been found to demonstrate deficits in executive functioning tasks, memory, and attention (Kozlowska et al., 2015). Conversion symptoms also can be triggered on an arousal, hormonal, autonomic, or cardiovascular level. For instance, children with conversion disorder have been found to have higher arousal, a greater startle reflex, and inability to habituate compared to healthy children (Kozlowska et al., 2011). Similarly, children with nonepileptic seizures had lower heart rate variability and increased cortisol levels compared to healthy controls (Bakvis, Spinhoven, & Roelofs, 2009). In sum, this research shows that it is more than just an emotional process that drives the development of conversion symptoms.

In addition, research has examined the role of physiological and autonomic arousal in children with other somatic symptoms. Children with psychogenic movement disorders, nonepileptic seizures, and syncope have intensified physiological responses in situations associated with a perceived threat compared to healthy peers (Kozlowska et al., 2011). In addition, the autonomic nervous system and limbic hypothalamic–pituitary–adrenocortical system have been shown to be hyperresponsive to stressful events in children with somatic symptoms (Gunnar, Bruce, & Hickman, 2001). Increased physiological reactivity also has been associated with internalizing symptoms during childhood (Bauer, Quas, & Boyce, 2002; Boyce et al., 2001). Children experiencing impairment related to somatic symptoms may also have an increased focus on both internalized physical *and* emotional symptoms (Beck, 2008).

There are many identified biological factors associated with chronic pain syndromes, as well. Specifically, neurological processes including functional differences, structural changes, and attention play significant roles in pain perception. Regarding functional factors, while traditional theories of neurological pain perception focused solely on the somatosensory cortex, functional magnetic resonance imaging (fMRI) technology has enabled the discovery that pain perception occurs in many areas of the brain (Coghill, Sang, Maisog, & Iadarola, 1999), which expand over time as the brain continues to experience pain in a process called central sensitization (Woolf, 2011). Abnormal changes in pain pathways and sensory processing have been found to affect both the initiation and maintenance of chronic pain conditions (Diers et al., 2008). Simply put, the more pain the body feels, the more areas the brain recruits to think about it, which increases the overall perception of pain.

Neuroimaging work in children with chronic musculoskeletal pain has shown that there are also structural changes associated with chronic pain in some brain areas, such as the amygdala, which can be reversed through integrated therapies (Simons et al., 2014). fMRI research in children with IBS demonstrated both structural *and* functional changes in the brain compared to healthy children, and these changes related to pain intensity and functional impairment (Hubbard et al., 2016). Finally, research on attention has shown that some people seem to be biologically wired to attend to pain, thereby increasing the amount of pain felt, whereas others are biologically wired to attend *away* from pain (Legrain et al., 2009). Overall, research shows good evidence that chronic pain is a real, true signal produced by structural and functional changes in the nervous system and attended to differently by some people than others that can be changed through treatment.

In sum, research demonstrates that there are biological factors underlying somatic symptoms. This evidence has significantly advanced the thinking about and understanding of somatic symptoms, enabling us to go beyond the initial assumptions of "it's all in their heads" to realizing that biological factors *do* play a role in somatic symptom presentations, although they may not be the "easy" factors to identify through standard medical testing. How to explain these biological contributions to somatic symptoms to children and families in the clinical sense is reviewed in Chapters 3 and 5.

Psychological Factors

Psychological factors and coping ability also play a strong role in the development and presentation of somatic symptoms. Theoretically, the cognitive-behavioral model posits that the symptom experience results from an interplay between cognition, emotion, and behavior in response to or in association with symptoms (Beck et al., 1979; Lazarus & Folkman, 1984), whereas psychodynamic theory assumes symptoms are unconsciously produced from a desire to avoid a situation or inability to express distress (Husain, Browne, & Chalder, 2007).

Anxiety and depression do not always preclude somatic symptom development. There is some evidence for anxiety and depressive symptoms predicting the development of somatic symptoms; however, further research is indicated to better understand the exact nature of this connection over the lifespan (Campo, 2012). Overall, there is variation in somatic symptom presentation, course, and outcome in terms of the association with psychological factors; there is not consistent evidence for specific psychological risk factors related to the development or trajectory of somatic symptoms (Beck, 2008). Clinically, psychological factors associated with somatic symptoms must be accounted for, though do not assume that children will have a more or less difficult course based on the presence or absence of comorbidities.

Regarding research on specific somatic symptoms, investigation into the role of cognitive and emotional processes in children with conversion disorder revealed two patterns: employment of cognitive inhibition to manage strong emotions (i.e., masked their emotions) and development of "exaggerated" responses that resulted in getting comfort from caregivers (i.e., overshowed their emotions; Kozlowska et al., 2011). In this way, extreme forms of emotional expression have been associated with functional neurological symptoms. These processes occur on a subconscious level, but associations are built over time and the body and mind learn that symptoms allow escape in situations with high levels of perceived threat. In providing treatment, the goal is for children to unlearn this connection that has been reinforced.

Among children with syncope, children with a history of unexplained fainting had higher rates of internalizing symptoms than children without a history of fainting (Byars, Brown, Campbell, & Hobbs, 2000). In adults with syncope, despite similar reports of psychological distress, those with unexplained syncope (i.e., who did not have symptoms on the tilt-table test), reported greater perceived distress than those with a positive tilt-table result (Rafanelli, Gostoli, Roncuzzi, & Sassone, 2013). Another study of adults with syncope showed an overall high rate of psychological distress, including anticipatory fear of syncopal episodes and negative consequences of fainting, which led to severe disability (McGrady, 1996). These types of psychological stressors likely fuel the arousal of physiological changes that underlie cardiac symptoms. In that sense, this process can be viewed as a self-fulfilling prophecy: just *thinking* about the feared event produces enough physical arousal to actually make it happen. It is important to teach children with syncope or any type of cardiac-based somatic symptom about these connections between psychological and physiological states, as it will help them understand why strategies for both responses improve symptoms and impairment.

Another psychological factor that is highly relevant in its contribution to the onset and maintenance of somatic symptoms is coping. Coping can be defined as a process that includes the thoughts and actions used to manage demands of situations that are perceived as stressful (Lazarus & Folkman, 1984). There are many theories of coping and ways to categorize coping responses. For example, coping responses can be voluntary (e.g., goal-directed behavior) or involuntary (e.g., change in heart rate), emotion focused versus problem focused (e.g., "I cannot handle this" vs. "There is nothing I can do"), engaging versus avoiding, and repressive versus sensitizing (Blount, Davis, Powers, & Roberts, 1991; Compas, Connor-Smith, Saltzman, Thomsen, & Wadsworth, 2001). Across all definitions, both cognitively and behaviorally driven coping responses to stress have been found to affect children's adjustment to somatic symptoms overall.

In a study of children with abdominal pain, passive coping efforts were most strongly associated with high levels of somatic and depressive symptoms compared to active or accommodative strategies (Walker et al., 1997b). In other words, children who elected to rest or retreat or who felt defeated in the face of symptoms were the most likely to continue struggling. This finding has been replicated in children with chronic pain syndromes: more active coping styles and fewer catastrophic thoughts and actions in the face of pain were associated with less impairment and better psychological outcomes (Vervoort, Goubert, Eccleston, Bijttebier, & Crombez, 2006). Overall, what children think and feel in response to their symptoms relates to their overall adjustment; research supports the adoption of an active coping style and resilient thinking pattern to improve children's experience with all types of somatic symptoms.

Finally, while some case examples have suggested that there is a common personality type among children with somatic symptoms (e.g., perfectionistic or "Type A"), systematic, population-based research has not found a specific personality type consistently associated with somatic symptoms. Participants in a retrospective study on nonepileptic seizures completed personality inventories, and the most frequent personality traits identified were inhibited, submissive, and introverted, consistent with other research in the field of coping indicating a more passive/avoidant coping style among children with somatic symptoms in general (Plioplys et al., 2014; Sawchuk & Buchhalter, 2015).

Social Factors

In addition to the influence of biological and psychological factors, social and contextual factors also contribute to somatic symptoms, including modeling of illness behavior in the family as well as exposure to adverse events at home or school (Beck,

2008). Behavioral theory explains how contextual factors influence somatic symptom presentations. For example, through classical conditioning, children can acquire conditioned responses to initially neutral stimuli, and through operant conditioning, behaviors are reinforced if followed by pleasant consequences or the successful avoidance of unpleasant consequences (Skinner, 1953). Social learning theory provides explanations for how social influences contribute to symptoms, such as the modeling of a family member whom the child sees receiving attention or reinforcement for symptoms (Bandura, 1986). And finally, structural models focus on how the family environment is involved in the development and maintenance of symptoms, illustrating that all people—especially children—rarely function alone and are influenced by the larger system; if something in the system allows the symptoms to happen or the system benefits in some way, symptoms will be more likely to persist (Minuchin et al., 1975). Thinking in these behavioral and systemic terms allows you to consider assessing and intervening with challenges a child may be facing in the family, school, or peer environment.

In general, stressful social–environmental factors, including school difficulties (e.g., starting/changing schools, poor academic performance), difficulty getting along with peers and teachers, and bullying, are associated with high somatic symptom reports among children (Due et al., 2005; Eminson, Benjamin, Shortall, Woods, & Faragher, 1996; Taylor, Szatmari, Boyle, & Offord, 1996). In one study, children's most common life stressors were identified as peer insecurity, family conflict, learning difficulties, and bullying (Sawchuck & Buchhalter, 2015). Stressful life events can negatively impact symptoms: children with higher levels of impairment from abdominal pain were those who had experienced more negative life events in the past year (Walker & Greene, 1991b).

Although there is some evidence from retrospective adult reports of somatic symptoms and a history of childhood abuse or trauma, it is difficult to demonstrate the same links concurrently in childhood and adolescence (Eminson, 2007). Certainly among children who have been through abusive situations, there is often somatic symptom involvement (Friedrich & Schafer, 1995); however, research does *not* suggest that the reverse is true, and there is not support for the notion that a majority of children with somatic symptoms have been abused. Although it is important to assess for trauma history when meeting children with somatic symptoms, as in any psychological intake, it is not considered as a primary associated concern.

Overall, research has shown that biological, psychological, and social factors interact to produce and maintain somatic symptoms. This evidence base lends support to the importance of the biopsychosocial model in understanding and treating somatic symptoms, addressed in the next chapter. Throughout the book, keep in mind that there are always unique differences and individual factors that contribute to each child's symptom presentation. This is consistent with research on individual responses to stress. While this theoretical and research review focused mainly on the negative biopsychosocial aspects of somatic symptoms, there are also areas where children may show positive qualities. Two children may undergo the same stressor, but one is back at school the next day and the other is in bed with a stomachache. There is resiliency in addition to pathology; it is as important to understand the areas where children *are not* doing well as it is to understand areas where they *are* succeeding.

MYTH BUSTING

There are many providers in the health care and therapeutic fields who wonder about the "realness" of symptoms or the legitimacy of somatic symptom disorders. It is a natural response to question a new concept when first learning about it, particularly for a construct that is gray and murky at best. Discussion of what somatic symptoms *are* is just as important of what somatic symptoms are *not*.

In this chapter, the ways in which somatic symptoms are real have been identified and supported through the scientific literature. Children do have pain and they do feel dizzy. They do experience leg paralysis and gait imbalance. They are not intentionally producing symptoms and the symptoms are involuntary. No matter the cause, *the child has the symptoms*. Skipping ahead to the treatment section, it would be evident that regardless of what is causing the symptoms, everyone's focus, especially the mental health provider's, is to return children to normal function. Ultimately, this is what makes any physical symptom better and easier to cope with. This is true whether a child has a gait disturbance related to conversion disorder with no associated injury, or a gait disturbance related to chronic pain from a (now-healed) broken ankle. It is true whether a child has syncope that was diagnosed via tilt-table test with orthostatic signs and treated with medication, or a child who did not demonstrate clinically significant cardiac changes but continues to experience dizziness. And it is true for a child with nausea and abdominal pain that arose after a nasty viral infection but never went away, as it is for a child with anxiety who throws up each morning before school with no such infectious history.

When questioned by colleagues who wonder about working with children with somatic symptoms, we say, "We work with children with medical problems that are real, but are not from diseases, to help them understand their symptoms and learn coping strategies to get back to their lives." In going beyond questioning the reality of symptoms, accepting that they are real, and understanding the related factors that affect children's lives, a mental health provider can help children overcome *both* the symptoms and impairment.

Despite the very best descriptions of somatic symptoms and efforts to explain this type of intervention, at times it is hard for parents, health care professionals, and even other mental health providers to believe that children are not producing these symptoms on purpose. Sometimes the message conveyed to children and families is that the referral to a therapist is being made because the symptoms are believed to be "all in your head." Unfortunately, this sets mental health providers up for failure, as they are not any more in control of the symptoms than the child. Usually, the idea that somatic symptoms are made up or untrue is due to confusion between malingering and secondary gain. It is important to address these myths about somatic symptoms, as they out there in the public consciousness. The majority of children with somatic symptoms do not falsify symptoms, but there can be secondary gain in symptom reinforcement.

Malingering/Factitious Disorders

In some circumstances, it can be the case that children are not actually experiencing the symptoms they are reporting, but are in fact making up their symptom presentation. By definition, a factitious disorder is the falsification of medical or psychological symptoms where the person is taking deliberate action to misrepresent or actually cause illness or injury to him- or herself (or others, as in Munchausen syndrome by proxy) in order to satisfy a need, such as the need for attention or nurturance (American Psychiatric Association, 2013). Malingering, while not classified as a psychiatric disorder, shares the same definition as factitious disorder, with the addition that symptoms are reported primarily for personal gain or reward. While there is no methodologically sound way to estimate the incidence of self-induced factitious disorders or malingering in children, the clinical opinion is that it is uncommon in clinical settings (Bass & Halligan, 2014). Because the evaluation of illness falsification requires careful behavioral analysis using medical records, it is a time-consuming and challenging task that is rarely pursued. It is recommended that clinicians believe children's symptom reports unless there are warning signs present that require further evaluation. Children who falsify illness in themselves are also distressed and require a biopsychosocial treatment approach for recovery, similar to children with somatic symptoms. Additionally, it's possible for these disorders to coexist. Finally, children with either diagnosis may have a parent who interferes with care to such an extent that a suspected child abuse report is required.

Unintentional Secondary Gain

It is not a key feature of somatic symptoms that children seek secondary gain based on their symptoms. However, it is certainly the case that this *unintentionally* happens. For example, a child with multiple symptoms (nausea, vomiting, fatigue) may discover that her parents fight less when she is in the hospital; thus, while the child may not *make* herself vomit to the point of hospitalization, she is reinforced for having symptoms because of the family harmony her illness achieves. In this way, bodily responses can be unintentionally classically conditioned.

Sometimes, when these patterns are noted, it is suggested that perhaps children are making up their symptoms or getting sick "on purpose" in order to receive the benefit that has been identified. Acknowledge that while these secondary gains and reinforcement patterns exist and may maintain the symptom presentation, they are not the sole reason for the symptoms in the first place and the child is not producing symptoms intentionally. Children with somatic symptoms often have an extremely high, sustained degree of symptoms and impairment; it is not our experience that children sit around plotting their next distressing malady just so they can stay home and get that new video game they have been wanting. The impact of somatic symptoms on family relationships and children's behavior is reviewed in Chapter 9, as are strategies parents can use to uncouple these associations and form a healthier pattern of interaction with their children.

CHAPTER SUMMARY AND TAKE-AWAY POINTS

■ Somatic symptoms are common in primary care and specialty care settings and are seen in every body system. They are common among school-age children 6 to 18 and happen in both boys and girls in childhood, with higher incidence in adolescent girls. Somatic symptoms are impairing and associated with psychological distress and high levels of health care utilization.

- The most common somatic symptoms include headache, fatigue, dizziness, aching muscles, limb pain, nausea, abdominal pain, and neurological symptoms (e.g., changes in eyesight, balance, sensation, or gait). Somatic symptoms are real, they are not intentional, and they are involuntary.

- Theory and research demonstrate that somatic symptoms are produced and maintained by the contribution and interaction of biological, psychological, and social factors.

CHAPTER 3

The Biopsychosocial Model
of Somatic Symptoms

Now that we have established a basis for understanding cognitive-behavioral treatment and the nature of somatic symptoms, this chapter will address how they are best understood from a conceptual standpoint and how to explain them to children and families. The assessment and treatment of somatic symptoms should be firmly grounded in the biopsychosocial model of medicine, which accounts for the contribution and interaction of biological, psychological, and social factors in the presentation of *all* physical symptoms, organic and functional. It might seem that this should be obvious—of course all symptoms are the result of physical, emotional, and contextual experiences. However, medicine was not always practiced this way, and somatic symptoms in particular were not always understood within this framework.

THE BIOMEDICAL MODEL

The traditional conceptual model of symptoms and disease that Western medicine was founded on, the biomedical model, simply does not have a medical explanation for somatic symptoms and, as a result, does not provide treatment guidance other than a recommendation to seek psychiatric attention (Engel, 1977). Unfortunately, this is where the old adage "It's is all in your head" was born, and persists, to some extent, to this day. Positively, in recent years, a new model of symptoms and disease has taken the place of the biomedical model; the biopsychosocial model improves the care of organic conditions by acknowledging that psychosocial factors play a role in those presentations, as well as better accounts and provides a foundation for treatment of somatic symptoms (Drossman, 1998). To best illustrate how the biopsychosocial approach enhances the ability to understand and treat children with somatic symptoms, first consider the model that came before it.

Simply put, the biomedical model separates "mind" and "body." The model is based on the belief that identifiable medical causes for illness, such as injury, disease, and infection—and only those causes—lead to a person's experience of physical symptoms. The biomedical model is the foundation of Western medicine, firmly rooted in the physical sciences of molecular biology, physics, and chemistry (Engel, 1977). It distinguishes mental processes from physical ones, so that symptoms must be fully accounted for by disease or injury; in the absence of an identifiable medical cause, anything else is simply *not* of medical origin or concern (Wade & Halligan, 2004). Following from this rationale, medical care focuses on assessment, treatment, and cure of organic, identifiable, disease-based symptoms. For example, a quintessential biomedical success is illustrated by what happens when a child falls and cuts her arm. She gets patched up by the doctor, ointment is applied to prevent infection, and the wound is expected to heal without complication. A clear biological insult was identified, the treatment was directly targeted to the injury, and the eventual result is cure, with only a small scar remaining to remind the child of the whole ordeal. In this way, the biomedical model clearly explains and successfully treats organically based medical issues and is responsible for the development of many innovative and successful medical treatments.

Despite these significant biological advances, there were two clear challenges to the biomedical model. One was the inability to account for psychosocial factors that influence all illness experiences, both organic and functional. The model did not take psychosocial factors into consideration in the experience of any symptom, and was thus much more focused on disease than illness. The other challenge was the absence of a mechanism to explain and treat symptoms without an identifiable disease-based etiology. Somatic symptoms were categorized as nonmedical in origin, and therefore as mental or emotional in causality; thus, there was no role for medicine or medical providers in the care of patients struggling with somatic symptoms. In the case of patients for whom the symptoms started or continued in the absence of clear injury or disease, they left the physician's office with a clean bill of health and a very confused mind. A different approach was needed and warranted for treatment of patients regardless of symptom origin, and the biopsychosocial model was there to meet the challenge.

THE BIOPSYCHOSOCIAL MODEL

The biopsychosocial model is similar to the biomedical model in that it is also grounded in the physical sciences; however, it goes beyond this perspective to incorporate the behavioral and psychological sciences (Engel, 1977). In contrast to the dualism of the biomedical model, which separates physical from mental, the biopsychosocial model is multicausal, connecting mind and body so that symptoms, any kinds of symptoms, arise from *both* mental and physical processes. By definition, the biopsychosocial model "integrates biological science with the unique features of the individual and determines the degree to which biological and psychosocial factors interact to explain the disease, illness, and outcome" (Drossman, 1998, p. 262). In addition to disease and injury, psychological, social, environmental, behavioral, and physiological factors are all recognized as contributing and interacting factors in the subjective experience of symptoms (Drossman, 1998; Engel, 1997; Gatchel, Peng, Peters, Fuchs, & Turk, 2007; Wade & Halligan, 2004). "Subjective" is a key word, as this signifies the importance of considering a patient's own experience of the illness rather than the disease observed under the microscope. In other words, a disease or injury is only *one* way in which symptoms may arise (Stone et al., 2005). Physicians practicing within the biopsychosocial model consider multiple causes and treatments for symptoms, including physical, social, emotional, and behavioral factors, for all types of symptoms presentations. Using the previous example of the child who fell and cut her arm, a biopsychosocial treatment approach would still ensure that she is stitched up and given ointment to prevent infection in order to address the biological nature of her concerns, but emphasis is also placed on ameliorating any emotional distress she may have about her injury and on social support by staff and family members. Not only does the child receive the same great medical care, but the psychosocial aspects of illness are also addressed to enhance her treatment and recovery.

A great example of the benefits of the biopsychosocial model comes from a child life specialist we know who does international work with a group that performs operations on children in need of cleft palate repair in impoverished nations around the world. Her role is to familiarize children with the anesthesia masks prior to surgery through fun games and activities (think: anesthesia mask as a bubble blower!). She is an essential part of the medical team because the group has found that *children have better surgical outcomes when they are not scared prior to surgery*. Fear is a common reaction among children who present for these surgeries because most have never even seen a doctor, let alone been whisked away from their parents for a major medical intervention. Biologically, fear produces high levels of cortisol and epinephrine, and this presurgical physical state does not allow children's bodies to maximize their healing potential. Simply attending to children's psychosocial needs by familiarizing them with the equipment through the universal language of play, in a comfortable environment and with the support of their parents prior to the procedure, allows them to go into surgery feeling calm and relaxed as they enter a now-familiar situation. The result is better surgical outcomes. That is a true story of the biopsychosocial model in action that even the most biomedically oriented medical provider cannot dispute.

Since its entrance onto the medical scene, the biopsychosocial model has revolutionized all aspects of medical care. Most importantly, for our purposes, it changed attitudes toward assessment and treatment of somatic symptoms. With its mind–body approach, the biopsychosocial model provides a conceptual framework from which to understand and treat symptoms that start or continue in the absence of injury or disease. It "provides the rationale and support for explanations and treatments that direct their focus to the non-medical reasons why people may feel ill" (Wade & Halligan, 2004, p. 1400). Some might say this approach combines Eastern philosophy with the science of Western medicine. In some senses, it represents the best of both worlds by incorporating recent scientific advances in the field of medicine with early medical and holistic practices.

In addition to the benefits afforded to a child with somatic symptoms who is treated within the biopsychosocial model, also consider the enhanced experience of the family, particularly for parents receiving explanation of children's somatic symptoms. Not surprisingly, parents have certain expectations about receiving information relating to diagnosis, treatment, and prognosis when seeking medical care for their children (Korsch, Gozzi, & Francis, 1968). When these expectations aren't met, they feel uncertain about their children's health, and their uncertainty is associated with the perception of greater symptom severity, emotional distress, and protective parenting behavior (Stewart & Mishel, 2000). A biopsychosocial approach better addresses parents' expectations about the medical encounter, reducing their uncertainty and improving their ability to understand their children's symptoms and provide them with better support (Williams, Smith, Bruehl, Gigante, & Walker, 2009).

While application of this model to somatic symptoms has many benefits, the biopsychosocial framework improves care for *all* symptom presentations, including injury and disease, and improves understanding of the experience of *any* illness for both children and their parents. For all of these reasons, the biopsychosocial model is now the cornerstone of the philosophy underlying contemporary medical assessment and treatment.

APPLYING THE BIOPSYCHOSOCIAL MODEL TO SOMATIC SYMPTOMS

The application of the biopsychosocial model to our understanding of somatic symptoms represents a big shift in thinking for health care providers as well as for children and families. The biomedical model has dominated medicine for most of the modern era, and that mentality has translated over into public opinion as well. While the new generation of medical providers has been thoroughly trained in the importance of adding the "psychosocial" to the "bio," the general public is still catching up to this way of thinking. Mental health providers should be prepared to encounter parents, and even some children themselves, with deeply rooted beliefs that symptoms come from either the mind or the body. Children and families in this position benefit from education about the evolution of medical care and from hearing real-life examples that illustrate the importance of psychosocial factors in treating children with injury or disease, like the evidence for improved surgical outcomes for children who received psychosocial intervention. Patience is key—providing this education takes additional time, but it must not be omitted, as it is the basis for children and families to buy into the treatment that follows.

The biopsychosocial model is a more detailed and better developed take on the "mind–body connection," a term with which many are familiar, and this is one way of introducing it that may create some familiarity for those who are otherwise unaware. Engaging in a mind–body dialogue with children and families in this manner allows for discussion of the involvement of other factors that come along with physical symptoms without creating or furthering the message many children with somatic symptoms have received that "it is all in their head." *It is extremely important for a clinician believe in the reality of the child's symptoms. It is equally important to say, "I know your symptoms and distress are real" to children and families the very first time you meet them.* Their symptoms are not in their head; they are real, biologically based, distressing, and impairing. In our practice, time and time again children have told us that the most important words we have spoken to them in treatment were "I believe you."

The fact that there is not a test to "show" or "prove" the reality of children's suffering through existing medical technology does not mean that their symptoms are not real, or possibly organically based. A very famous example of this comes from the history of ulcer treatment. Prior to the discovery of the *Helicobacter pylori* bacteria in 1982 (which by most people's count is not that long ago!), the commonly held belief was that "stress" alone caused stomach ulcers. Simply put, ulcers were just another type of somatic symptom. With the discovery of *H. pylori*, the medical community discovered that in fact *germs* were the primary cause of ulcers—up to 90% of ulcers in fact—and new biological therapies were delivered as a result to target the source of the problem. Emotional stress certainly makes the experience of having ulcers worse and is still considered a contributing factor to a person's vulnerability to *H. pylori*, but stress is no longer implicated as singularly *causing* these problems in the first place.

While the *H. pylori* discovery well illustrates how something considered to be purely psychological in nature was found to also have a significant biological component, there are also a number examples of diseases once believed to be purely *biological* in nature that are now best understood from a biopsychosocial context. A good example of this is in the world of cancer. Everyone agrees that cancer has a strong physical basis in terms of the presence of disease and the need for an equally strong biological treatment. However, these days, everyone also agrees that the way people feel about having cancer and how they are supported socially are core parts of the successful treatment of cancer. Imagine meeting a child with cancer and telling his or her family that there was no need for psychosocial support—this would rarely happen. This is another good example of the benefit of the biopsychosocial treatment approach for even the most biological of diseases.

Medical tests and procedures are changing and becoming more innovative all the time. What biological causes for somatic symptoms will be discovered in the future, causing us to look back and wonder how they were ever considered *solely* as the result of emotional stress? This is another reason to consider *all* symptoms using a biopsychosocial model. Even when all of the medical tests come back normal, this does not necessarily mean that the child has no biological abnormality, it just means that we do not have the test to identify it at this point. This can be frustrating for children, families, and providers alike, who all wish there were more medical knowledge about these symptoms and the associated biological treatments right now.

The job of the mental health provider is to guide children and families through this challenge by sharing what we *do* know about the biology of somatic symptoms, that they are real even in the absence of a test saying so, shifting attention away from a futile search for the "cause" and focusing on the psychosocial factors that are intertwined with the physical experience. Ultimately, this approach best enables children to cope with symptoms, whatever may be causing them, by giving them permission and teaching them how to return to normal functioning. We have on many occasions told families that although they may continue their search for an elusive cause, our treatment will remain unchanged *regardless* of new diagnoses. As long as we know that the symptom is not dangerous, which has been determined by the time children see us, any symptom will improve if the focus shifts from sickness to wellness and function. The first step in teaching children and families about this approach is to increase understanding of symptoms in the context of the biopsychosocial model, which can be done right from the start through the assessment.

CONDUCTING A BIOPSYCHOSOCIAL ASSESSMENT

For health care providers, the biopsychosocial model provides a framework for assessment and treatment and can also be used as a tool to educate children about their condition. A key to the biopsychosocial explanation of somatic symptoms is to describe that physical symptoms exist *and* they are affected by psychosocial factors. It is very helpful to explain this model to children and their families when assessing somatic symptoms, and typically, when shown that all factors are on an equal footing, they quite readily recognize the contribution of each one. To make this conceptual model more concrete, draw it as an actual figure, such as the "Biopsychosocial Assessment Tool" (in the Appendix), which can be used as a guide to discuss each of these areas in the assessment while filling in the child's own experience.

When conducting an assessment within the biopsychosocial model, start with the biological factors. Beginning here provides a concept and language with which families are comfortable and familiar, not to mention the primary reason why they are seeking treatment. Specifically, the biological component covers how the symptoms are experienced (e.g., pain, dizziness, physical impairment) and can be used to understand the child's experience as well as to generate discussion of how these symptoms are produced from the physiological functioning or malfunctioning of the body, several models of which are covered later in this chapter.

Once the biological experience is established, children and families can be encouraged to consider the psychological and social factors that coexist with the experience of somatic symptoms and to feel more comfortable doing so. The psychological component focuses on the emotional factors (e.g., thoughts, feelings, and actions) that affect or contribute to symptoms, and the social component focuses on how different contextual factors relate to symptoms (e.g., family, school, friends, community interactions and reactions). Step-by-step instructions are provided on how to carry out the specifics of a biopsychosocial assessment with the child in Chapter 4.

After each symptom area is addressed, the interplay between all three factors can be considered in terms of the impact on the child's overall health and well-being by pointing out the intersection between the three areas on the "Biopsychosocial Assessment Tool." Through this process, children recognize that the interaction of all three factors results in poor overall health and well-being, and this can then be used as a way to generate motivation to target each area as part of a cohesive treatment plan to improve overall health. The biopsychosocial assessment also provides a way to understand the pattern to children's symptoms by hearing them describe the various factors that comprise and affect their symptom experience, which will guide the focus of treatment.

Another interesting perspective can be gained by turning the biopsychosocial model on its head, so that instead of looking at the negative side of these three factors, which add up to overall poor health, you consider the positive side of each factor, which can result in wellness. Thus, instead of symptoms, the biopsychosocial model can be used to focus on resilience, consisting of physical strength and perseverance, a positive mental attitude and coping ability, and a supportive social context. Either perspective, the positive or the negative, sets the stage for effective treatment buy-in, which is the ultimate goal of the biopsychosocial assessment.

As a brief example of this approach, a child identified the following biopsychosocial factors in her somatic symptom presentation:

- Biological: intermittent dizziness, headache, and nausea.
- Psychological: anxiety, frustration, and loneliness.
- Social: family arguments, missed school, and fewer social events.
- Intersection: poor overall health.

During the assessment, as each area was highlighted, the interplay that each factor had with the others was discussed—how the anxiety increased the headaches, which in turn promoted school absences that increased family arguments and the child's frustration, all of which resulted in increased symptoms. By laying out all of these factors and showing how they were intertwined, the family had an experience that validated the layers of challenges they had been facing and began to understand how the experience of illness was affected by and contributed to the physical manifestations of the problem. It is also helpful for the provider to discover these negative patterns associated with symptoms and begin thinking about how to switch the focus to a more positive pattern. Through this experience, the family began to see that the solution would require addressing more than just the physical nature of the issues at hand. They were able to see that reducing symptoms and improving strength through exercise, mentally addressing symptoms in a more confident manner, and normalizing daily function with support would be a path to improved function and eventual symptom improvement.

The rest of the book will focus on putting the ideas that arise during the assessment into practice. Next we provide several specific applications of the biopsychosocial model that are useful in educating children and families about the biological origins of somatic symptoms, which allows for further understanding of the role of psychosocial factors as well.

EDUCATION WITHIN THE BIOPSYCHOSOCIAL MODEL

The key to understanding the biopsychosocial model is to first address how biological processes are affected by psychological and social factors, as this will help you as the mental health provider teach children how their symptoms are related to their thoughts, feelings, and actions. This section illustrates how three major physiological responses play a role in the presentation of somatic symptoms: (1) the autonomic nervous system (ANS), (2) anticipatory anxiety, and (3) pain. Think back to the example of the relentlessly ringing fire alarm from the first chapter. We examine several ways in which that fire alarm—minus the smoke—can start and keep ringing in the human body. Understanding these processes is key for being able to effectively educate children and families, a topic that is covered in detail in Chapter 5. First, we want *you* to have a good understanding of these connections through the examples presented here. In addition, these examples are suitable to draw on in educating children and families. We recommend that you provide education about the first topic, the ANS, to every child you see with somatic symptoms, as that provides core information that is applicable for all presentations, and that you add education about anxiety and pain as needed.

Autonomic Nervous System

The major player in the experience of any kind of physical symptom is the ANS. The ANS is a division of the peripheral nervous system and the largely unconsciously controlled force in our body that connects the brain (part of the central nervous system) to the internal organs and regulates critical everyday functions, such as respiration, circulation, and digestion. The ANS has three branches, two of which play a major role in energy distribution in the body. The sympathetic branch controls the "fight-or-flight" response and springs the body into action, initiating increases in heart rate, breathing, and muscle tension. The parasympathetic branch controls the "rest-and-digest" response and relaxes the body, facilitating physical restoration with decreases in heart rate, breathing, and muscle tension. The ANS is always on and constantly balances those two branches to enact a series of physical responses that give us energy when we need it (sympathetic) and back off when we do not (parasympathetic). An excellent book describing the ANS and the relationship of the stress response to chronic illness is *Why Zebras Don't Get Ulcers* (Sapolsky, 2004).

The ANS is something every human being has, and it is wired to enact responses automatically depending on the situation, largely to promote survival. The degree to which a person experiences sympathetic or parasympathetic activity has a direct impact on any physical symptoms he or she experiences; this is especially true for children with somatic symptoms. Many times, in the case of somatic symptoms, the problem is not the ANS activity itself—we all have these responses, after all—but that the ANS activity is either out or proportion to what is needed in the situation, it does not turn off after the perceived stressor has passed, or the experience is interpreted as a dangerous response when it is in fact a normal process. For example, when sympathetic activation starts but does not stop, like that pesky fire alarm that continues ringing long after the flames are out, the prolonged response creates problems of its own by perpetuating symptoms like increased heart rate or muscle tension. Turning on the relaxation response calms down the body and reduces symptoms; however, that is very difficult for a person to do under conditions of extreme or chronic activation, which is the case for many children with somatic symptoms.

In addition to the challenge of coping with the symptom itself, autonomic symptoms are made worse by negative emotions, largely because emotions *also* activate the sympathetic nervous system, adding fuel to the proverbial fire. For example, children who are anxious are more likely to pick up on aspects of their situation that are worrisome or uncertain because they are activated and on high alert; however, this vigilance maintains apprehension and fear, which leads to amplified somatic symptoms. One way to teach children about this connection is to ask them to think about the last time they were really excited about something and if they noticed any corresponding physical sensation in their body. Most children will answer that they were jumpy or had butterflies, which is a good way to illustrate the connection between symptoms and emotions.

Overall, teaching children the connection of the ANS to somatic symptoms and emotion enables their understanding that this is a *normal process* that is just working *abnormally*, and they can learn to recognize and take control of it. Two examples that can be used teach children about the ANS are the Caveman and the Car. These examples are presented in the same language used to describe this process to children. Again, this is education we provide to all children with somatic symptoms.

The Caveman

"To understand the autonomic nervous system and why it is important for human survival, let's go back for a minute and imagine the days of the cavemen. Imagine that a caveman is out for a nice walk through the rocks and trees, and all of a sudden, a saber-toothed tiger jumps out at him! This is a dangerous situation and his body knows to protect him from danger, so he has an *immediate* physical reaction. His body activates to give him super strength to fight off the tiger or to run away and survive another day. Phew! The tiger leaves him alone, he sees that he is safe, and he goes back to his cave to relax for the evening. This process of activation and relaxation is automatic—he didn't even have to think about it—and it is one that still happens automatically in our bodies today. It is regulated by a system in our body called the autonomic nervous system (the ANS), which is controlled by the brain.

"There are two parts to the ANS that control how we get energy in our body. The part that makes us active is called the sympathetic nervous system, which controls the *fight-or-flight response* [see "The Fight-or-Flight Response" worksheet in the Appendix], and this helps us survive in times of danger or gives us enough energy in times of excitement. It does this by speeding up our heart and breathing rate so we can pump more blood and oxygen to our muscles to be strong, putting our digestion on hold so we can use all of our energy for moving, making our pupils in our eyes big so they can take in all of the information around us, and making our hands (and feet!) a little sweaty so we have good traction to pick things up or run. All of these responses are helpful for making our body the most effective it can be for action, and we do not even have to think about turning it on, it occurs automatically for us in situations where we perceive that something is happening. The part of the ANS that slows us down and lets us relax is called the parasympathetic nervous system, and it controls the *rest-and-digest response* [see "The Rest-and-Digest Response" worksheet in the Appendix], which calms us down when the danger is gone and allows us to rest when it is time to sleep. It does the *opposite* of the fight-or-flight response; it makes our heart and breathing rate go slower, our muscles get loose and relaxed, our stomachs digest our food to build up our energy reserves, and our hands and feet get warm and dry.

"These two systems work together all day long to keep us in balance, just like a seesaw or a teeter-totter: one side goes up to give us more energy while the other goes down to take a break, and then they take turns and the opposite side takes over to do the work. For the caveman in our example, the ANS really helped to get him out of this situation. His fight-or-flight response turned on to give him the energy to escape the danger, and then when he was safely back in his cave for the night, his rest-and-digest response turned on and allowed his body to relax and save up enough strength for tomorrow.

"Now these days, of course, we no longer have to worry about saber-toothed tigers jumping out at us (thank goodness!), but we do need to keep an eye out for cars when crossing the street or for the sound of a fire alarm, and our fight-or-flight response is still helpful in those situations to alert us and give us the energy we need to protect ourselves. But the problem is that sometimes the fight-or-flight response is not so helpful. For many children, their fight-or-flight response gets turned on if they are worried or nervous about something that is not *physically* dangerous, like taking test at school, or even when they get very excited about something, like going to a fun birthday party. It can even turn on when kids have had a long day, are tired, dehydrated, or are playing in really hot weather. It is not their fault that this system turns on! Remember, the fight-or-flight response is *automatic*, and whenever our body perceives that something is happening (either dangerous or exciting), it turns on the fight-or-flight response to give you more energy to act. But for situations that are not *physically* dangerous or are just plain fun, the activation that is felt from the fight-or-flight response doesn't help us out, and actually, it can make the situation as well as our thoughts, feelings, and body responses worse.

"As you can probably imagine, it is really hard to concentrate and take a test when your heart is racing, your muscles are shaking, and your hands are sweaty. It is also really hard to enjoy a birthday party when your stomach is hurting and you have to run to the bathroom. Another challenge about the fight-or-flight response is that sometimes when it turns on, our bodies forget to turn it off, and that can make our bodies feel really bad over time. What started out as a helpful way to warn us of danger or give us energy to have fun sometimes turns into feeling pretty bad, and as you can probably guess, that is something that happens to a lot of kids who have somatic symptoms. The good news is that we can learn ways to turn that fight-or-flight response off at times when it is not helpful, learn how it is normal but not dangerous to feel this way, and make your body feel more relaxed instead of activated."

The Car

"To understand how your body works and how this affects the symptoms you feel, imagine that your body is like a car [see the "Learning to Drive the 'AUTO'nomic Nervous System" worksheet in the Appendix]. And just like a car, your body has two pedals that control how fast or slow it is going. The gas pedal speeds a car up; the system in our body that does this is called the sympathetic nervous system, which controls the fight-or-flight response. In a car, when we push on the gas pedal, it increases the amount of fuel that goes to the engine, which speeds up the motor and increases the rate that the tires are spinning, and the effect is that it makes our car go faster. In our bodies, when the fight-or-flight response activates, it is like hitting the gas—epinephrine (also called adrenaline) and other chemicals are released to make our bodies go faster, which we feel through our breathing and heart going faster, our muscles tensing up, and digestion slowing down to divert energy to the parts of our body that need to act. This body response allows us to react to an uncertain or exciting or dangerous situation, just like a car speeding up to pass a truck on the highway.

"But what about the brakes? When the danger or excitement has passed, we need to slow down again. The parasympathetic nervous system controls the rest-and-digest response, which is our body's brakes. Pressing on the brakes allows a car to slow down once it has passed the truck by slowing down the motor and making the tires spin less. The rest-and-digest response in the body does the very same thing by slowing down the heart and respiration rate, turning on the digestion process again, and stopping the production of epinephrine so we can relax. This allows our body to restore our energy and save up our strength for the next time we might need it, and it makes us go to sleep, just like a car pulling into the garage for the night.

"Like a car smoothly traveling on the highway, avoiding drastic changes in speed by having just enough gas and just enough brakes, our bodies also respond best by having a balance of activation and relaxation. Sometimes, however, this balance is difficult to strike. Have you ever felt like your gas pedal got stuck and you were speeding down the highway without any brakes? If this happened in a car, you would feel out of control or maybe even get pulled over because you were speeding. Most people have felt that way in their bodies, when our whole system is going very fast and it feels like our bodies have completely forgotten about the idea of having any brakes at all, and you feel like you are going to crash. The result is that we end up being in a constant state of fight-or-flight, except there may be no danger or excitement in sight, or at least not the kind that requires that much of a reaction. The physical symptoms of a body racing at top speed like an out-of-control car can be dizziness, nausea, headaches, jitteriness, muscle tension, or feeling hot and sweaty, all of which are produced and maintained by an overactivated nervous system. Often, these types of symptoms are a function of a nervous system that has gotten stuck on 'go' and forgotten how to hit the brakes. We will work on recognizing when your body is stuck on the gas and learning to find the brakes again."

Anticipatory Anxiety

Teach children about the role of anticipatory anxiety in somatic symptom presentations when applicable to their clinical presentation and symptom pattern. From the point of view of behavioral theory as it applies to anxiety and somatic symptoms, the process of anticipatory anxiety and avoidance can be described in terms of negative reinforcement (Figure 3.1). It is a response pattern that leads to *temporary* relief of anxiety and somatic symptoms, reinforcing the negative thought process, emotions, and physical response, leading to avoidance. Children may begin the process by waking up in the morning and thinking, "Ugh, I really don't want to school. What if I pass out in gym class again?" This thought pattern may lead them to expect that this is going to be a hard day, which increases somatic sensations and worry, increases ANS arousal and dizziness—and now they feel exactly as they feared they might. These cognitive, emotional, and physiological responses feed into the need for escape— there is no way they can go to school feeling this way—and if they are allowed to stay home and avoid the feared thing, they get a feeling of (temporary) relief. In this way, anticipatory anxiety leads children to plan a day of symptoms *before they have even gotten out of bed.* Their bodies are on alert, they scan to find symptoms, which are present once they turn their attention to them, their minds fill in the blank that those symptoms are a threat, and they plan for avoidance. The absence of the feared thing happening produces enough relief to reinforce this pattern of events happening tomorrow, and the next day, and the one after that.

This type of short-term strategy may produce relief in the moment, but it certainly does not result in long-term gain if children are missing out on life events, and it only further solidifies the symptom presentation from a physiological and psychological standpoint. That process is also strengthened when children are positively reinforced for *not* doing something, such as the day of missed school resulting in a special day with a parent. The cycle just becomes stronger: not only does the child experience the emotional relief of not having to think about getting symptoms at school that day and the physical relief of the symptoms abating in the moment with the removal of the immediate stressor, but now the child also associates avoidance with a positive parental interaction. The longer cycles like these have gone on, the stronger they are and the harder they are to break. Anticipatory anxiety in somatic symptoms is like a monster that demands to be fed—the more you feed it, the more it expects, it grows bigger, and it threatens to never leave you alone until you address it. So much about teaching children to cope with the anxiety associated with somatic symptoms is teaching them to face the monster—whether they pass out or whether they do not, a mental health provider's job is to help the child feel like he or she can make it through that situation. That is the only way to break the cycle.

The key to success for children is recognizing this process of anxiety and avoidance, seeing how it is linked to somatic symptoms, and retraining the brain to think differently. Some children are able to do this on their own, and these are the ones that do not seek out treatment; they have symptoms but do not experience significant impairment due to a combination of internal resilience factors, effective parenting or schooling approaches, and biological factors that better regulate symptom intensity. The children who end up in a mental health provider's office have likely had more difficulty understanding the cycle of anxiety and avoidance. Thus, it is important to explain these connections to them. Although examples based on their own symptoms and situations are always the most effective, a general example that can be used is the following:

> "Now that we have a better understanding of how the ANS works, it makes sense that in the presence of danger, our body would prepare to react and survive. But

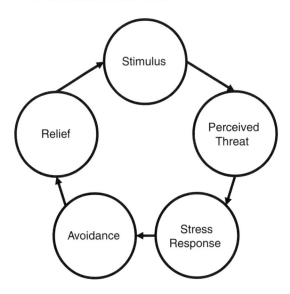

FIGURE 3.1. Avoidance cycle.

what happens when we just *think* about a fearful event? The same fight-or-flight response activates, *even when danger is not there*, and can get stuck there in the 'go' position, making our bodies speed up and feel bad, and it might make us miss out on something we really want or need to do."

To personalize these examples, think about times this might have happened to children you work with, like before a big test, when they are shooting free throws to win the big game in a crowded gym, when they have a bad headache, or when they are thinking about what other children will say if they pass out. In these situations, children's bodies might be too activated and energized to actually perform very well, and then their worst fear comes true when they do not do as well as they wanted to. Consider how you feel when you are excited; now think of how you feel when you are running late to catch a flight. Many of the same physiological reactions are present when you feel joy and also when you feel fear. Our brain determines what emotions to assign to a situation; our body just knows whether or not something is happening. Teach children to recognize when they are in situations in which just *thinking* negatively results in *feeling* badly and develop different strategies to change their thinking or alter aspects of the situation, which can improve their body responses as well as the confidence they need to function well. Here are two specific examples of the anticipatory anxiety and avoidance process that can be used to explain these connections to children, one that we call the Hallway and the other we call Pea Soup.

The Hallway

"I am going to tell you about a girl your age who has a lot of somatic symptoms like you: dizziness, headache, and sometimes her balance gets really tricky and she either falls down or passes out altogether. When she started having those problems, she and her whole family understandably felt very worried, so they took her to her pediatrician. The pediatrician felt like she was probably OK and told her she should stay well hydrated and take more breaks when running around outside. Just to be sure, the doctor also sent her to a specialist to check out her heart and another to check out her brain, which was a little scary for her to hear. The specialists also believed that she was OK and said she might grow out of it. This did not help her out very much because she still had the symptoms, and it was still scary for her to have these experiences and for her parents to watch it happen. And, as we discussed, when something is scary, the fight-or-flight response turns on, which made all of these symptoms worse.

"She tried to keep going, but getting around the hallway at school was becoming more and more difficult because she never knew when she might feel dizzy and fall. She found herself thinking about her symptoms all the time, which made her fight-or-flight response turn on even more. Pretty soon, she could just *think* of what it would be like to have the symptoms and the *same* activation started. Each morning, she thought, 'What if I feel dizzy and fall down at school tomorrow?,' which activated her nervous system *and made it more likely that she would actually have these symptoms*. Pretty soon, she avoided walking in the hallways at school altogether so she could stay safe, but the problem was that if she could not walk in the hallway, she could not go to school. Although her body felt like she was doing the right thing in the short term by staying home, she would have problems in the long term by missing so much school. And the whole process was started through just *thinking* about walking in the hallway! Our brains and bodies are connected, and learning about these associations can help us undo these patterns that seem like a good idea at the time but are bad for us in the long run."

Pea Soup

"Another way to understand the role of anxiety and associations in ANS arousal is to think of something that has caused a physical reaction for you in the past that you now have a negative association with, maybe something that made you nervous, made you throw up, or caused you pain. I bet you can think of a negative experience that is associated with a physical symptom, such as feeling nauseous and throwing up after eating a particular food that was spoiled. You might notice that you avoid that food to this day—case in point being split pea soup! Think about something that you have experienced as we go through this example.

"After we have eaten something and gotten sick, biologically, our bodies and minds remember these experiences so we can avoid getting sick in the future. This is done through our ANS, which activates when we see that food again or even if we just think about eating it. Although it is unlikely that we will actually be sickened by that dish a second time, our body remembers the time that it did and creates a response to make us avoid taking a chance. Luckily for us, there are lots of other options for lunch than split pea soup. But what if there were not? In that case, we would have to unlearn the negative connection that was made between symptoms and the food, and relearn positive associations to enable us to eat lunch. However, you can certainly appreciate how that would be hard to do; after all, would you be willing to eat a food that previously made you sick? It would be really difficult, especially at first, because while logically you would know that this food is not likely to be poisoned, your body would be trying to tell you otherwise. Breaking associations like this is a hard concept for our human minds to grasp, as our bodies are conditioned to attend to these experiences as a way to alert us to threat. CBT helps with this by teaching coping skills to calm the body down at times when it is becoming activated and to relearn how to think about the situation in more helpful and realistic ways. In this case, we could learn to take a deep breath, think about positive experiences with the food, and remind ourselves about how many times we previously ate the food with no trouble at all.

"This is the same process that happens for somatic symptoms—the body remembers previous times when it has felt poorly, and associates symptoms to situations in an effort to avoid that process again in the future. Because of that, even just thinking about a time when the symptoms occurred can make them happen, just like getting sick at the idea of eating pea soup! However, for you, the activities that somatic symptoms get associated with usually cannot be easily avoided, like school or sports or seeing friends. Therefore, we teach you the same process of retraining the brain to get used to doing those activities again and feeling confident about returning to normal functional patterns."

Pain

Besides modification of factors related to the anxiety and avoidance cycle, there are also factors that can be modified to change a person's pain experience. To help children with painful somatic symptoms you need to understand and teach them about the role of the nervous system and the gate control theory of pain.

First, consider the role of the nervous system in the experience of pain. Many children (and adults, even) may think that pain is a symptom that comes only from the muscles or organs around the place that hurts, so a child with chronic stomachaches might think that only the GI system is producing pain. While it is true that pain is being felt in that location, the actual *experience* of pain is happening through the nerves in those organs or muscles, and ultimately, all pain is processed by the brain. Once children understand this, they can better understand why they will be learning pain coping techniques that are, in effect, brain-based techniques to think about and respond to pain in a different way. It will help them to understand why the ANS plays a role in pain, too, with sympathetic activation increasing the experience of pain, because that is also a process directed by the brain. This biological understanding of pain allows children to buy into treatment by realizing that brain-based coping tools *are* directly related to pain, even if you are not teaching them something to do with the actual part of their body that hurts.

The second factor to understand is the gate control theory of pain, and how this theory can be used to modulate pain perception (see "The Gate Control Theory of Pain" worksheet in the Appendix). The gate control theory represented a significant advance in the biological understanding of pain processing, stemming from the observation that two people could have the exact same painful thing happen but demonstrate very different responses (Melzack & Wall, 1967). Prior to the inception of this theory, scientists did not have a good way to understand the factors that led to these different reactions. Melzack and Wall posited that there is a process of communication between the spinal cord and the brain that functions like a gate opening and closing, and pain signals have to pass through that gate in order to get to the brain. If the gate is open, all of the pain signals pass through and the person experiences the full amount of pain that is being communicated. However, if the gate is closed, the pain signals do not pass through, and although pain signals are present in the body, they do not succeed in carrying their message to the brain; therefore the person does not feel pain. The gate can be partially opened or closed as well, and pain perception changes based on the degree to which pain signals are able to get through.

With this concept in place, it was possible to understand the reason that people have different pain experiences because there are many factors that affect the position of the gate. Attention to the signal, emotional state, cognitive processes, ANS involvement, and contextual factors such as social support or the specific situation all affect the position of the gate and change the pain experience, even when the pain stimulus is exactly the same. It is important to understand all of the factors that affect the position of the gate for children with somatic symptoms, as those are key points of intervention and areas for coping skills training during treatment. After establishing this concept with children, the phrase "Will that close or open the gate?" can be used throughout treatment so that they can better understand their pain experience and the ways they can improve it.

Here is an example of how to explain the way pain works in relation to the nervous system and introduce the gate control theory of pain to illustrate these points (see Figure 3.2 and the "The Fight-or-Flight Response" worksheet in the Appendix to aid in the illustration of this pain education).

The Nervous System

"First, we will learn about the purpose of pain and why we have it in our body in the first place. Pain is a signal that travels through the nervous system and is processed in the brain. The job of the nervous system is to communicate messages back and forth from all different parts of the body to the brain, including sensations such as touch, temperature, and itch. One of the most important sensations the nervous system communicates about is pain, because that is a warning signal in our body that usually indicates that something dangerous is happening that we should respond to in order to protect ourselves.

"To better understand this, say that someone injures their toe, stubbing it against the wall really hard. What happens? First, a little nerve ending picks up a signal that something has happened. But the toe is not really the smartest part of the body and therefore cannot figure out anything more than that something

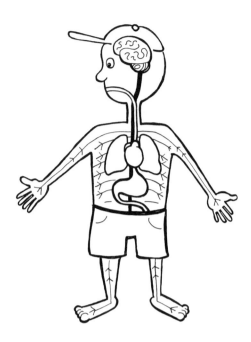

FIGURE 3.2. A body diagram to illustrate the nervous system.

has happened. So the nervous system does what it was made to do—the small nerve in the toe picks up the signal and *communicates* it, first by sending it up the nerves in your leg, then to the superhighway of nerves in your spinal cord, and finally all the way up into the brain. The brain picks up the message—I imagine it says something like 'Oh, look! A message from the toe!'—it reads the message, and you know what it says in response? That's right—OUCH! The brain sends a signal back down to the toe to move it away from what is hurting it. It is not until the signal is processed by the brain that a person feels pain—*it takes the brain to feel pain.* We call this pain 'protective' because it warns us that we are hurt and makes us stop what we are doing so we can prevent further damage and heal. Whereas acute pain is helpful, pain that goes on and on without any injury or damage to warn us about, like chronic pain, is unhelpful and is what we call 'nonprotective' pain.

"Chronic pain is the result of a mixed-up connection between the brain and body. It is the result of pain signaling that has gone wrong, not structural damage or injury. One way to think about it is as an alarm system that was designed to help us, like a smoke alarm, but now it is ringing even there is no fire. Sometimes we say the fire is out, but the alarm is still ringing. Chronic pain is like the smoke that is still hanging around in the air, not causing any danger but still setting off the bell! Another way to think about it is that chronic pain is a software problem, not a hardware problem. The machine is OK and you do not need a new computer, but there is a glitch in the software causing it to malfunction."

The Gate Control Theory of Pain

"We used to think it was easy for pain to get communicated to the brain: some harmful event happens or a chronic alarm keeps ringing, a signal is sent to the brain, and it is processed as pain. Now we know that it is more complicated than that, and there are other factors in the body and environment that affect how signals are received by the brain. The best theory of pain perception in the brain that describes how this works is called the gate control theory. Basically, when pain signals arrive to the brain, they have to pass through something like a gate, just like you would find across a road. Now, in our bodies it is not a real physical barrier—it is more like a series of chemicals and nerve impulses between the spinal cord and the brain, but for our purposes we will think about it as an actual gate that can open and close.

"When the gate is open, all of the pain signals are allowed to come through and your brain experiences the full amount of pain that is being communicated. If the gate is partially closed, pain signals still get into the brain but in a slower fashion, lessening the pain experience. If gate is closed all the way, pain signals are not able to carry their message into your brain at all—and in that case, you do not feel any pain. It is possible for pain signals to be there, but as long as they are not processed by brain, you do not feel pain.

"Now, if you have acute pain due to injury, you want to have the gate open to feel the pain and protect yourself from further damage. Imagine touching a hot stove—it would be important to notice that so you could remove your hand! However, if you have chronic pain, such as headaches and stomachaches, which are real signals but not alerting you to acute danger, then it is *not* helpful to have that gate open. In this case, the goal of treatment is to learn how to close the gate on unhelpful pain signals.

"There are some situations, thoughts, feelings, and actions that are more likely to open the gate, like paying a lot of attention to pain, the fight-or-flight response being turned on, feeling nervous or upset, and stressful experiences at school, with friends, or in your family. And there are a lot of situations, thoughts, feelings, and actions that close the gate, like taking attention away from the pain signal through distraction, turning on the relaxation response, and getting the right kind of support from school, family, and friends that improves function. A good example of the other factors that can open and close the gate is imagining that you got an envelope in the mail, and as you opened it, you got a paper cut right across your finger. Ouch! Now, if you found a brand new $100 bill in the mail, your thoughts, feelings, and actions would be so positive that you'd hardly even notice the pain from that paper cut. But if you found a bad report card being sent home to your parent, your thoughts, feelings, and actions would be so negative that you'd notice the pain from that paper cut a lot. Same cut, two totally different pain experiences because of the different influence of thoughts and feelings on the pain gate.

"Pain is also worse under conditions of sympathetic activation. Pain is a signal that is supposed to protect the body from damage, so when your body feels pain, the ANS *automatically* activates and opens the gate to allow the pain signal into the brain to figure out what is going on. In the best-case scenario, the sympathetic nervous system turns off once the brain and body respond to the danger. But as we know, with chronic pain, the signal doesn't stop ringing, so the brain never gives the all clear, which means the sympathetic nervous system stays on, and the gate stays open. We will work on stopping this response by learning pain coping techniques that can push on the brakes *and* close the gate. When you learn how to relax or distract yourself or think about a tough situation in a different way, those strategies have a *biological* effect on how pain is perceived, and this is how pain gets better over time."

CHAPTER SUMMARY AND TAKE-AWAY POINTS

- Somatic symptoms are best understood from a biopsychosocial standpoint in that physical, emotional, and contextual factors co-contribute to symptom presentation.

- Assessing children within the biopsychosocial model establishes the nature of this collaborative framework for understanding symptoms.

- The ANS, the role of anticipatory anxiety, and the gate control theory of pain are three specific ways of applying a biopsychosocial explanation to common somatic symptoms.

PART II

Assessment and Education

INTRODUCTION

The first three chapters reviewed what somatic symptoms are, why they are a problem for children and adolescents, and how to understand them through a biopsychosocial framework. The next two chapters focus on how to apply the biopsychosocial model to assessment and education of children with somatic symptoms. Overall, the focus of this initial phase of treatment is *not* to dig deep for a clear psychological stressor that is the sole cause for symptoms. By the time they get to a mental health provider, children have been asked ad nauseam what stress-causing factors in their lives have given rise to their symptoms, or worse, they may have been given the suggestion that something traumatic happened to cause their symptoms, insinuating that their symptoms are purely psychiatric in nature. As mentioned earlier, on a rare occasion, there is a clear, significant stressor that started off the chain of events; however, more often there is not, and it is far more constructive to understand all of the factors that interact to produce children's symptom experiences.

The goal of the assessment and education process is to put down the magnifying glass, help the family identify areas in which the child is experiencing dysfunction as a result of symptoms, and explore in a unified manner the psychosocial factors associated with the physical symptoms to discover how you can all work together to restore a more typical level of function. The nice thing about approaching treatment in this way is that it moves away from the idea that there is something psychologically "wrong" that led to this symptom presentation. Once that question is off the table, the conversation naturally shifts to a more productive focus on coping and function. Paying less attention to the problem and more attention to the solution reduces reinforcement of symptoms and the cycle of illness and increases reinforcement of adaptive behavior and resiliency. In this way, the dysfunctional associations between symptoms and impairment are clarified, and then education provides children with the framework to create new, more productive associations.

Assessment and education are truly the first steps of intervention that allows children to create more adaptive responses to symptoms, leading to functional restoration and symptom reduction, as reviewed in Part III. Each phase of intervention requires consistent application of the biopsychosocial model to help children make new connections between physical, psychological, and social factors influencing symptoms to realize ultimate success. Chapter 4 includes information on how to conduct a thorough assessment at the initial visit, highlighting the way this baseline interaction can be used to both successfully elicit the necessary information *and* lay the foundation of treatment within the biopsychosocial model. Chapter 5 describes the education phase detail, including examples of how to illustrate the factors underlying somatic symptoms to children with the most common symptom presentations and their families. The establishment of a solid biopsychosocial understanding of children's symptoms in the assessment and education sessions cannot be overemphasized; it is the cornerstone of the building that will ultimately be capped by the child's success.

CHAPTER 4

Assessment

A thorough assessment is the start of all good psychological interventions as a way to understand all of the variables before beginning to solve the equation. This chapter includes instruction on how to conduct a clinical interview with children with somatic symptoms and their families. This is an essential first step in getting a clear picture of the child's presenting challenges, both physical and psychological, the level of impairment related to symptoms, and the areas of resiliency and support. It is also an opportunity to set up the education and treatment phases of intervention by establishing a solid biopsychosocial framework.

A good biopsychosocial assessment introduces the child and family to the language of the mind–body connection, which permeates all phases of the intervention, and gains buy-in from the child and family for intervention right from the start (Kozlowska, English, & Savage, 2013). Taking the time and care to establish this foundation lessens the possibility of the family not understanding or agreeing with the focus on nonmedical investigation and intervention. Incorporating families into this framework early on is an important part of the assessment process, and tips on how to accomplish this are woven in throughout the following chapters. Finally, the chapter includes a review of somatic symptom questionnaires that can provide an objective angle to assessment and a good way to establish a baseline from which to measure changes in symptoms, coping, and function over the course of treatment.

SETTING UP THE ASSESSMENT

There are some unique aspects to conducting an assessment for children with somatic symptoms that are important to note at the outset. As described in the previous section, most families presenting to a mental health provider's office will not have sought out psychological care because of mental health concerns, but rather because of the child's physical symptoms and health concerns. Although it is also necessary to do a thorough interview from a mental health standpoint, it is best to start with an accurate assessment of the physical symptoms, as this is the presenting problem. Taking this approach in the first interview will also improve children's and family's buy-in for ongoing intervention, as they will feel confident that their primary concerns are being addressed, thereby eliminating any potential fear that a solely psychological approach is being taken. Even for families that may be more psychologically minded and are open to this approach, beginning with assessment of physical symptoms and associated impairment is still appropriate for evaluation of a child with somatic symptoms.

After you have a thorough understanding of the physical symptoms and health challenges at hand, the psychological factors can be assessed. This must first be done in the context of finding out what psychological struggles are associated with the physical problems, rather than focusing on or assuming there must be some deeply buried psychological trauma or emotional experience causing the physical problem. *This is a critical distinction between a somatic symptom assessment and a mental health assessment.* Going into the assessment trying to discover the "true cause" of the physical symptom will only further a mind–body dichotomy that is ultimately unhelpful in treating the child. In fact, mental health providers are in a unique position to *correct* any misinformation that a family might have in terms of what to expect at a mental health visit and to provide an alternate view to the child's current symptom presentation in the context of the biopsychosocial model. Providers can accomplish this by getting a good understanding of the somatic symptoms, how the child is coping with them, and the impact on overall function *before* venturing into the assessment of comorbid mental health concerns. This approach is also helpful for children and families who arrive in your office already with a good understanding of the mind–body interaction in that they feel confident a shared approach is being utilized. Presented in this way, children and families often offer up the role of stress and negative emotions in children's symptom presentation before being directly asked about it. This is a good sign that families are engaging with the biopsychosocial framework, in that they are not defensive about considering the role of stress in their children's symptom presentation.

Overall, using the first interview as a tool to communicate the biopsychosocial framework and rationale for treatment is more powerful than just using it to gather information. It is a good first step in shifting children and families away from the view that "it's all in your head" to the more integrated perspective of the interaction of physical symptoms with children's emotional and social experiences, which you can provide simply by organizing the interview like this:

1. Biological (onset, frequency, duration, triggers, sleep, impairment)
2. Psychological (thoughts, feelings, actions)
3. Social (family, community, peers, activities, school)

This order allows for effective assessment of all the factors associated with the child's symptoms that interact to produce distress and difficulty in the child's life. Tackling the domains in this manner is the most productive way to guide the interview, allowing for fluidity and flexibility when there is natural overlap between domains (e.g., social factors may come up in the biological section when assessing impairment, or psychological factors may be discussed in the context of symptom triggers).

Logistically, the length of the assessment can be flexible in terms of what works best in your practice setting. The suggestions made for sessions throughout this book are based on the 50-minute patient hour. For the assessment, it is reasonable to spend 10 minutes on the introduction, 10 minutes on each section of the biopsychosocial model (for 30 minutes total), and 10 minutes on the conclusion, where recommendations for treatment are covered. The introduction and conclusion place more emphasis on you providing information about the biopsychosocial model, while the assessment of the three factors is much more conversational and interactive, with a focus on the child, with the parents' support as needed, reporting on the presenting problem.

The Role of the Family

Inclusion of the family throughout the child's treatment process is essential. Children live in a context, and treating them only individually does not take into account the larger world in which they live. For school-age children through adolescents, both parents and children are intentionally included together in the first two visits for the assessment and education sessions. Delivering the same information to as well as gaining information from both parties is advantageous, and also allows for observation of and learning about the family dynamic. As treatment progresses, more individual time with the child is recommended to promote self-management, a core component in building the confidence the child needs to get back into aspects of typical functioning where parents would not normally be present for support (e.g., school, peer interactions). However, parents need to know what their children are learning so they can support their new coping efforts, so including families either at the beginning or end of intervention sessions is recommended. This arrangement strikes a nice balance, allowing children to learn interventions independently to build resilience, while enabling parents to be aware of what the child is learning so they can reinforce practice at home.

While including families in children's treatment is imperative, it can also be a bit tricky in terms of managing parents who have good intentions but are anxious and tend to take over the reporting. Be mindful of how much time the parent spends giving information versus the child, and balance the interaction as much as possible. One way of setting up this parent–child interaction for success is to communicate at the beginning of the assessment that it is best for all parties to provide information by saying:

> "In the first few sessions, I like to talk to parents and kids together so I get a chance to get to know both of you, you get a chance to get to know me, and we can all talk together about how we understand these symptoms you are having and what we can work on in treatment. To make sure I hear from everyone, sometimes I will ask questions to _____ [the child], sometimes I will want to hear from your parent(s), and sometimes from everyone."

In this way, both the child and parent know what to expect and the stage is set so that everyone can participate and be heard. Then be sure to follow through on this promise by eliciting information decisively and with direction from the child or parent during the interview. One way this can be done is to be mindful of making direct eye contact when asking questions. For instance, if the child is anxious or quiet, or may otherwise not be inclined to answer right away, directing eye contact to the child, giving him or her some time to come up with a response, and not looking at the parent while waiting for the child to answer are simple but powerful techniques that communicate to everyone exactly whose voice needs to be heard in that moment. When needed, verbal redirection can be given if someone answers out of turn, such as thanking a parent for his or her perspective, then turning the conversation back to the child by saying "What do you think?" or "Did your mom get that right?"

Depending on the dynamic between the parent and child, you might consider interviewing them together at the beginning of the assessment, then separately at the end. This is particularly useful for a shy or quiet child, and also for adolescents who may be reticent about speaking openly with their parents present. Similarly, parents also benefit from the individual time, as they may feel more comfortable sharing their fears or perceived negative qualities about the child that they otherwise would have avoided discussing in the child's presence. The challenge to splitting up the parent and child is that it adds significant time to the assessment, as often questions are repeated, and you may need two sessions to accomplish the work you could typically do in one. If this style is preferred, extended time may be needed for the new visit (e.g., 60–75 minutes).

INTRODUCTION

To start off the initial interaction on a good foot, take the lead to let children and families know how the first meeting will progress. As with any first meeting, there may be some anticipatory anxiety, even more so in the case of children with somatic symptoms whose family never imagined they would end up in the office of a mental health provider. The parent of a child we worked with once summed it up to us by saying, "Let's be honest, no one wants to sit in a psychologist's office." This illustrates perfectly that many families may have preconceived notions about what it is like to talk to a mental health provider, many of which may come from television shows or pop culture notions of what therapy entails. While it can be frustrating to hear families share this sentiment, this perception exists, so be mindful of ways to engage children and families to have a different and positive experience. Maintain a kind, open, upbeat attitude from the start to set children and families at ease, explicitly address the reason they are there, and inform them of the structure of the interview so they know what expect. In our practice, we often begin like this:

DOCTOR: Welcome! I am a pediatric psychologist here at the clinic/hospital.

MOTHER: Hi, this is Johnny and I'm his mom, Susan.

DOCTOR: It is nice to meet you both! Since today is our first session, I will tell you about my background and about how today's visit will go, and then I would like to hear what you want to focus on so we can start getting to know one another. Sound like a good plan?

MOTHER: Yes, that sounds good.

DOCTOR: Wonderful! If you have any questions as I am talking, please feel free to ask them at any time. So as I mentioned, I am a pediatric psychologist, which means I am a doctor who specializes in talking with children who have health concerns and their families. Johnny, I understand that you have been dealing with stomach problems for quite some time now, and I can imagine it has been really hard to understand why it is happening or know what to do about it.

MOTHER: Yes! This has been so hard. But we are not really sure why we are here—it is something that our physician recommended, we do not think Johnny is making it up or has any mental-type problems—but we decided to go ahead with the appointment because if there is anything you can do to help Johnny feel better, well, any kind of help would be great at this point.

DOCTOR: I hope that I can be of some help, too. It can be confusing to understand why a psychologist is recommended when you are dealing with a health concern, so let me explain a bit more about what I do. Johnny, let me go back and get your answer, too—has this been hard to deal with, having these stomach problems, understanding why they are happening and what to do about them?

JOHNNY: Yeah, I guess. I don't feel good a lot of the time and I don't really know why.

DOCTOR: Thanks for telling me that. This is why you are here, so we can talk about ways for these problems get better. Before health problems happen to kids, most people do not know that there is a doctor like me who specializes in talking to kids and families about these types of concerns. In fact, there are a lot of people like me who do this kind of work, and you all are not alone in going through this. I've worked with many kids who are dealing with the very same health problems you are having, Johnny, so I know from them just how hard it can be to understand why your body is feeling this way and what to do about it. We can work together to understand why this has been happening and find some solutions to cope with it so you can get back to just being a kid.

MOTHER: Well, that is reassuring. That sounds great. Sounds like just what we need.

DOCTOR: Well, I am really glad that you decided to come to the appointment and give it a try. Let's talk about Johnny's health and then we can talk about getting him back on track.

It is useful to introduce the biopsychosocial framework for understanding symptoms at the beginning of the assessment. This reassures children and parents that you understand the symptoms are real before you ask specific questions about the presentation. And it leads nicely into a more thorough description of the three factors that will be the focus of the assessment. We talk about it like this:

DOCTOR: Johnny, as we talk about the symptoms you've been having, one thing I want to tell you right away is that I know the symptoms you are having are real. Your symptoms are physical, meaning that they are in your body, also called somatic symptoms. They are not made up, or all in your head, or only the result of feeling stressed or anxious.

MOTHER: That's a relief! We were worried that's why our physician sent us here.

DOCTOR: I understand why you might have thought that! These symptoms can be very hard to understand, and unfortunately some families get that message from their doctors when there is not an organic diagnosis or clear medical explanation for the symptoms. Let me tell you a little bit more about how we understand somatic symptoms. The brain and the body work together, so whenever the body is not feeling good, the brain is not either, so it is common for all people—kids and grown-ups alike—to feel stress or negative emotions when they are sick. Now, that doesn't mean that stress or negative emotions *cause* your symptoms, it just means that they go along with them, because our bodies are wired that way. Let's think of an example of when that may have happened for you, Johnny. Have you ever felt worried or upset over something, maybe with a friend or at school that led to you having a stomachache?

JOHNNY: Yeah, that happens at school, like when I have to take a test. I get really worried about tests anyway, and now I notice that my hands get sweaty and I think I am going to throw up. My stomach feels terrible for the rest of the day.

DOCTOR: That's a very good example of how the brain and body are connected; just thinking about a tough situation like taking a test in school can make your body have a very strong reaction that in this case just makes your stomach feel even worse. Thinking about how the brain and the body work together in this way is what we call a mind–body approach, and this is how we will talk about Johnny's health. We will focus on how three big parts of life work together that can make people feel good or bad: the first are the *biological factors* or physical symptoms we feel in our bodies, the second are the *psychological factors* or the thoughts and feeling we have in our minds, and third are the *social factors* or the interactions that happen with our families, friends, and school [reference the "Biopsychosocial Assessment Tool" in the Appendix]. We will use this to get a better understanding of how you have been doing, and most importantly, it will help us figure out some ways for you to feel better.

BIOLOGICAL FACTORS

Once the purpose for the interview has been established and the rationale is set up for the role of each area in the biopsychosocial framework, a discussion of the biological factors associated with the presenting problem can begin. For this assessment area, the overall goal is to gain an understanding of the child's experience of the primary symptoms, as well as any secondary or associated symptoms. If a new physical symptom is reported during the course of the assessment, beyond what is noted by the referring provider, ask if that is a symptom has been reported to their medical provider. If not, recommend follow-up with the appropriate provider about the concern. As we review in more detail in Chapter 11, it is important for mental health providers to collaborate with our health care colleagues in the treatment of children with somatic symptoms, and we want to encourage families to continue that communication as well.

During the assessment, it is best to direct these questions to the child as much as possible, since the child is the one experiencing the symptoms. If parents are answering too much for the child, you can encourage the child to respond by saying something to the effect of "Johnny, your mom is giving me a good idea about what she sees you go through, but I also want to hear from you, because you are the only one who knows how it feels on the inside." Typically, we assess physical symptoms by asking questions in the following categories, jotting down the most important details in the "Biological Factors" portion of the "Biopsychosocial Assessment Tool" for the child and family to see:

Primary symptom: "What is the health concern that bothers you the most?"
  • Headache, stomachache, dizziness, numbness, gait disturbance
Associated symptoms: "Does anything else happen when you feel [symptom]?"
  • Nausea, fatigue, feeling hot or cold, heart racing, other somatic symptoms
Quality: "How does it feel?"
  • Throbbing, stabbing, spacey, tingling, painful, difficult, weird
Frequency: "How often does it happen?"
  • Constant, intermittent, several times a day, weekly
Duration: "How long does it last?"
  • All day, several minutes to hours
Exacerbating factors: "What makes it worse?"
  • Activity, eating, physical position, time of day, school attendance
Alleviating factors: "What makes it better?"
  • Medicine, rest, distraction, nothing
Triggers: "Is there anything that brings on the symptoms?"
  • Foods, stress (physical or emotional), time of day, activity, random
Sleep: "Do your symptoms affect your sleep?"
  • Delayed onset, awakenings, sleeping more, sleeping less, napping
Appetite: "Do your symptoms affect your appetite?"
  • Weight gain, weight loss, poor appetite, food avoidance, overeating
Impairment: "What do your symptoms get in the way of doing in your life?"
  • School attendance, sports performance, social interaction, exercise, self-care
Diagnosis: "What have the doctors told you this is?"
  • Abdominal pain, chronic headache, tachycardia, conversion disorder, spells, nothing, "it's all in my head"
Treatments: "What treatments have you tried for the symptoms?"
  • Medicine, physical therapy, complementary or alternative therapy

If the child presents with both organic and somatic symptoms, assess whether there are differences in symptoms, triggers, or situational events between sets of symptoms (e.g., how nonepileptic vs. epileptic seizures present) to get a better understanding of how to develop the treatment plan for the somatic symptoms, and ensure the family knows how to treat the organic episode appropriately. In both situations, it will be beneficial to engage in a functional approach for the child no matter the cause of the symptom, with the major difference being whether medical intervention is required.

The child's and parent's responses to these questions should result in a good initial understanding of the physical nature of the health concerns. At this point in the assessment, the child or parent can be asked any follow-up questions, if there is anything else that is important to know about the symptoms, or if there are other somatic symptoms in addition to the primary complaint. A successful assessment of biological factors should result in an appreciation for the child's actual experience of the symptoms. Ask yourself if you have a good idea of how the child feels during a symptom flare; if the answer is yes, move on to the next section. If there is something that is missing in the understanding of symptom presentation, go back and clarify it before moving on.

PSYCHOLOGICAL FACTORS

Once the biological factors have been assessed, it is appropriate to then move on to a discussion of the psychological factors. A nice transition into this section usually comes from identified exacerbating factors or triggers reported in the biological assessment, as children and families typically offer up stress, school, or negative emotions as something that makes symptoms worse. Rather than saying, "Now we are going to talk about the psychological factors affecting your physical symptoms," we recommend making a more natural transition such as this:

> "Now, Johnny, as you mentioned just a minute ago, feeling worried about a test at school is something that makes your symptoms worse. This is a great example of how even thinking about something difficult, like school, and negative feelings, like worry, make your symptoms worse. Let's talk more about the ways you feel stress and negative emotions, and any other situations that are hard to deal with."

Think of this part of the assessment as similar to how assessment of a child with an anxiety or depressive disorder is approached. To stay consistent with the core of the presenting problem, which is the health concern, assess the psychological factors associated with the symptoms first:

> *Symptom-related mood changes*: "Do you notice any changes in your mood or feelings when you have your symptoms?"
> - Quiet, irritable, nervous, withdrawn, agitated, sad

Then, to gain a more thorough history of psychological functioning aside from the current health concerns, consider a transition such as this:

> "That makes a lot of sense that you are feeling irritable and not quite yourself when you are having these symptoms. Remember, your brain and body are connected, so most people have those types of emotions when their bodies do not feel

good. Now, do you have any troubles with worries or feeling sad besides these times when you have symptoms? Or in the past, before you started feeling sick?"

Briefly cover the following specific categories, which are recognizable as standard in terms of obtaining a psychological history. For each category, suggestions are provided for how to ask that question with specific emotional assessment examples underneath. Feel free to use your own style in terms of assessing mental health concerns:

Anxiety: "Are there things you worry or feel anxious about?"
- Fear, nervousness, anticipation, stress

Depression: "Are there things that make you feel sad or upset?"
- Sadness, irritability, isolation, grief

Anger: "Are there things that make you feel mad or frustrated?"
- Anger, arguing, poor frustration tolerance

Behavioral: "Do you have a hard time following the rules or paying attention?"
- Opposition, aggression, inattention, hyperactivity

Trauma: "Have you had any scary or difficult events happen to you, like accidents or people hurting you?"
- Abuse history, traumatic event experience

Psychosis: "Do you see or hear things that other people don't see or hear?"
- Auditory or visual hallucinations

Harm: "Have you ever had thoughts about or tried hurting yourself or someone else?"
- Self-harm, suicidal/homicidal ideation or attempts

Treatment history: "Have you ever seen a counselor or therapist before for mental health concerns or for somatic symptoms?"
- Past or current diagnostic and treatment history

The goal of the psychological assessment is to gain an understanding of the child's emotional experience of the health concerns, and to find out if there are comorbid psychological disorders above and beyond the child's health concerns. For instance, Johnny may feel sad, angry, and worried in association with his symptoms *and* have a history of generalized anxiety (e.g., worries about the safety of his family, interacting with peers, leaving the house). As much as we have emphasized that it's important not to consider a somatic symptom assessment from a solely psychological approach, comorbid psychological problems must not be ignored, as they could negatively contribute to somatic symptoms as well.

SOCIAL FACTORS

Finally, now that the child's experience of symptoms is established and a good understanding of the psychological factors has been obtained, discuss the ways in which the current symptoms have impacted the child's social functioning to get a sense of how his or her life and development have been affected, as well as any factors in the child's environment that have contributed to the maintenance of symptoms. As with the lead-in to the psychological factors section, there may be familiar information to guide this part of the discussion. We like to make an introduction such as this:

> "The last area for us to talk about is how you have been getting along and inter-acting with your family, friends, and school since you have had these symptoms. Earlier, you mentioned that you have not been able to attend school as much as you would like (or be on your sports team or see your friends) since these symptoms started. That happens for a lot of kids who are having health problems. Let's talk more about the activities you have missed out on or are not able to do because of your health, and also find out about the ways that other people have tried to help you."

Areas of specific assessment in the social category are as follows:

Family: "What has changed in your family since you have had these symptoms?"
  • Strained interactions, arguments, more "special time" with family when sick, reduced expectations for chores, a change in family activities
Friends: "And how about with your friends? Are you spending as much time with them as usual? Are they helping you out or are some making it harder for you?"
  • Bullying, less time spent with peers, special attention from peers due to illness, difficulty staying the night with friends, fewer social events, friends not understanding of health challenges, not telling friends about symptoms, feeling left out
School: "Tell me about school in terms of how you are doing with getting to school, keeping up with your work, and anything the school is doing to help you with these health concerns."
  • Attendance, grades, school support, education plan, history of learning disorders
Extracurriculars: "Is there anything else you do or did after school or in your community such as sports, music, clubs, or hobbies? Has anything about that activity changed due to your symptoms?"
  • Sports, music, theater, dance, art, clubs, youth groups
Culture/Faith: "Are there any aspects of your culture or faith that have changed or been helpful related to your health concerns?"
  • Spiritual beliefs, attendance at religious events, cultural understanding of symptoms, support

At the end of this section, you should have a good understanding of the ways in which the child's social network has changed or responded to the symptoms as well as the larger impact the symptoms have had on the child's development in terms of limitations to function. This part of the assessment is also an opportunity to find out valuable information about what will serve as a motivator for the child to engage in treatment and get back to his or her life, such as finding out about a social activity he or she is not currently doing but would like to do. You may also discover information about activities that the child may not be doing because of the symptoms that he or she did not like in the first place. This may present an additional barrier to getting back to regular activities beyond the challenge of symptoms in that the child may be experiencing secondary gain.

As you wrap up the social section, review the "Biopsychosocial Assessment Tool" (in the Appendix) that you have been writing on throughout the interview, and see if there are any areas for which you need further information. As your last assessment question, ask the child and family, "Is there anything else I should know?", to offer an open-ended way for them to add information they may not have shared.

ASSESSMENT MEASURES

In addition to the clinical interview, formal assessment tools and standardized measures can provide an objective rating of the child's baseline functioning, which can serve to increase understanding of his or her experience and the family's perception of symptoms, as well as provide a baseline from which to monitor treatment success as the child progresses through therapy. If possible, send the measures to the child and family before their first visit or ask them to arrive 15–20 minutes early for their appointment to complete them in the waiting room. It will help your conceptualization and recommendations if you can score the measures prior to the visit, then review the information with the child and family during the initial session (after you wrap up the interview portion), but if not, include a review of what you learned at the beginning of the second session.

There are a lot of ways that measures can be incorporated into assessment and treatment; there is not one correct way, and it is recommended that you work within the easiest and most productive system for your practice. Some providers choose to get a brief measure each time the child is seen for treatment to track symptoms over time, which can be helpful from a symptom improvement standpoint because that information can be incorporated into practice in real time. Other providers rely on a baseline to end of treatment model, which is also a nice way to show improvement at two points in time or provide another piece of information later on in treatment to help make decisions about the course of therapy. And finally, a third way of using this information is just at the initial visit to round out the understanding of the child's experience. Overall, ensure that measures are helpful, succinct, and worth everyone's time. The measures reviewed in this section are appropriate for school-age children and adolescents via self-report.

Symptoms

Somatic symptoms can be measured in a number of ways. There are symptom specific measures, such as the Numeric Rating Scale (von Baeyer et al., 2009), for rating pain on a 0–10 scale, with 0 being no pain, each number higher representing progressively more pain, and 10 being the most pain one could imagine. Pain ratings using this scale can be given for highest level, lowest level, average level, and current pain in a specific time period (e.g., last week). A comprehensive measure of children's somatic symptoms is the Child Somatization Inventory (CSI; Walker, Beck, Garber, & Lambert, 2009), which asks children to rate the degree to which they are bothered by a number of somatic symptoms from all body systems and produces a total score. The Behavior Assessment System for Children, Third Edition (BASC-3; Reynolds & Kamphaus, 2015), is a more general measure of the parent or child's report of the child's physical, behavioral, and emotional symptoms.

While getting a standard measure of symptoms is an obvious way to think of assessing this population, consider that much of what will be done in treatment is focusing the child *away* from symptoms, and if you add a measure of symptoms, it will be in effect doing the opposite of what you are trying to do. There is not a right or wrong solution to this one—include a measure of symptoms mindfully if desired, and utilize it for getting an idea of how the child is doing, but do not spend too much time focusing on every aspect of his or her response.

Impairment

Of all of the measurement categories, a report of physical impairment is most valuable, as a primary goal of treatment is to improve function. A well-established measure of functional impairment is the Functional Disability Inventory (Walker & Greene, 1991a). This is a brief, 15-item measure asking children how much physical trouble or difficulty they have completing typical child and adolescent daily tasks due to their health concerns (e.g., attending school all day, doing something with a friend, walking). The measure has been validated and normed on a broad group of children with a variety of health concerns, including established clinical cutoffs for children with chronic pain conditions indicating minimal, moderate, and severe ranges of functional disability (Kashikar-Zuck et al., 2011). It is also a well-utilized measure in clinical trials of children undergoing CBT for somatic symptoms and is sensitive to change in function over time. Another well-established measure of physical impairment is the Pediatric Quality of Life measure (Peds-QL; Varni, Seid, & Kurtin, 2001), which has many illness-specific versions and assesses impairment across multiple domains of children's lives.

Stress and Coping

Gaining insight into how a child is coping with symptoms or stress in general is useful. There are numerous questionnaires to assess coping; the most psychometrically sound measures are presented, with a focus on child self-report rather than observational measures, as questionnaires are a more efficient manner of collecting data in a clinical setting. If you are interested in exploring these areas further, Blount and colleagues (2008) reviewed measures of stress and coping in the child and pediatric research literature, identifying measures that were well established, with sound psychometrics, and had utility in broadening understanding of coping.

Regarding stress in general, the Children's Hassles Scale and Children's Uplifts Scale (CHS, CUS; Kanner et al., 1987) are two subscales of a child self-report measure of daily demands and rewards in the last month for children ages 8–17. There are many measures of anxiety, depression, and behavioral concerns for children and adolescents; it is beyond the scope of this work to review them all. If there is a measure of psychological functioning that you use in your practice, it would also make sense to use it in the assessment of children with somatic symptoms.

Regarding coping, there are measures of both general coping and coping with pain. Well-established general coping measures include the Coping Strategies Inventory (CSI; Tobin, Holroyd, Reynolds, & Wigal, 1989). The CSI is a 32-item self-report (age 7 and up) or parent report (age 3 and up) measure assessing coping cognitions and behavioral response to stressors, categorized as engagement and/or disengagement styles. The Ways of Coping Checklist (WCCL; Vitaliano, Russo, Carr, Mailro, & Becker, 1985; Folkman & Lazarus, 1985) is a 68-item self-report measure for children, adolescents, and adults measuring behavioral and cognitive coping skills.

There are two well-established measures of coping with pain. The Pain Coping Questionnaire (PCQ; Reid, Gilbert, & McGrath, 1998) is a 39-item self-report measure of coping with pain, including headache, stomachache, muscle pain, joint pain, back pain, earache, and menstrual pain, for children ages 8 and up. The Pain Response Inventory (PRI; Walker et al., 1997b) is a 60-item self-report measure for school-age children with abdominal pain, with three areas of pain coping measured, including active, passive, and accommodative.

Finally, finding out how parents respond to children's symptoms can also be instructive. The Adult Responses to Children's Symptoms (Van Slyke & Walker, 2006) is a parent self-report measure of adults' solicitous, protective, distracting, and monitoring behavior toward children during times of illness.

PUTTING IT ALL TOGETHER

Once all of the biopsychosocial factors have been addressed in the context of the interview and any formal measures have been conducted and reviewed, the interview ends by putting all of the pieces together to establish a shared understanding of the child's symptoms and commitment to engage in treatment. While much more description of symptom origin will be provided in the upcoming education session, it is important to present a brief biopsychosocial conceptualization of the child's symptoms and impairment using the child's own examples that were provided during the interview. In addition to this verbal description, it can be helpful to provide the symptom-specific fact sheets (see the Appendix) to children and families for information regarding diagnosis and treatment from a biopsychosocial model so they have something concrete to take home and refer back to prior to the next session.

DOCTOR: So, Johnny, now that we have talked about all of those areas that affect your health—how it feels physically, what you think about it, and how other people help you—let's talk about how we understand symptoms working in the body so we can figure out the strategies that will help you do more of the activities you want to do, which is what makes the symptoms less bothersome.

JOHNNY: OK.

DOCTOR: When we think about health problems, we must understand how the whole body is affected by that experience. You have been focused on the biological factors happening in your body and you have been going to doctors to fix the problem, which makes sense because symptoms usually mean danger or problems in our bodies. You had tests and evaluations to find the cause of those symptoms, but when those were done you were told everything is "normal" although you still have this stomachache. That is unsatisfying, because there is no quick or easy answer! You know it is not normal to feel sick all the time, and everyone wishes there was a quick test or procedure that could tell you why your problems are happening and, most importantly, fix them!

JOHNNY: Yes, that would be nice!

DOCTOR: What we have talked about today is how it is not *just* the biological ways we think about symptoms, but also psychological and social factors, how you feel and who supports you, that are important. All three of these factors come together to influence how your body feels, *not any one of these alone.* Although your medical tests came back normal, we know your pain and physical experience as you described it to me today is real, and what we have learned is that it is not the type of pain that comes from the bones or the muscles, which medical tests are designed to find. It is the type that comes from the nerves and the body feeling out of balance, which again is real, just not the kind of symptom we can easily find in the medical tests we have. The psychological part of your symptom experience is that the symptoms are very stressful and frustrating to deal with and make life a lot harder in many ways, as you told me about today. You have also noticed that anytime you feel worried or sad about something that also increases pain and symptoms. This is the way that symptoms and emotions work hand in hand. Then, we considered the social world you live in that involves your family, friends, school, activities, and church, as well as the experiences you have had when people interact with you in a way that can either help you or make things harder. In this way, all three worlds work together, your physical experience, how you think and feel, and how other people in the world interact with you. It all adds up to feeling the way that you have felt in your stomach. Does that make sense, how we think about those factors working together?

JOHNNY: Yeah, it does. So what can I do about it?

DOCTOR: Good question! Let's talk about what to do about it. The solution to these health problems that come from the intersection of these three factors is learning tools from each area to get back on track, like ways these factors can work together to make life better instead of making it worse. The biological tools are ways of taking attention away from symptoms, learning to relax your body, distracting your mind from the symptoms, and learning healthy habits to take care of yourself. The psychological tools are ways of understanding the link between emotions and symptoms and learning how to use your thinking so you can have more positive experiences. And lastly, the social tools are ways to get you back into your activities and teach people to help you focus on your function instead of focusing on the symptoms. Function improves *before* symptoms get better, so in all three of these areas, we want you to focus on what you *can* do instead of the ways you do not feel good or what you feel you cannot do. After you notice a reduction of your disability or impairment is when you will notice a change in your symptoms.

This is an alternative way to talk about the biopsychosocial model as it applies to treatment:

DOCTOR: When we talk about coping strategies, we use the biopsychosocial model. Basically, this is a way to understand how physical factors (like how your body is feeling) interact with psychological factors (like your emotions) and the social situation you are in (like being by yourself, interacting with others, or being at school). They all intersect in the middle and can come together to help you or they can come together to make life worse. Lately, you have been in a situation where they are all coming together to make life worse. Finding ways to work on each area to come together and *improve* the overall experience for you is what we will work on. For example, physically you could be feeling tired and having a stomachache, emotionally you could be feeling frustrated, and socially you could be with people who do not know how to help you. While you might be able to handle one of these challenges, the combination of all three areas feeling badly is going to make the experience much more difficult. So, when you find yourself in that kind of situation, we want to focus on what we *can* do in each area, and then those improvements combine together to create a much better experience for you. For example, physically you could drink water, move around, have a snack, relax your muscles, take your medicine, or distract from the signal. Emotionally, you could think of what is going well in your day, remember your motivations, and do an activity that makes you feel positive emotions. Socially you could reach out to the people around you to ask for support or change something in the environment that will better support you. That is what we work on together in treatment and what we call learning coping tools.

MOTHER: That sounds like a really good plan.

DOCTOR: Great. This type of coping skills training is called cognitive-behavioral therapy, or CBT for short. The studies we have done on CBT show that these strategies are effective in helping kids feel more in charge of their symptoms and get back to doing the activities they enjoy doing in their lives. And that is exactly what we want for you—to get back to doing what you love to do and not have these stomach problems hold you back anymore.

Finally, conclude the session by eliciting goals, describing how treatment will move forward, and letting the family know what to expect at the next session:

DOCTOR: Thanks to both of you, we had a great start today in terms of talking about what has been a challenge for Johnny, and it has given us some great ideas of how we can work on different strategies to get back on track. Johnny, what are three activities you would really like to do that you feel you cannot do now because of your health?

JOHNNY: I want to play with my friends again, I want to do well in school, and I want to have something to do that makes my stomach feel better.

DOCTOR: Johnny, those are wonderful goals. Mom, what do you think about that?

MOTHER: Oh yes, I would like him to do all of that, especially school. He is usually such a good student, and it has been so hard for him to struggle with tests and even just staying there are all day when he doesn't feel well.

DOCTOR: It sounds like we have a lot of important activities to get you back to, Johnny. I would like to suggest that you come back to work with me on a weekly or every-other-week basis to learn the coping tools that we talked about today. At the next visit, you and your mom will meet with me together again and we will talk more about how we understand these symptoms and how they work in your body. After that, we will have individual sessions for you to learn the coping tools, and we will include your mom at the end of those sessions so she can also learn the tools and help you use them at home. Does that sound like a good plan?

MOTHER: Yes, that sounds great. How many sessions total should we schedule?

DOCTOR: Let's start with five or six sessions. We can always add more or take away a few as needed. Johnny, between now and the next session, I want you to focus on what you *can* do even when you have these stomachaches.

JOHNNY: OK. I will keep a list. I can do that.

DOCTOR: Perfect. It was so nice to meet you both, and I will see you next time!

CHAPTER SUMMARY AND TAKE-AWAY POINTS

- Using the biopsychosocial framework in the assessment helps the child and family understand the connection between the mind and the body from the first session.

- Engage the child and family together in a review of the biological, psychological, and social factors affecting the child's symptoms in an interview format. Formal measures of symptoms, impairment, and coping can aid in your assessment and allow you to track change in treatment outcomes over time.

- End the assessment by presenting a biopsychosocial conceptualization of the child's symptoms and impairments and how you can use that information to improve coping and set goals for the future, focusing on a return to function. Logistically, tell the family what to expect in the course of treatment.

CHAPTER 5

Education

The goal of the second session is to continue building the treatment foundation from the end of the assessment by introducing the education process. Good somatic symptom education consists of providing "real-world" descriptions to children and their families that are easily understood and applied to children's experience. This chapter will cover how to thoroughly explain the somatic symptom presentation and establish the underlying reasons why symptoms are happening, which provides further rationale for treatment using the biopsychosocial approach. Education is the way for children understand the reason *why* we do the intervention. Without it, children may wonder why on earth breathing or thinking differently could change their symptoms, and then they will not be as likely to try out those coping tools. It essential to be thorough in providing this education because it will maximize the benefit of the strategies that are addressed in Part III.

The education session is the bridge between the assessment and treatment phases. As the concepts become more familiar to you, education may be woven into the assessment, or incorporated at different points during treatment rather than in just one session. In this chapter, our favorite clinical descriptions and comparisons of somatic symptoms are provided, and we encourage you to choose the words and examples that make the most sense for the child you are working with and the descriptions that best match your clinical style. Although there are many similarities in somatic symptom presentations, there are also some nuances, and thus both general and specific examples are presented. Tailor the delivery of this information to the individual child's experience. There is not a "one-size-fits-all" solution when it comes to education. In general, treatment of somatic symptoms takes patience, creativity, and flexibility.

At the beginning of the education session, set expectations that will shape interactions with the family as treatment progresses. First, set expectations for outcomes. *We never tell children we will cure them or remove their symptoms altogether.* This can be disappointing to hear, both for the children who struggle with these symptoms and for parents who watch children suffer. They want quick responses and permanent fixes; however, children and parents often resonate with the observation that these symptoms did not cause problems overnight, so it will likely take longer than that to recover. To the degree that these symptoms represent abnormal versions of otherwise normal body functions, they are likely to be part of the child's long-term experience. We often introduce this idea to families by sharing our treatment motto: *Slow and steady wins the race when it comes to treating somatic symptoms.* We tell children they will learn how their mind and body work together (or against each other), what they can change and what they cannot, how to cope with symptoms over time, and how symptoms don't have to go away completely in order for them to get back into their lives. In fact, since there are no guarantees on symptom remittance, the primary focus of treatment is on improving function. In doing this, families shift from the idea of passive treatment (i.e., "Take this and wait until you feel better") to the active approach to treatment (i.e., "You will be a participant in this work").

In addition, tell families that treatment will remain the same regardless of whether the family pursues other medical evaluations or solutions for the symptoms. Parents may ask, "But what if the doctor is wrong?"; "What if the headache is really a brain tumor?"; "What if the dizziness is a heart condition?" These are reasonable questions for parents to ask; after all, their job is to ensure the child gets the help that he or she needs. Our answer is that whether the symptom is somatic or organic in nature, it *still* causes impairment and the child will *still* benefit from learning coping skills in order to function better. The most important idea families should leave a mental health provider's office with is that the child will be working on developing symptom *coping* skills, not symptom *vanishing* skills. Focusing on how CBT teaches children how to manage current symptoms by addressing the biopsychosocial factors that contribute to impairment is a good way to remind families that the problem is being looked at from *all* angles. We recommend including the parents in the education session, too, as it allows them to hear the rationale for treatment and improves their buy-in as well. Finally, as reviewed in Chapter 11, it is critical to collaborate with the referring provider, especially at the beginning of treatment, to ensure that all reasonable organic medical causes for illness have been assessed and/or treated, as it will reinforce the assurance you are providing. While it is necessary to account for all aspects of treatment, including medical intervention, children experiencing impairment related to symptoms will *all* benefit from CBT, regardless of the biomechanics.

Finally, explain your role in treatment. Most importantly, you will be an advocate for children and families. You will be their team captain in their quest to return to their everyday lives. You will be the one who talks to the school and explains what they need. You will support the parents in striking the balance of validating children's experience while not paying too much attention to the symptoms. Be transparent with the family that your goal is not to make the symptoms disappear, but to teach children and families how to cope with the symptoms and reduce associated impairment. Above all, you will be flexible and respond to the individual needs of children and families.

INTRODUCTION

With those general points in mind, this is how we would introduce an education session, starting where we left off at the assessment visit:

DOCTOR: Welcome back! Now, last time, I asked you to think about something before the next session ... do you remember what that was?

JOHNNY: Um, oh yeah! You wanted me to tell you what I can do even if I still have stomachaches.

DOCTOR: Yes, that's it! Although we talk about what is not going well in your life, we also want to focus on what is going well for you, too, which might be hard to think about at first. So what did you come up with?

JOHNNY: Well, it was hard, because I can't do a lot of the activities I like to do and used to do, but I am still taking care of my pets and I also see my friends on days that I feel good.

DOCTOR: That's great news! Johnny, it is fantastic that you are still caring for your pets and seeing your friends. That tells me that you care a lot of about animals and about being a good friend, too. I want you to keep that up, and we will work together to find ways that you can do more of the activities you love, although you have these stomachaches. Last time, we talked about the biological, psychological, and social factors that all add up to you feeling sick, and how we will work together so you can learn strategies in each of those areas to get you back in your life. Today, we will talk about how I can help you do that as a member of your treatment team and we will also talk about how we can better understand why these symptoms are happening in the first place. Sound like a good plan?

JOHNNY AND MOTHER: Yes! Sounds good.

DOCTOR: I will work with you, your family, your doctors, and the school to help you cope with these symptoms so they cause less trouble. Some kids find that their symptoms get better, some kids find that their symptoms stay the same but they are less bothered by them, and nearly all kids learn ways to take care of themselves that they can use for symptoms or when they feel stressed. Most of all, we will work together to improve your overall function in your life, or your ability to do what you want and need to do.

MOTHER: That all sounds good—we definitely want Johnny to be able to do more—but I was hoping that this treatment would make the symptoms go away entirely.

DOCTOR: I know it can be really frustrating for kids and families who just want all of this to go away right now. Sometimes I say if it were that easy to make these symptoms get better, then we would not have the pleasure of meeting!

MOTHER: Ha! I guess so! We would have figured it out on our own and never needed you.

DOCTOR: Right! But, these symptoms have turned into quite a long-standing problem, and it makes sense that a long-term problem requires a long-term solution. Although CBT may not make the symptoms go away quickly or entirely, learning how the brain and the body work together and how to use coping tools makes the symptoms quieter or pop up less often, and in some cases, children do recover altogether over time. We want to figure out how Johnny can manage symptoms effectively and teach him strategies to use so the symptoms do not cause so much impairment.

MOTHER: I thought we should wait until he feels better to do be active again, but if I understand what you are saying, it's the opposite—*first* we have to get him back to his regular activities again, and then maybe symptoms will get better later on?

DOCTOR: That's exactly it. It does seem opposite! But that is how symptoms improve. We have to quite literally get his feet moving first before his brain and body learn to quiet the symptoms down and hopefully turn them off altogether. To do that effectively, you and Johnny will play an active role in treatment. Learning about coping is like going to a clinic to learn a new skill for sports, or taking lessons to learn a new instrument, or how to draw. It does not work well if you do not practice it. I will give Johnny homework each time for different strategies to try at home between sessions. Let's talk today about where these symptoms come from so we can figure out how to get back on track and why the treatment strategies will help you do that.

SOMATIC SYMPTOM EDUCATION

Recall from Chapter 2 that somatic symptoms are largely due to disorders of how the body functions, and typically not due to organic disorders in the structure or physiology of the body, like a broken bone or disease. Somatic symptoms are physical in nature and indicate that something is wrong, just in a different way than people are used to experiencing. In addition, somatic symptoms, just like organic disorders, can be affected by and have an effect on feelings and behaviors. To explain somatic symptoms generally and highlight how the mind and body affect the symptom experience, we provide a description like this for all children:

DOCTOR: Let's talk more about these symptoms you have that we call "somatic" or "functional" symptoms. As we talked about last time, these are real symptoms, but the difference is that they are not dangerous in the sense that your body is not being damaged in some way. With any kind of symptoms, we first have to understand how our brain and our body work together, because then we can figure out what makes the symptoms worse, and most importantly, what can make them better. For example, Johnny, sometimes you may notice that your stomach is really hurting you, does this make you feel sad or mad?

JOHNNY: Yeah, I get really angry and frustrated when my stomach hurts.

DOCTOR: Understandable. And as you said last time, you also notice the opposite pattern, that when you have a negative emotion, like feeling worried, you get a stomachache.

JOHNNY: Yeah, like when I'm taking a test in school that I'm kind of nervous about.

DOCTOR: So sometimes you notice the pain first, and sometimes you notice the emotions first, but they are both connected. They go together—the physical feelings, like pain, and the emotional feelings, like being worried or mad. I want you to know that negative emotions did not *cause* your problem with stomachaches— we know that you have abdominal pain and it is the nerves in your stomach that are causing these problems, which we will talk about more today—but negative emotions certainly do not make your stomach feel any better. That's an example of how we are going to talk about the way your mind and body are connected. We will learn about the ways that your mind and body can make situations, thoughts, feelings, and actions worse, because that gives us lots of clues about how to make them better. Does that sound good?

JOHNNY: Yes!

Through these discussions, children and parents often offer that symptoms are more likely to be present when the child is tired or stressed, or even when very excited or overstimulated. As part of the rationale for treatment, it is helpful to introduce the concept of healthy habits and good body care (which are a focus of level one intervention) during this education session. It is also an opportunity to discuss how these factors relate to the ANS as discussed in Chapter 3, which is part of the general education provided to all children with somatic symptoms. If children are tired, run down, hungry, or overwhelmed (even in a good way), they also have more sympathetic nervous system activity and greater difficulty coping with or paying attention to signals their body is giving them to slow down. Many children get used to functioning on less sleep and having higher levels of tension or arousal and "forget" what it feels like to be relaxed, which keeps their bodies activated and amplifies symptoms. In addition to providing the Car or the Caveman ANS training, we talk about the importance of good body balance through the example of charging a cell phone:

DOCTOR: Some of the skills we will focus on in treatment are maintaining healthy habits and taking good care of your body. For some people, it is really easy to do this; they get enough sleep, stay hydrated, eat healthy food, exercise, and get a good mix of school and fun with their friends. And this makes their body feel balanced. But some people have a hard time doing this; they might stay up late at night to get homework done, feel run down after a big soccer game, not be allowed to go to the water fountain at school, or spend all their time doing homework and not have as much time for friends or activity. Then when they do have time or feel OK, they really overdo it and almost have too much fun. And when you add it all up, all of that activity in either direction makes our body feel very out of balance. Let's talk about this connection by using sleep as an example: Why should everyone get enough sleep?

JOHNNY: Because then you aren't tired in the morning, and you don't oversleep so your mom doesn't yell at you to get up in time for school!

DOCTOR: Absolutely! No one likes to start their day in a rush after their mom yells at them. Getting enough sleep also rebuilds our cells, rests our brain, and recharges our bodies. What else needs charging every day?

JOHNNY: My cell phone.

DOCTOR: Yes! And what happens when the battery gets low?

JOHNNY: It will die and then I won't be able to text with my friends or play games.

DOCTOR: Exactly. Now, you might be surprised to hear that our bodies operate a lot like a cell phone. Getting good sleep, eating healthy food, drinking enough water, getting exercise, and balancing our daily activities are all ways that we "charge" our bodies so we can do what we want without running out of energy. When my cell phone gets low on battery, I only use it for certain tasks so it is doing less overall and then it lasts longer. The same thing is true with our bodies; if we are feeling run down, we have to choose what we are doing to save our energy for what we really need to do so we do not crash. What we will learn in treatment is how to improve your ability to "recharge" yourself and what you can do to take care of yourself when your battery is low, like taking breaks and planning ahead to make the most of your energy. For instance, stomachaches get worse when you run out of energy, so that's another reason to recharge.

JOHNNY: That makes sense. I never forget to charge my cell phone because it is so important, but sometimes I stay up late because I have homework. Then I feel really tired the next day, and I usually end up getting a stomachache.

DOCTOR: Great job making those connections. Sometimes kids get annoyed that they have to eat healthy meals or go to bed early because they think their friends do not have do that, too. But *everyone* needs to take care of themselves in these ways for good health; you just have an extra reason to do it to keep your body healthy because of the symptoms you have been having.

SPECIFIC SOMATIC SYMPTOM PRESENTATIONS

There are specific educational applications for each of the major somatic symptoms. While the approach is not appreciably different, there are fine distinctions between the symptom categories: cardiac symptoms, neurological symptoms, chronic pain, and GI symptoms. We have created three fictional cases to illustrate these clinical presentations; the patients described vary in somatic symptoms, age, background, impairment, and treatment needs. We will use these case examples throughout the book to illustrate the clinical application of biopsychosocial assessment, education, and treatment.

Cardiac Symptoms

Ashley, our patient affected by somatic symptoms related to syncope and a dysregulated ANS, is 16 years old and has symptoms that include chronic dizziness, syncope (passing out), nausea, fatigue, and headaches. Ashley was previously healthy; she began having intermittent headaches in middle school but managed them fine at that time and they did not impair her function. However, in the past 2 years, her headaches have become chronic and, even more troublesome, she has been having fainting episodes along with feelings of dizziness, nausea, and fatigue that have been significantly impairing. Ashley sees a neurologist, cardiologist, gastroenterologist, and physical therapist, and receives acupuncture. She has diagnoses of chronic migraine headache and syncope and is currently seeking further evaluation for POTS. She takes multiple medications but continues to have significant symptoms and associated disability.

Ashley was referred to a mental health provider by her cardiologist to address coping concerns, negative mood, and poor social participation. Ashley began online school a year ago due to difficulty with school attendance and is struggling to complete her junior year. She was previously a high-achieving student who was involved in sports through her school and in the community. She no longer participates in anything other than online school. Ashley lives with her mother and her mother's partner, and has an older brother who attends college. She reports difficulty sleeping, behavioral and social withdrawal, changes in appetite, and minimal exercise. She denies having generalized anxiety and depression but does feel that negative emotions worsen symptoms.

Ashley's symptom presentation is a good example of two interrelated processes. One is the association of negative physical and emotional symptoms with stressful situations that is mediated by the ANS, and the other is the effect that avoidance of symptoms has on impairment over time. First, when educating children about symptoms related to ANS dysregulation, such as syncope, you want to emphasize the dual role of that system: it affects physical *and* emotional symptoms alike by "stepping on the gas" or engaging the sympathetic nervous system, as we illustrated in the Car and the Caveman examples, which we recommend using in this education session. For Ashley, when she walked into school and started having significant symptoms, her ANS was activated and she felt a dual rush of what she interpreted to be negative physical and emotional reactions. This association became learned over a short period of time and promoted avoidance of school, like the Pea Soup example, which succeeded in her feeling better in the short term but only amplified negative emotions and symptoms in the long term.

Ashley's symptoms became so impairing that she removed herself from many age-appropriate activities. Although this seemed like a good choice at the time, this choice reinforced the avoidance cycle and taught Ashley that the perceived threat of dizziness or passing out must be managed by sitting, which by default meant staying home from school, sports, and social activities. Unfortunately, this inactivity only perpetuated her underlying autonomic dysfunction and chronic headache as well. Over time, her body became so deconditioned that now even small physical exertions are associated with symptoms, further reinforcing her belief that she will be safest if she just stays still.

When providing education, illustrate biological and behavioral connections to symptoms so children understand the associations of symptoms and avoidance, and why they need to be addressed. We start by explaining *perceived* threat, which is not necessarily *actual* threat; this is an important distinction. From a child's perspective, there are lots of perceived threats: exams, social interactions, needing to use the bathroom and not being allowed, feeling embarrassed, running late, meeting adult expectations, and so forth. All of these threats have an associated physiological response that, in the right circumstances combined with psychological and social factors, can contribute to the onset of somatic symptoms. However, this response is unhelpful, as there is no actual threat for which the body needs to prepare. We address this in treatment by teaching children to use the coping tools to balance their ANS and break the cycle of threat and avoidance.

In addition, it can be helpful to explain the biological reason behind cardiac symptoms. Our hearts do a lot of work on a daily basis, pumping blood around the body at the right time, rate, and rhythm as directed by the ANS (which can change at any given time based on level of activity). The body is generally good at keeping this system going without us having to think about it; it is essentially on autopilot. When children like Ashley present with dizziness or fainting, these symptoms are often due to their sympathetic nervous system being stuck in the "on" position; in essence, their body's "autopilot" is on the fritz. It is certainly distracting and annoying to feel dizzy, and it is pretty scary for children to pass out in the school hallway. However, once children know that these symptoms are an overactivation of an otherwise normal process, they can better understand how to balance their bodies and take control of these processes. Here is how we explain these concepts in an education session to our patient Ashley and her mother:

MOTHER: Dr. Jones referred us to see you, I guess, because Ashley has missed so much school that she changed to online school, which she really didn't want to do because she was a very good and active student, and he thought you might be able to help her deal with these problems. She has been diagnosed with syncope but the medications have not been helping. She has never seen a psychologist before and was nervous about coming here since she doesn't think anything is wrong with her feelings, and I don't either. Ashley and I think that the right medication will be found for her medical problems and then she will be fine. I think she worries people think she is making up her symptoms, since she does not have any injuries or disease, but she is not. Just look at her: she is so weak and unsteady.

DOCTOR: Many families are confused about the role of the psychologist in this situation. One of the goals of our treatment is learning how to manage the symptoms so that Ashley can return to her previous level of functioning. We have many well researched strategies that can positively change function, which improves symptoms over time. I imagine it has been very hard to have such a loss of activity, to go from being a good student to not being able to attend school. I would like to talk about the way we understand Ashley's symptoms and how they relate to ANS dysfunction, and then focus on the strategies that come from that understanding to help Ashely improve her function.

ASHLEY AND MOTHER: OK. That sounds like a good start.

DOCTOR: In terms of the diagnosis of syncope, we know that these are real symptoms that are *involuntary,* meaning they are not under your control, Ashley. They are related to changes in the cardiovascular and autonomic nervous systems. Syncope is when your body is more sensitive to environmental and positional changes, like being in a hot shower or standing up too quickly, and as a result you have symptoms like dizziness and even passing out because of your body's ineffective regulation of heart rate, blood pressure, and getting the right amount of oxygenated blood to your brain. Then let's throw on the challenge of what happens if you just *think* about what happens when you stand up. The ANS activates, like stepping on the gas, and without even moving, guess what?

ASHLEY: I get dizzy.

DOCTOR: Yes. Many people with syncope want to avoid these triggers altogether and don't even go to places where they could happen. While that is an effective a way to get out of a tough situation in the moment, in the long term, this takes you out of a lot activities you would like to do, like school, and it does not train your ANS to rebalance itself. But it is hard to know how to do it differently when you feel bad. Ashley, I bet there are a lot of mornings when you want to get up, but it feels like you just cannot do it?

ASHLEY: Yes, exactly. It seems like the hardest thing in the world to just get up and get dressed, although that sounds so simple. I lie in bed dreading it because I know I will feel terrible or even pass out as soon as I put my feet on the floor.

DOCTOR: We have many strategies that we can work on to reduce the impairment related to dizziness and passing out and help the body regulate itself: physical skills, ways to deal with emotions, and ways for other people to help you.

ASHLEY: That sounds fine except for the emotions part. I don't know why all the doctors keep asking me what I am worried about or what caused all of these symptoms. I wasn't worried about anything until I got these symptoms! I'm not doing this on purpose.

DOCTOR: Of course not; it is clear that you are dealing with a number of physical symptoms. Because the brain and body are connected, physical symptoms end up affecting our emotions as well. So the way we think about it is that stress and negative emotions don't start these physical problems in the first place, but they certainly make them worse.

ASHLEY: Yeah, I guess I see what you are saying.

DOCTOR: Our goal in treatment is for you to take small steps to rebuild your function, which improves management of symptoms and rebalances your body and mind. Let's talk about how we do that. What would happen if I decided to *run* a marathon tomorrow? I would probably make it about a half mile (I am not a well-trained runner), get frustrated or injured, and give up. I think I would never be able to do it. But what if, instead, I decided to *train* for a marathon tomorrow? My first step would *not* be to run 26 miles, but to do research on training programs, get good sneakers, and maybe just do a light jog around the block. All of a sudden, my goal seems much more manageable—I am thinking about it differently and feeling differently. That is what we will be doing together; a combination of learning, training, and managing obstacles in small steps to reach your goal that will change the way your mind and body respond. The way you think about that goal, how you feel about it, and what kind of help you get from others all make a big impact on how successful you are in reaching it.

ASHLEY: That makes sense. When I was playing soccer, our coach always told us how well we played or how hard we ran could be affected by how we were thinking about our skills. But it is really annoying that people keep telling me I am too emotional or too stressed. It makes me feel like they're not listening to me, or just dismissing my problems. I *want* to be back at school.

DOCTOR: The goal is for you to manage symptoms effectively so you can do that.

ASHLEY: Well, I want to go back to school, but I just can't because I feel so bad. And I can't stand the way my teachers and other kids look at me, like they feel sorry for me or think I'm faking. No one understood or helped me. Teachers took forever to get me make-up work, and then I would get so behind there was no way I could catch up. Because I was failing some classes I wasn't allowed to do anything fun like go to the football games. So I just stopped going. What was the point?

DOCTOR: That sounds like a tough situation, Ashley. It is a good example of the social aspects of coping with these symptoms, which can be really tricky. Many teens with somatic symptoms say that people tell them they look fine or that they must not be sick. The stressful experience of just being in those unpleasant social situations is actually enough to bring on those lightheaded symptoms, which sends the message to the brain that the situation is dangerous and it is better to just stay home, and your body learns that cycle of avoidance. It makes sense in the moment because your body is trying to protect you, but it doesn't help you over time because you are getting more deconditioned and your symptoms get worse.

ASHLEY: I understand what you are saying, but with all of those problems at school it really seems impossible to go back while I'm still sick.

DOCTOR: I know it seems overwhelming, but that is why you are here! We will work together on how to manage these symptoms and improve function.

Neurological Symptoms

The patient in our next case example is Alex, age 13, who presents with a functional gait disorder, including symptoms of poor balance, weaving gait, and numbness/tingling in both legs. He has no prior history of medical concerns; his symptoms came on suddenly after a track meet a few months ago. He initially visited his pediatrician, who referred him to a neurologist. After a diagnostic hospital admission and full workup, including MRI and blood work, the neurologist determined that his gait imbalance was not organic, meaning he did not have a brain tumor or disease causing the impairment. Alex was diagnosed with conversion disorder, discharged home from the hospital and back into the care of his pediatrician, and referred to a physical therapist and mental health provider. He is not taking any medication and walks as much as he can at home but uses a wheelchair in the community due to ongoing gait problems.

Alex is in eighth grade, lives with his biological parents, and has a younger brother. He was previously a well-functioning adolescent, with no identified social or emotional concerns aside from being relatively introverted. He earns average grades in school, is on the basketball and track teams, and is in robotics club. Alex's symptoms have kept him from participating in sports, gym class, and family activities. He missed school while hospitalized and anticipates difficulty getting around the building when he goes back due to the continued trouble he has with walking.

When educating families about conversion disorder or functional neurological symptoms, keep in mind that children experience significant, obvious impairment related to their symptoms and can sometimes go a long time without a diagnosis, so this can be an especially confusing situation for children and families. We have at various times described conversion symptoms as the body's way of "waving a white flag of surrender," "a bad coping skill," or "the body's way of telling us it needs a break." For children with less emotional expression and resiliency, conversion disorder represents a very basic coping mechanism: the brain gets overwhelmed with a strong emotion it cannot otherwise process, and the body expresses it.

For a child such as Alex with conversion disorder, we would draw on the anticipatory anxiety educational example presented in Chapter 3. The presence of symptoms brought on by a poorly recognized anxiety process removes the perceived threat. The nature of the threat can range from something seemingly minor, such as picking out the right outfit in the morning, to something more challenging, like wondering whether your ACT score will be good enough to get into college, which can both lead to avoidance. Symptoms represent the body's most instinctual and involuntary response to threat in order to survive and escape. Our job is to teach children more effective coping and emotional expression skills to keep their bodies working for them in the face of stressors and break the cycle of anxiety and symptoms.

Now, imagine that Alex comes back after the initial assessment with very confused parents. During the first visit, you learned that the family had been given the diagnosis of conversion disorder, but they did not understand much about it. Today, they tell you that they are worried about that diagnosis after doing a web search for conversion disorder, as the information they found suggests a significant trauma may have occurred. As we previously mentioned, many children who have experienced a trauma have somatic symptoms, but not all children with somatic symptoms have experienced trauma. The family explains that Alex is a happy, previously healthy boy who never seems stressed by much of anything, is a good athlete, and does fine academically. Further, his dad communicates skepticism about this psychological approach, as he feels that there are medical explanations for Alex's symptoms that he has been researching on the Internet. Many times, families will come into the second session having done some research and will have follow-up questions such as this. Be open to talking about these questions in a nondefensive manner. The education session provides an opportunity to further discuss the diagnosis in addition to providing education on the process of anticipatory anxiety related to Alex's presentation.

DOCTOR: Let's start today by talking more about the diagnosis of conversion disorder. What did your referring doctor tell you about it? What have you read?

MOTHER: Well, Dr. Smith said that they ran a lot of different tests that are normal and said she thinks that it might be functional or a conversion disorder. But I looked that up on the Internet, and Alex did not have anything traumatic happen; he has a good life, so that doesn't seem to make any sense. I am worried that we are missing something in his brain or an infection that they did not find. I mean, how could there just not be an explanation for his symptoms? They came on all of a sudden, and his legs still shake when he tries to walk! That can't just happen because of your mind, can it? I don't think he is stressed. No offense, we just feel like something is being missed. We are getting a second opinion.

DOCTOR: I certainly understand what you are saying and am glad you are bringing these concerns to my attention. There is so much confusion about diagnoses like functional neurological symptoms or conversion disorder because there is no positive test—it is based on ruling out a lot of other diseases. You are welcome to get another medical opinion if you would like. This is good timing for us to have this discussion, because today I would like to talk more about conversion disorder with you to help you understand where it comes from and how the coping skills can help Alex. I think you will find that many of these strategies and approaches will be beneficial regardless of exactly where the symptoms are coming from.

FATHER: OK, thanks for understanding. It is just really hard to know what the right thing to do is, and of course we do not want to miss something that could help him.

DOCTOR: I understand. In terms of conversion disorder, there are a lot of definitions you might find on the Internet that suggest this comes from a really bad thing or trauma happening in a child's life. However, the research tells us that there are no consistent risk factors like that for what causes children to develop conversion disorder. What is consistent is that children often have a harder time identifying or expressing emotions, which then gets paired with a physical problem. Many times, when families are sent to a mental health provider, it can feel like the medical team is suggesting that there is no "medical" cause for the symptoms, even though this is usually not the case. For example, if you cannot walk because you have a broken leg, then there's a clear reason for that. But if you cannot walk although your legs and your brain look perfectly intact, it is hard to know what that means, and in that case the message from the doctors can feel like "Well, then it is all in his head."

ALEX: It did seem like the doctor thought I was making it up.

DOCTOR: Alex, a lot of kids in your situation have felt that way and I know it is hard, because it sends the message that the symptoms are under your control. But we know they are not: these symptoms are involuntary and not directly controllable. Some of the newer research on brain processes in kids with conversion disorder suggests that the signals somehow get crossed in the brain and voluntary muscle control is affected. That is a fancy way of saying we do not know what started this chain of events off exactly, but we know for a fact that Alex is not doing this on purpose. Sometimes a hard test at school combined with an overwhelmed body can be enough to cause symptoms, or a slow buildup of negative emotions and a tense body over time.

MOTHER: Well, Alex does push himself in school and sometimes gets worried about how he is doing in sports; middle school has been a tough transition for him.

DOCTOR: It often is! Alex, how do you deal with challenges in sports or school?

ALEX: Usually I just try to keep going and work harder. But it doesn't always work, because I sometimes study really hard but I still don't get a good grade or I practice a lot but still miss a shot in basketball.

DOCTOR: Those are great examples. Let's talk about how people cope with challenges like that, and I think you will see a lot of connections to what you just described. I like to think of our body's ability to cope by comparing it to a beverage container with a spout, maybe like one you might find at one of your basketball games.

ALEX: We do have those! Ours are pitchers filled with sports drinks.

DOCTOR: Yes! So imagine that pitcher is like our ability to cope with challenges and the spout is our way of relaxing. If the pitcher is empty, you are feeling great. But then you think about your math test and that adds a little liquid, or having to clean your room, and that adds a little more, and then you have a really big track meet coming up, and that adds even more. None of those events are very big or scary by themselves, but a little liquid gets added to your ability to cope with challenges each time. Then imagine that there is more liquid added for all of the regular stressors that come along with being a teenager, like getting homework finished, staying up too late, social drama at school, and trying to figure out who you want to be when you grow up. All of a sudden, that container is full to the top and we have not let any out from the spout. Now what will happen if we put something else in there—can you think of any recent stressful events?

ALEX: Well, before I stopped running track my coach kept telling me I wasn't working hard enough, but I really was trying my best.

DOCTOR: Let's add it—now what will happen to our already full container?

ALEX: It overflows.

DOCTOR: Exactly. And that's how we think about conversion disorder; the overflow of the liquid is your body's way of saying, "Help! I need a break!" Sometimes I tell families that conversion disorder symptoms are like a very basic coping skill; you don't have them on purpose, but they serve to get you out of the challenging situation in the moment, like an escape hatch. Just like our Pea Soup example, sometimes all you have to do is *think* about putting liquid into the container and it will overflow!

ALEX: That has happened to me—I thought I was going to have a hard time walking in school one day and I then I did. I had to go home early.

DOCTOR: That is a good example of what we call anticipatory anxiety or a self-fulfilling prophecy, which is when your mind and body convince themselves they cannot do something before you even try it out. But it is not very helpful because it keeps you from doing what you want and need to do in your life, like play sports and walk through school successfully. We want to give your body the message that it can *change* its coping process to handle those challenges more effectively. Learning coping skills is like learning to use the spout to let some of that liquid out of the pitcher before it overflows.

FATHER: I see what you are saying and that makes sense for some situations that we see Alex struggle with, but overall Alex is not stressed; he is a happy, easygoing child. And these symptoms do not always occur in stressful situations.

DOCTOR: Good point. We think about stress in a few different ways than you may commonly hear about. Stress can be physical, like not getting enough sleep or doing too much activity on a hot day, or emotional, like feeling overwhelmed in school or worried. Kids with conversion disorders sometimes have a hard time using coping skills, have not faced a stressful event in their lives before, or are not very practiced at identifying and dealing with their emotions. Sometimes, symptoms happen at the same time as stress, before, after, or can be hard to predict. Or they might occur when kids are more tired or when they have a lot of small stressors build up and reach a boiling point.

MOTHER: Alex does have trouble with that; he tends to hold everything in and then just explodes over something small, a lot like that pitcher spilling over, actually!

DOCTOR: Right. So this does not mean that Alex is "bad at managing stress," it just means that we need to teach Alex to understand these connections and cope more effectively. Once these new coping skills are in place, he will experience less impairment related to his conversion symptoms.

FATHER: Well, that does sound helpful. I guess no matter what is causing this to happen, we want him to go back to doing his usual activities.

Pain and GI Symptoms

Johnny, whom we have already introduced to you in earlier chapters of the book, is a 10-year-old who presents with intermittent gastrointestinal (GI) distress, alternating diarrhea and constipation, as well as chronic abdominal pain. He has been having these problems off and on "all of his life," but the episodes became more severe after he had an acute illness earlier this year. Johnny now has stomachaches three or more times a week, with pain lasting for at least an hour at a high intensity. Johnny was first seen by his primary care provider and treated for suspected acid reflux; however, his symptoms persisted. He was referred to a pediatric gastroenterologist, who did a series of tests, including an endoscopy and colonoscopy; all of those tests came back as normal. He was given diagnoses of chronic abdominal pain and IBS. He was prescribed a tricyclic antidepressant (amitriptyline), and it was recommended that he follow a high-fiber diet. Despite this, he continues to have pain and GI distress.

Johnny is in the fourth grade and used to be a good student, but this year he misses school at least 2 days per week, is behind in his work, and gets lower grades than usual. The pain keeps him from doing a lot of activities he used to do, including seeing friends in the neighborhood and playing on his soccer team. Johnny has been described as having an anxious temperament throughout his development, and worry is a trigger for his current symptoms. He was referred to a mental health provider by his GI physician to address anxiety and the role it plays in his experience of abdominal pain.

When delivering education about pain and GI symptoms to children and families, build on the biopsychosocial message that you provided during the assessment. Pain and GI distress are the result of a combination of physical, emotional, and social experiences. The goal is to provide education about the role of the nervous system in pain perception as well as the gate control theory of pain as presented in Chapter 3, which we recommend using in the pain education session. It also can be useful to refer to the research presented in Chapter 2 to inform children and families that we know a lot about how pain operates in the brain: brains change in structure, activity, and attention under conditions of chronic pain. The good news is that these processes can be reversed through learning and applying the skills of CBT.

In addition to pain-specific education, the ANS education from Chapter 3 is also an important part of the education we use with children with pain and GI symptoms. In particular, it is important to relate sympathetic activation to opening the pain gate, and this is especially the case for GI symptoms due to the strong brain–gut connection through the ANS. This is the biological explanation for why pain, GI distress, and emotions are connected; as we like to say, anxiety doesn't cause a chronic pain disorder or GI symptoms all by itself, but because it opens the pain gate through sympathetic activation, it makes it worse. Children and families find that explanation very validating because that biological connection illustrates the mind–body nature of that experience well. We describe those processes like this:

DOCTOR: As we have talked about today, Johnny, your abdominal pain is real; it is a signal processed by the nervous system and allowed into your brain through the pain gate. But the difference is that your pain is not acute pain, which is pain from damage or injury that our body is designed to warn us about. It is chronic pain, which is pain that has lasted for 3 or more months and is no longer a helpful signal. Unlike acute pain, there may or may not be something that you know about that started it off, and there certainly has not been anything you have found to fix it. Now, you have had stomach problems for a long time, but ever since you got sick this year, you've had pain every day without knowing why. This is actually a very common way that children develop abdominal pain.

MOTHER: I didn't know that—why would a sickness cause this abdominal pain condition? He is not sick anymore, but the pain is still happening almost every day.

DOCTOR: Good question. The idea is that when the body is sick, our ANS that we talked about earlier activates in order to fight it off and allow us to heal. Sometimes I think about it as if this room we are sitting in is like our body, and when a sickness like a virus comes in, our body responds by turning on all of the lights, the heat/air conditioning, the computer, whatever it can find to turn on to try to chase the sickness out. And then the sickness finally leaves … but guess what the body forgets to do?

JOHNNY: Turn off all the electronics!

DOCTOR: Yes! And for children who have had trouble in their bodies already, with headaches or dizziness or in your case stomachaches, that makes the nervous system *stay* activated, and whatever trouble you had before seems to get worse and go on for a long time. And because of those problems, you did what anyone would do by stopping your activities, resting, and not going to school. But, unfortunately, those strategies that we naturally use for acute pain make chronic pain worse, and you know this for sure because you have tried all of those strategies, but you still have pain. And not only do you have pain, but you have GI symptoms too which also get worse the longer your body stays out of balance. I am here to tell you that you did nothing wrong in your response to pain—no one ever knows the first day they have pain that it will be chronic. But now that we know what it is, we can learn a different way to deal with it.

JOHNNY: OK, I think I understand, but how do I do that?

DOCTOR: Great question. What we want to do in treatment is to find ways to get out of the chronic pain cycle, reset those misfiring pain signals by getting you functioning again, and retraining your brain to stop paying attention to these unhelpful signals. We do this through finding ways to close the gate on pain. Johnny, can you guess what affects the position of the gate?

JOHNNY: Maybe how I eat? Like if I eat too much junk food the gate will open?

DOCTOR: Yes! The biopsychosocial factors that we talked about before affect the position of the gate, including physical factors such as eating. Let's do a few more examples. What if you are all by yourself or really bored. What happens to pain?

JOHNNY: Oh, the pain gets worse. That's happened to me.

DOCTOR: Yes! And why is that?

JOHNNY: Well, because there is nothing else to think about. I focus more on the pain.

DOCTOR: That's exactly correct, the gate opens in situations when you are not active or distracted. What about feeling strong emotions—like when you are feeling worried about a test in school, what does that do?

JOHNNY: Oh, definitely opens the gate, we talked about that one last time.

DOCTOR: That's a good example of how negative emotions do not *cause* pain conditions in the first place, but they do affect the position of the gate, so that is how stress and pain go hand in hand. This also has to do with the ANS: remember that negative emotions push on the gas pedal in your body and make it activated, and activation is also something that opens the gate and makes GI symptoms a whole lot worse. That's another reason we want to find the brakes, so we can close the gate and calm down the GI system. Now let's talk about something that can make the gate partially closed. Medication is one example of that—it helps a bit, but pain signals are still getting through. Is that what has happened to you?

JOHNNY: Yeah, I take medicine, but I'm never sure if it really works.

DOCTOR: I know that's disappointing, but that is the experience for most kids. We just do not have a medication for chronic pain that will close that gate all the way. So now let's think about what would close the gate completely. Have you ever been doing something so fun that you do not notice pain?

JOHNNY: Yeah! That just happened to me the other day. I was playing a new video game with my friend and didn't even notice my stomach, but then after the game ended it really hurt and I had to go home.

DOCTOR: That is a good example of distraction closing the gate! Believe it or not, those pain signals were there all along, but because you were focusing attention on your game and having fun with your friend, the gate was closed. And that's exactly what we want to do! Doing regular activities like going to school, is another thing that closes the gate because there are a lot more distractions and things to focus on in school than there are at home. What we will do in treatment together is to find more ways like that to close the gate.

Whether the children in your office have trouble walking like Alex, are struggling with dizziness and passing out like Ashley, or have pain and GI distress like Johnny, by the time they get to you, their somatic symptoms have already become negatively associated with different situations. Somatic symptom education is a way to teach children and families about these connections, and through that process, they realize that there are ways to undo these connections to establish healthier and more functional patterns. In summary, although each of these patients has different symptoms, they all share a similar presentation in that they have impairment in their day-to-day activities due to somatic symptoms. These case examples are used throughout the book to further illustrate how to engage in all of the interventions that are presented.

COPING TOOLS

Once the general and specific aspects of education are in place and everyone is operating from the same understanding of where somatic symptoms come from and how they are interfering with children's lives, the session can be concluded with the positive description of what will be worked on in treatment to turn those negative patterns around. We describe coping skills that address somatic symptoms as tools in a toolbox, and just like real tools, all coping skills are not meant for all symptoms or situations. Children will be introduced to them, practice them, and learn when and where to use them, when they are most effective, and which ones they like the best. Some children might find that one of their best coping tools is prevention, including good sleep, hydration, and exercise. Others might find that they prefer activity-based coping skills (like pleasant activities or seeing friends), and yet others might find that quiet distraction and relaxation skills work best (like listening to music or imagining being in a calming place). The best recommendation is to do something, anything, when having symptoms. The next section of the book is focused on the tools that can be used to address symptoms now that the child and family have a good understanding of them. A nice way to wrap up the education session is with a summary of the content of the session and a description of treatment using this coping tools language.

DOCTOR: Today we have talked about the way we understand your symptoms and how we can use that information to make your function better, which is the first step in getting better from somatic symptoms. The first part of treatment is going to address the biological factors or how your body feels. We will do this through healthy habits, relaxation, and pacing your energy through the day. Then we will focus on the psychological factors, like the thoughts and feelings that affect your symptoms, and develop positive coping actions to get you back to activities that you enjoy. We will also talk about the social factors, such as how to manage symptoms in different situations, like at home or at school, and how people can help you with that. My goal is the same as your goal, to get you back to school and hanging out with your friends. We will not move too fast—remember, slow and steady wins the race—but I will have you do some challenging activities that may feel hard at first, so we will talk a lot about how to do that. Starting next time, you and I will work one on one in these sessions and include your parents at the end so they know what tools you are learning and can help you practice at home.

JOHNNY AND MOTHER: That sounds good.

DOCTOR: We like to talk about these strategies as "coping tools," and if there is one thing we know about tools, it is that they do not do us any good when they just sit in the box! And just like any other tool, sometimes they will work across multiple situations, sometimes in just one, and sometimes you do not feel like using a certain tool at the moment (or cannot!) and want to try something else. If that happens, I want you to feel like you can talk to me about what makes it hard to use them or ways we can tailor them to fit your life and your schedule. We can problem-solve together, because it is important that you feel like you can actually use the tools we are learning in session. This is what we will do at your next session.

CHAPTER SUMMARY AND TAKE-AWAY POINTS

- Set reasonable expectations for treatment, *not* promising to make the symptoms disappear, but instead to teach children coping skills that will allow them to manage their symptoms, reduce impairment, and increase function.

- Provide general and specific somatic symptom education to children and families to set the stage for why the treatment strategies will be helpful in addressing symptoms and impairment. Case examples throughout the book show common somatic symptom presentations—including cardiac symptoms, conversion disorder, chronic pain, and GI disorders—to illustrate delivery of education and intervention.

- Coping skills training can be framed as learning coping "tools" to put in the "toolbox" that must be used in an active fashion outside the sessions by the child and family to effectively to treat somatic symptoms and related impairment.

PART III

Intervention

INTRODUCTION

In the first two parts of the book, the conceptual understanding of somatic symptoms and the approach to assessment and education were addressed, representing the first two introductory sessions of treatment. In this section, the core of the treatment will be reviewed as we present the strategies that help children manage somatic symptoms. The next three chapters cover somatic symptom intervention. They are organized into three levels that build on each other and allow for delivery of effective coping tools children can use to manage symptoms and improve function.

For straightforward somatic symptoms, intervention can be delivered in the order in which the levels are presented in this section, with each level representing content for two sessions for a total of eight sessions altogether, including the first two sessions of assessment and education that have already been reviewed. For children with more complex symptom presentations, three or more sessions can be spent on each level, and levels can be repeated as needed. The focus of level one and two interventions is on physical, emotional, and behavioral factors, consistent with a behavioral activation model of CBT for depression or exposure therapy for children with anxiety; we then move on to the cognitive factors in the third level of intervention. This structure represents a general progression from a focus on physical well-being to a greater understanding of the role of emotions and cognitions. When children are disabled by somatic symptoms, they benefit from increasing their baseline level of activity first; before getting into the more technical work of understanding the connections of thoughts, feelings, and actions, children just need to get their feet moving.

This approach to intervention works in a true biopsychosocial fashion in terms of the physical, emotional, and social factors building on one another to improve overall health and well-being, with a jump start from the physical side. When children physically reengage in their lives, they also feel the psychological benefit of having positive experiences and coping more effectively with symptoms. This reestablishes more developmentally typical social interactions, which feeds back to a biological benefit of increased activity and less focus on symptoms. In this way, children break out of the negative cycle of sickness into a new pattern of wellness. As children progress through each level, there is typically more and more engagement in therapy, which further enhances treatment outcomes through a growing commitment to the approach. Overall, the focus of these intervention sessions is to improve function, which is the ultimate way to successfully manage symptoms.

Treatment strategies discussed in this section relate back to empirical research on somatic symptoms as well as the factors that perpetuate them in the biopsychosocial model. Specifically, biological factors can be improved by engaging in a regular daily schedule to enhance adherence to behaviors that improve overall health and function, as well as by learning relaxation skills that close the pain gate and push on the brakes of the autonomic nervous system to create a less symptomatic and more restful physical state. Psychological strategies teach children how to identify and manage negative thoughts and feelings connected to physical symptoms. Increasing social interaction improves engagement in activity, which reduces symptom signals through distraction and trains the brain to think of the body as feeling "normal" while receiving supportive and functional messages from peers, family, teachers, and the community. All of these processes work together to retrain the nervous system, so that it is no longer attending to the misfiring of symptom signals, getting stuck in a cycle of anticipatory anxiety, and engaging in chronic ANS activation, but instead feeling physically balanced and attending to positive influences and developmentally appropriate experiences. Quite naturally, children are motivated to continue using these strategies because they benefit by feeling better, so it becomes less like "having to do homework" and more like "getting to live a healthy and productive life." The increase in confidence is exponential.

The treatment information provided for each level of intervention is designed for both readers who are learning the basics about working with children with somatic symptoms and those who have experience with this patient population and are looking for creative solutions to challenging cases. In each chapter, the basics are presented, followed by the application of the strategies in more complex ways. If the initial concepts are familiar, read further to review the challenges of applying the interventions in more complicated clinical situations.

Individual sessions are recommended for each level of intervention, but family support in all of these areas is crucial in shifting children's attention *away* from symptoms and disability and *toward* function. At the end of each chapter in this part, specific parenting strategies are reviewed, with the idea that parents should be included at the end of each session so they can learn about what the child is practicing and find out how to facilitate the child's engagement in those strategies at home. In addition, Chapter 9 in Part IV covers specific parenting and family-based strategies that can be targeted in the course of treatment to support the cognitive-behavioral techniques that are taught to the child and ensure the home environment is changing to support a more functional pattern for everyone.

To explain the delivery and progression of treatment as clearly as possible, we divide the various strategies—physical, emotional and behavioral, and cognitive—into three separate levels; however, it is somewhat artificial to think of providing a psychological intervention in such a rigid fashion, given that in real life treatment requires more fluidity. Therefore, clinical judgement should be used with regard to delivery of the strategies; think about the most beneficial order for the child and the symptom presentation. Younger children often do well with behaviorally based interventions, and adolescents engage readily with the cognitive strategies. Level of impairment is another consideration; children with less impairment may need only a session or two at each level of intervention and do well with a shorter course of treatment overall, while children with more impairment will likely require repetition of all parts of the intervention over a longer time span. Taking those factors into account, it is our recommendation that treatment proceed in the order in which we have presented it and that you adjust the amount of time you spend on each level as necessary per your clinical judgment.

Children with significant comorbid anxiety or depression may have a slower start to treatment because it may be harder for them to identify and express their emotions, and they may be caught in maladaptive patterns of expressing emotions physically. We recommend that you begin treatment by allowing them to process negative emotions, validating their physical and emotional experience, and helping them identify their emotions, while introducing behavioral activation steps. The intervention level also depends on the temperament and developmental level of the child, which can often be determined from the initial sessions. Some children have good insight; may readily notice how thoughts, feelings, and actions relate to physical responses; and may move quickly through the beginning levels of intervention. Other children may not have a sophisticated understanding of the role of thoughts and feelings in their physical presentation and may be more defensive or even confused by those ideas; therefore, they would be better served by more time engaging in a behavioral approach. As with any treatment course, attention must be paid to children's ability to meet the demands of treatment and readiness to change and maintain behavior. There is no hard-and-fast rule in terms of when to move up a level; this decision requires clinical judgment to determine whether children have successfully incorporated the skills and are demonstrating readiness for the next level. In addition, the symptom measures reviewed in Chapter 4 can be repeated to provide a point of reference. Overall, consider level of impairment, age, comorbidities, the complexity of the presentation, and response to treatment when thinking about how to proceed through intervention.

Regardless of the strategies on which the session focuses, allow the child to pick a goal by the end of the session related to the content of that session. If the child has hard time picking a goal, make it multiple choice based on what you know is motivating for the child. At the end of the session, the last question before the child leaves the office is always "What do you want to work on for next time?" Remember to check in on the assigned homework at the beginning of the next session. This ensures that the child is actually incorporating the strategies into his or her life, allowing you to address barriers to completion, and provides reinforcement for trying out techniques. Emphasize to the child that the strategies build on one another, so that when he or she finds what is working, he or she needs to continue doing it.

Finally, a major challenge of treating children and adolescents with somatic symptoms is that the behavioral engagement that reduces somatic symptoms means engaging in the *very same* situations that have been avoided and that led to greater impairment and disability in the first place. During the intervention chapters, keep in mind that the role of the mental health provider is to help children and families confront those challenging situations, because while it feels better to avoid the bad thing in the short term, it is detrimental in the long term. Remind children of activities they like, but have not been able to do, as motivation to tolerate the distress of *not* avoiding their somatic symptom triggers anymore. The role of treatment is not to plunk them down in difficult situations and tell them to just "handle it"; instead, it is to train them on how to use coping tools to address the challenges they feel in those situations with an understanding that it is safe and OK to do so in order to get to a better functional outcome and break the symptoms and avoidance cycle.

CHAPTER 6

Level One: Physical Factors

As discussed in the introduction, the intervention sessions begin with a behavioral approach that is focused on improving physical factors, with psychosocial supports. Similar to the rationale of the order in which the assessment was conducted, addressing physical factors first is most closely tied to the initial presenting concern of the child. Strategies improve children's physical experience of somatic symptoms, including healthy habits, symptom monitoring, and functional daily schedules. Typically, healthy habits and symptom monitoring can be presented in one session, and the functional daily schedule in the next.

Physical coping tools give children the ability to regulate their bodies, which represents a significant step forward after they have felt out of control on account of the somatic symptoms. To achieve this, carefully choose physical outcomes for treatment children *can* have direct control over, which means not picking the symptom itself. It is tempting to pick symptom reduction as the chief biological outcome; however, neither a mental health provider nor children with somatic symptoms have direct control over symptoms. Therefore, pick from the multitude of factors children *can* change about their physical experience. Start by having children engage in daily healthy habits to promote good overall physical well-being, focusing on exercise, sleep, hydration, and nutrition, in addition to a manageable goal children can be proud of accomplishing on a daily basis.

Addressing physical factors allows children to appropriately attend to their bodies to (1) get more clarity about their exact symptom patterns and (2) remind them that they can think about their bodies in a *positive* way. This can be accomplished through symptom monitoring strategies, which clarify symptom patterns, further inform treatment, and improve children's body awareness. In general, children with somatic symptoms typically have poor body awareness. This might sound counterintuitive at first, because as previously discussed, children with somatic symptoms are often *hyperaware* of their bodies. However, this heightened level of awareness is not normative; while they *are* attuned to their bodies, they are stuck on one very negative channel, to the exclusion of awareness of the positive or even neutral signals. Some of this is natural—after all, not many people wake up thinking of everything that feels *good* in the morning—but this awareness is taken to an extreme for children with somatic symptoms. Addressing this pattern of hyperawareness through the symptom monitoring strategies improves children's body awareness in ways we *want* them to attend to their bodies.

Healthy habits and symptom monitoring can be included as part of a daily schedule aimed at increasing activity and normalizing function. Introducing a daily schedule early on is another way to break the cycle of relying on symptoms to determine children's actions. Instead of symptoms dictating activity, the schedule does, and children can avoid making the "wrong" choice from a functional standpoint. Equate this to why we do not ask small children "if" they want to go to bed—every tired parent knows never to ask a small child a question that he or she can say no to! Instead of "Do I want to do my exercises today?"—which it is easy to guess the answer to—it becomes "Time to do my exercises." Children know that is part of their plan and don't question whether it feels like the right time or not. Incorporating healthy habits and symptom monitoring strategies into a functional daily schedule is a very efficient way to present these interventions.

Finally, while teaching children about the physical coping tools, address the role the family plays in engaging children in more positive physical self-care as well, which includes providing support for the child to engage in healthy lifestyle patterns at home (e.g., interacting around health and wellness instead of symptoms and sickness) and reducing focus on symptoms by limiting the family's symptom-focused check-ins. Each of the descriptions in this chapter includes the content of the treatment strategy followed by examples of how the strategy could be explained to children and families.

HEALTHY HABITS

The rationale for improving children's healthy habits in the context of somatic symptoms is similar to that for coping with other health conditions. For instance, for a person with diabetes, giving insulin does not fix all of the problems of diabetes, and it is widely accepted that there are lifestyle considerations to attend to, such as diet, exercise, hydration, skin care, and stress management. Similarly, for a person with an anxiety disorder, just taking anxiety medication does not solve anxiety; changing thoughts and using relaxation are essential tools to effectively manage anxiety. The same is true for somatic symptoms, although sometimes that idea gets lost when the family does not understand what condition the child has and is hoping for a pill or procedure that will provide a cure. Suddenly, very basic activities that children and families used to engage in go right out the window. After all, if parents believe that children have a serious medical condition or worse yet, do not know what is making children sick, the *last* thing on parents' minds is keeping children on a functional daily track. Instead, children are in the sick role, staying home from school, resting, eating when they feel like it or not at all, and disengaging from regular aspects of their lives. While this approach works well for children with acute illnesses, who get better in a few days, it does not work well for children with somatic symptoms. Not only do their symptoms persist, but this passive, nonfunctional approach is exactly the *opposite* of what is beneficial for improving the neurological function and physical biomechanics of somatic symptoms. The outcome is that children do not get better, in fact, they likely get worse, which takes a toll on their whole life. Teaching children the importance and safety of reengaging in a normal daily pattern of healthy behaviors is a critical first step in treatment.

Therefore, the first level of treatment begins with the basic coping tool of putting children on a healthy everyday track by attending to their exercise, sleep, hydration, and nutrition, with the understanding that these are behaviors *every* human being should do as a matter of course to stay healthy and alive. In fact, if we *all* did them, we would all feel better too, regardless of whether we have somatic symptoms or not. Normalize how everyone needs to take care of themselves in these ways to assure children that this is not something special that only they have to do. This mentality gets children out of the mind-set of being sick and having to do something extra or unfair, and into the mind-set that they are well and therefore *get* to keep themselves healthy, generating feelings of hope and normalcy. Another way to describe engagement in healthy habits is to refer to the education offered earlier on the ANS, and on how the automatic "driving" feature is not working well for them, so they have to "take the wheel" and learn to hit the "gas and brakes" in the right ways to make sure their "car" drives the best that it can. Of course the analogy is that children have a lot of control over their bodies, and by taking care of themselves and appropriately regulating their everyday tasks, they can steer their lives in the directions in which they want to travel. It is also a way to illustrate that *not* engaging in healthy habits is equivalent to creating a condition of physical stress in the body, which further exacerbates somatic symptoms. Here is an illustration of how that information could be presented to a child such as Alex, our case example patient with conversion disorder:

DOCTOR: OK, Alex. The first tool we are going to learn about today is how to keep your body healthy when it has not been feeling good. Remember the example of your body being like a car, and the ANS is the part of your body that controls how fast or slow your body goes?

ALEX: Yeah, I remember that. My gas pedal is stuck so my car is going too fast, and that doesn't make me feel very good.

DOCTOR: You got it! Kids with somatic symptoms have bodies that are like cars that are driving too fast. When that happens, our bodies forget to do their regular jobs, like telling us when we are hungry or thirsty, when we are tired, and when we need to exercise, because all of our energy is spent speeding down the road. That's a problem, because doing those healthy behaviors makes us feel better by slowing us down to a regular speed. So, instead of waiting for our bodies to tell us we need to do those activities to stay healthy, what do you imagine we need to do instead?

ALEX: Tell ourselves that we just need to do it and not wait for our bodies to tell us?

DOCTOR: Yes, we have to do it *anyway*. We cannot ask ourselves if we *feel* like it, because our bodies will give us the wrong answer. We have to do these healthy behaviors anyway because it is important. Let's talk about activity. When is the last time you exercised?

ALEX: Well, I was supposed to do my physical therapy exercises last night, but I felt really shaky so I skipped it.

DOCTOR: I understand that: many kids who have problems with their muscles feeling shaky have a really hard time exercising, but that is the best way to retrain your brain to move your legs more confidently and to build up strength. In fact, *not* exercising is a physical stress on our body, which pushes on the gas pedal and makes everything feel worse.

ALEX: Yeah, I guess I hadn't thought of it that way.

DOCTOR: From what you know about the human body, can most humans just say, "OK! I exercised yesterday, I don't ever need to do that again"?

ALEX: No way! People should exercise every day, or at least a few times a week. I used to exercise a lot when I was on the track team.

DOCTOR: You got it. Same thing with drinking water, eating, and sleeping. We cannot do any of those activities once a week and call it good. We have to do them every single day—it is part of being a human being, after all! Let's talk about ways we can make sure you are doing each one of these healthy habits every day, no matter how you are feeling, so we can get your body back to driving at the right speed.

As with the car analogy for ANS regulation, you can also use the pain gate example or anticipatory anxiety leading to symptoms to match the education style you present to the child (e.g., not caring for ourselves is equivalent to a stressor that would raise the pain gate and engaging in healthy habits will close it, physical stressors lead to anticipation of symptoms and healthy habits break the cycle of anticipation). Once the rationale has been established for the importance of healthy habits, use the cell phone example to remind children of the energy these tasks provide on a daily basis and the importance of a regular pattern:

> "Just like our phones, we have to recharge our bodies on a daily basis, whether we feel like it or not, so they are ready for action the next day. The way we do that is to make sure we have enough to eat and drink, that we do some movement and exercise, and that we sleep enough at night every single day. Once this is part of the daily routine, just like plugging your phone in at night, you will not even really need to think about doing it anymore. It will just become something you do every day anyway, like brushing your teeth or putting your shoes on before you walk out the door. That is what we all have to do on a daily basis to take care of our body."

As far as what healthy habits to recommend for children, typically you can follow the general pediatric guidelines based on a child's age for exercise, sleep, hydration, and nutrition. If there are any specific recommendations that have been made by a child's doctor or there are limitations based on their symptoms, account for those during development of the child's plan. In general, children with somatic symptoms have very few limitations, and most are able to use the normative recommendations for their age. Some specific recommendations are made below for both standard tips that we provide in our practice, as well as modifications for children with different symptom presentations. After introduction of healthy habits, give an overview of what will be targeted in each healthy behavior category and discuss any potential barriers to reaching the goals. Remember, you will have some clues about how much children are engaging or not engaging in these healthy habits from the assessment, which will allow you to focus on the areas in which children need your support as well as provide reinforcement for healthy behaviors that they are already doing well. For each of the four healthy habits, the general recommendations are reviewed, noting specific points for certain somatic symptom presentations when applicable.

Exercise

The Centers for Disease Control and Prevention (CDC) recommends that children engage in 60 minutes of exercise-based activity on a daily basis and offer a helpful online activity resource (*www.cdc.gov/physicalactivity/basics/children*). For children with low impairment, this will likely be achievable if they are in school and have a physical education class; for children with high impairment, this might be 60 more minutes a day than anything they have been doing in the past year. The CDC recommends engaging in both aerobic activity that increases cardiovascular activity, such as walking, running, biking, or playing sports, as well as muscle strengthening, such as sit-ups, push-ups, or core exercises, during this 60-minute time frame. Children have the most success in reaching this physical activity goal when they are engaging in something fun with peers or family and when it is part of the daily routine. For children with somatic symptoms, make sure they get the go-ahead from their medical providers that it is safe and OK to engage in a program of exercise, because without the proper medical clearance and reassurance, it will be very difficult and perhaps impossible for them to increase their activity.

For children with cardiac symptoms, there are some exercise recommendations that are important to note for safety, given that they often experience dizziness with prolonged standing or postural changes. Although they may find it hard to do at first, children with these conditions particularly benefit from exercise, as it improves their physical conditioning and symptoms of dizziness over time, especially exercises that strengthen the legs. There are also ways that they can stand that reduce dizziness, such as crossing one leg over the other, ensuring that the knees are not in a locked position, and shifting weight or rocking from one foot to the other. All of these strategies improve the legs' ability to continue pumping blood throughout the body despite the physical stress of standing, which will reduce dizziness. It is beneficial for children with significant dizziness to begin exercise in seated positions (e.g., recumbent bike) or in the pool to combat any potential danger of falling and suffering a setback or believing that exercise is unsafe.

Children with chronic pain syndromes, such as headache, painful GI disorders, or musculoskeletal pain, as well as conversion disorder are *strongly* encouraged to exercise to improve biomechanical properties of their bodies (e.g., joint protection, conditioning, balance, endurance). Exercise benefits pain and gait disturbances and creates positive neurological effects that regulate ANS function and release endorphins, both of which normalize nervous system dysregulation that contributes to pain and conversion symptoms. Children with these conditions usually do not have activity limitations based on their symptom presentation, although this can be surprising to them because pain is typically a signal that means you *should not* move and gait imbalance or disturbance usually means that you *cannot* move. Telling them that it is safe for them to move (based on their medical providers' assurances) and picking the right activities (e.g., stretching, seated exercise, swimming, short bouts of walking) are critical to ensuring a steady path to increasing function for children who have become physically disabled by their symptoms.

Children and families will need special instruction to pace physical activities as they get going. A common way we do this is to encourage them to set aside an hour of time each day that they are going exercise to make it a priority. Within that hour, encourage them to build up their activities based on their level of conditioning—*not* symptoms—so that they start small and work up to more activity and higher intensity. For instance, a family may decide to take a walk every evening for their hour of movement. If they have not done this in a long time, recommend small intervals, such as first doing 5 minutes at a slow pace, 5 minutes at a moderate pace, then taking a 10-minute seated rest break, then repeating that pattern two more times for the remainder of the hour. Once they have mastered that, they can incrementally increase walking time and decrease break time until they can walk briskly for the full hour. Caution children about doing too much too fast when initiating exercise at the risk of *overdoing* activity and flaring symptoms, which could backfire if children conclude "See! Exercise makes it worse" when pacing was really the problem. The goal is for children to feel *good* after exercise, have fun, and continue engaging in physical activity. If you are at all in doubt about the exercise recommendations you should make for children you are working with, collaborate with their health care providers or encourage families to reach out to their team directly to clarify any concerns. With few exceptions, exercise is a core part of the recommended treatment for children with somatic symptoms.

Sleep

The American Academy of Sleep Medicine (AASM) recommends that school-age children (ages 6–12) get 9–12 hours of sleep per night and adolescents (ages 13–18) get 8–10 hours of sleep per night (Paruthi et al., 2016). Children in these age ranges are not advised to nap during the day, and adherence to good sleep hygiene habits is recommended. You do not have to worry about whether to consult with children's medical providers—good sleep patterns are *always* a good idea for children, and particularly for children with somatic symptoms, who quite often have disrupted patterns of sleep. Standard sleep recommendations include keeping a consistent bedtime and wake time (even on weekends) so that children are going to bed at night and getting out of bed in the morning at the same time every weekday (plus or minus an hour for weekends), creating a peaceful sleep environment (dark, quiet, neutral temperature room), and establishing a good bedtime routine (no physical or stressful activity for at least 2 hours before bedtime, no caffeine, having a relaxation or wind-down period, limiting screen time an hour before bed).

Sleep regulation does not happen all at once, but over a matter of days or even a few weeks, children usually sleep more soundly by implementing these strategies. Bodies like the predictability of sleep routines—parents understand this if they are reminded of the bedtime routines they carried out for their infants to ensure good sleep that benefitted the whole family. The same principles hold for what children need to do when they have somatic symptoms; because their bodies are not giving them the proper sleep and wake signals on which they used to rely, they need those external supports to rebuild a good sleep routine. Many of the recommendations about good sleep, and good healthy habits for that matter, are all about getting back to the basics.

Overall, there are no special sleep recommendations for different somatic symptom presentations, but there are some general patterns of sleep disruptions for children in this population. First, children with somatic symptoms of any type often feel worse in the morning and better in the afternoon or evening. This leads to later wake times and bedtimes than usual, and sometimes naps during the day, all of which are highly disruptive to regular sleep patterns and daily functioning. Second, most children have problems falling asleep and staying asleep due to symptoms, which leads to disrupted sleep schedules. Sometimes children use electronics or other distractions while in bed in an effort to relax, but this strategy keeps them up even longer due to the mental stimulation, positive reinforcement, and effect of the light emitted from electronic screens. Because of these challenges, we strongly recommend that children adopt regular sleep routines and environmental supports *despite* these difficulties. This means that even if children have had a very difficult night of sleep or do not feel well in the morning, they wake up *anyway* at the set time, stay up all day and be active, go to bed *anyway* at the set time (even if they are not tired or are having a difficult time with symptoms), and discontinue all electronics or reinforcing activities at night, aside from quiet relaxation, to establish a positive sleep pattern over time. Sleep hygiene requires firm boundaries on the mental health providers' part, as children and families are easily swayed to fall back into bad habits when a child is unwell at night. While all healthy habits are equally important to improve children's overall physical wellbeing, sleep may edge the others out in terms of the significant benefits that children feel once they reestablish these sleep routines.

Finally, something that is surprisingly common among children with all types of somatic symptoms is that the *whole family* has shifted their sleeping routines or even locations based on children's symptoms. One of us actually received a therapy referral solely on the basis of a family sleep problem: a young patient was referred to us because her family was tired of sharing her uncomfortable bed with her at night. It was either buy a new mattress or try CBT! Upon meeting the family, it became clear that while the disrupted sleep was the family's most pressing concern, the reason for it was the child's nightly abdominal pain complaints that resulted in her parents sleeping in her bed so they could comfort her as she cried out in the night. Turns out, a somatic symptom was the sole cause of this family sleep problem. After a short course of treatment, the child was able to independently cope with her symptoms and the parents returned to sleeping in their own (more comfortable!) bed. If there are sleep disruptions for the child, regardless of age or gender, find out more information about factors in the bedtime routine that could be targeted during intervention, as well as who is sleeping where, so the whole family can get back to getting a good night's sleep.

Hydration

Generally speaking, children are encouraged to have eight 8-ounce servings of fluids on a daily basis, a bit less for children who are younger (six glasses) and a bit more for children who are older or more active (10 or more glasses). Caffeinated beverages are not recommended for children under the age of 18 due to their negative cardio-vascular effects (Temple et al., 2014). For nutritional purposes, also be mindful of the amount of sugar in drinks such as sodas or even "healthier"-sounding drinks like smoothies or sports drinks, which often have more sugar than one might expect. A good rule of thumb is that at least half of children's fluid intake for the day should be water, and the remainder should be other healthy, noncaffeinated beverages.

Dehydration is a significant factor contributing to poor physical health in many children with somatic symptoms; thus, hydration can be a very "simple" thing to do that improves children's symptoms. Strategies include keeping a paper chart that children can check off on a daily basis or using an app that accomplishes the same function, having a schedule for hydration to follow to throughout the day, using an alarm on the phone to sound a drink reminder every hour, and having a favorite glass to drink out of at home or carrying a water bottle to school (which children may need a permission slip to do, as many schools do not allow water bottles). If children are resistant to drinking water, make water tastier and more appealing (e.g., using flavor packets, putting in fresh fruit, using a fun cup or straw, flavoring the water with small amounts of juice).

Good hydration is especially important for children with headache and syncope, as dehydration leads to changes in circulation that bring on symptoms. Children with those conditions often have higher fluid recommendations of up to 100 ounces of fluids per day from their medical providers, along with higher salt intake recommendations to increase the body's absorption and retention of water. This can be done through eating a salty snack when drinking water (which is particularly beneficial prior to exercise or in hot weather, as sweat results in rapid loss of water, especially in children) or through adding sports drinks to fluid intake regimens. This is a significant amount of fluid for anyone to take in, let alone a child or teen, and they benefit from special consideration of how to increase and track daily hydration. For example, you can use a chart indicating how many 8-ounce cups the child is currently drinking, and then add one 8-ounce cup each day or week until the goal is reached. Slowly adding a cup a day or week tends to be less overwhelming than measuring out 80 to 100 ounces of liquid on day one. Talk with the family about keeping fluids readily stocked in the home as well as having additional water bottles/sports drinks/juice boxes in the car or backpack or school classroom or nurse's office, so that the child has fluids available at all times.

Finally, all children with somatic symptoms need to take in water *slowly* over the course of the day instead of gulping it in big boluses, as it will be viscerally uncomfortable to have a large quantity of water in their GI tracts if they drink it all at once and they will not absorb what they need if it is taken in such a large quantity. This can be practiced in session by getting a cup of water together during the session, modeling how to take frequent, slow sips to finish the cup by the end of the session or using a timer to go off at regular intervals as a reminder to drink. For children who have symptoms in the morning, including dizziness, headache, gait imbalance, or nausea, recommend hydrating before they even put their feet on the floor. Keeping a bottle of water by the bed along with a salty snack and sitting up and eating or drinking for a few minutes before getting out of bed is beneficial. Our bodies become dehydrated overnight, and children with somatic symptoms will be especially sensitive to these effects in the morning. Hydrating and replacing salt lost overnight replenishes cells and improves ANS function, including circulatory benefits, which minimize symptoms associated with changing positions from lying down in bed all night to standing.

Nutrition

In general, we recommend that children adhere to standard nutrition guidelines of eating healthy, balanced meals every day and small, healthy snacks. Current national standards for nutritional guidelines provide a basis for making recommendations for healthy eating habits. The U.S. Department of Agriculture (USDA) website has a variety of tools that provide general information about the five food groups (protein, vegetables, dairy, grains, and fruit) as well as personalized options for how to balance these into a healthy daily diet based on age, gender, weight, and activity level (*www. nutrition.gov/life-stages/children*). A nice visual representation of this information is found in the "My Plate" graphic illustrating the composition of a healthy meal (*www. fns.usda.gov/sites/default/files/MyPlateAtHome.pdf*).

For children with somatic symptoms, there are specific ways that healthy and consistent eating patterns are beneficial. First, regarding eating consistency, when anyone has not eaten for a long period of time, blood sugar drops, and because this is experienced as a physical stressor by the body, it can trigger somatic symptoms in children who have them. Attend to this healthy habit particularly for children with chronic headache or orthostatic intolerance, as blood sugar dips are common triggers for the onset of or a spike in pain or dizziness. In addition to low blood sugar, irregular eating patterns lead to GI dysfunction, which can be a trigger for symptoms in children with FGIDs. Paradoxically, children who are nauseous and have abdominal pain do not feel like eating anything; however, eating is *exactly* what they need to do to get their GI system functioning normally again. Make sure children eat reasonably sized meals; otherwise they will feel the negative effects of having their blood sugar and GI function swinging from too low to too high, which can induce somatic symptom exacerbations as well. This is a pattern with children who do not eat in the morning or at lunch but then come home to a huge snack and a huge dinner, which induces discomfort at night that then keeps them from eating in the morning, and the cycle goes on.

Nutritional content is important to address as well. Many children with somatic symptoms, particularly GI symptoms or headache, have a history of being "picky eaters" or have a restricted food repertoire based on symptoms. In these cases, there may be nutritional deficits playing a role in symptom exacerbation. You are unlikely to change a long-standing nutritional deficit or family pattern without additional support from the primary care provider and a dietician. If there are concerns regarding calorie intake or significant food restrictions, touch base with the child's medical provider to discuss this further. For some children, a lack of vitamins, such as riboflavin or other B vitamins, can increase symptoms such as headache; therefore, ensure that children are eating daily servings of protein, dairy, and green vegetables to provide essential nutritional elements. For children with GI symptoms or symptoms that are worse in the morning, such as dizziness or gait imbalance, suggest that they eat something small but palatable in the morning. Try the "something is better than nothing" policy, worrying less about the nutritional content of the meal that is most difficult for them to eat, and focus just on getting some energy (in the form of food) into the system.

Finally, particularly for children with FGIDs, there may be food restrictions based on allergies or intolerances (e.g., lactose, gluten). Ensure that children are abiding by dietary recommendations and are not triggering symptoms by poor adherence. Some children may not have been diagnosed with food intolerances per se, but have noticed that every time they eat a lot of pizza or ice cream their symptoms feel worse (e.g., lactose intolerance). Encourage them to discuss these connections with their health care providers in case there is an underlying medical reason for symptoms, and also to balance those foods out across their diet so that they are not overwhelming their system with a particular food all at once.

In general, we introduce these four healthy habits and then discuss with children how they are doing in each category using the "Healthy Habits" worksheet (in the Appendix). Write a goal in every category; give them lots of praise for the ways in which they are already taking care of themselves, and address areas that need to improve, spending more time there for education and goal setting. Some children have fitness tracking devices that record many metrics of daily function (including sleep, steps, hydration, etc.), which can be a motivating tool to inspire children to increase adherence to healthy habits, and a great way to check on how they are practicing skills between sessions by having them share their reports with you. Here is how we would set goals for healthy habits with Johnny, our patient with abdominal pain:

DOCTOR: There are four healthy habits that we are going to work on today: eat healthy foods and do not skip meals, drink eight glasses of water, spend 1 hour being active or exercising, and get 9–12 hours of regular sleep. Let's see which areas have been easier for you to do and then focus on the areas to improve. Let's start with hydration. How many glasses of juice, water, milk, or other drinks do you have per day?

JOHNNY: Well, I always drink juice if I have breakfast. Sometimes I do not have anything in the morning to eat or drink if my stomach hurts. I take a bottle of water to school but I'm not allowed to keep it at my desk, so sometimes I don't finish it. I drink a juice box at lunch. I always drink something when I get home from school and at dinner.

DOCTOR: If we add that all up, that's about four to six glasses of fluid on a good day when you eat breakfast and drink your water bottle, but on a tough day only three glasses. How many glasses of liquids do you think we recommend kids your age drink per day?

JOHNNY: Hmm, I don't know. Maybe five?

DOCTOR: Good guess! Actually, the answer is eight 8-ounce glasses. Drinking fluids, especially water, is one of the best ways to make your body feel good and balanced. Did you know that the human body is about 60% water?

JOHNNY: No! Weird!

DOCTOR: Because our body is mainly made of water, we have refresh it every day to keep our temperature regular, get rid of waste, and send blood and oxygen to all of our cells. When there's not enough water, our body doesn't work efficiently and that is hard on our whole system. If the goal is to drink eight glasses of water to keep your cells healthy, the good news is that on some days, you are really close to that! How do you think we could increase your hydration during the day to get to that goal of eight glasses, even on days you have symptoms?

JOHNNY: I could drink more water at school if I was allowed to have a water bottle.

DOCTOR: That's a great idea. I can write you a note to say that you are allowed to have a water bottle in school, which usually counts for two glasses. I bet you could drink that bottle of water during your morning classes, refill it at lunchtime, and drink it again in the afternoon. If you keep drinking liquids at every meal and when you get home from school, that would be eight glasses. Remember, being more hydrated will help your symptoms. What do you think?

JOHNNY: Yeah, that would work. I would like to have a note.

DOCTOR: Great. I will write one for you today. Which one should we do next?

JOHNNY: Well, exercise is easy because I go outside after school and usually play with my friends for an hour. Does that count for exercise?

DOCTOR: Definitely. Great job being so active. Do you make sure to get some activity on days that you do not feel good, too?

JOHNNY: Not really. I stay inside if my stomach is hurting.

DOCTOR: I understand why you have been doing that based on the signals your body has been giving you, but remember although those are *real* pain signals, they are not *dangerous*, and having pain doesn't mean you have to stop your activity. In fact, the *more* active you are, the more you can retrain your brain to stop thinking so much about pain!

JOHNNY: So, I should go outside and play even when my stomach hurts?

DOCTOR: Yes! It is safe and OK to be active when you have symptoms. Activity closes the pain gate, which makes the pain better over time. If you are having a hard time, you can pace yourself by taking breaks or playing a less active game than usual.

JOHNNY: OK. I can try that.

DOCTOR: Excellent. Let's talk about sleep now, because I think from our first meeting together you told me that you usually do a really great job with sleep.

JOHNNY: My lights have to be out by 9 P.M., and I wake up at 7 A.M. for school. On weekends I'm allowed to stay up until 10 P.M. but that's it. Sometimes I have a hard time falling asleep.

DOCTOR: Sleep is one of the most important healthy habits we can do for our bodies, and your bedtime allows you to get exactly the right amount of sleep each night for your age—10 hours. We want to keep the bedtime close to the same between weeknights and weekends, and you are doing a great job of that! We can use the relaxation strategies you'll learn soon to help with falling asleep. For now, keep up the great work on your bedtime schedule. OK, now we have eating, which I know can be a hard one.

JOHNNY: Yeah, when my stomach hurts I usually don't eat.

DOCTOR: Well, that is a tricky situation. Although it *seems* like the last thing your stomach wants to do is eat, it is actually the *best* thing to remind your stomach to get back to the business of digesting food and get out of the business of sending pain signals! When you haven't eaten for a long time your blood sugar gets low, which can make your stomach feel worse. Is there anything that you eat any time of the day that is OK on your stomach?

JOHNNY: Well, if I really feel bad at night, my mom usually gives me some saltine crackers or a granola bar, and I guess that is OK. I don't feel worse at least.

DOCTOR: Perfect. That's something that gives you a little bit of energy but doesn't make you feel worse. I call this the "something is better than nothing" policy. So if your stomach is hurting at mealtime, let's plan for you to eat some crackers or a granola bar. Then at your other meals, be sure to focus on the other food groups.

For children with more straightforward symptom presentations, this type of education and interaction will likely be sufficient to get them going on a good healthy habit pattern. However, for children with psychological comorbidities or who may be resistant to making changes or have more impairment, it may be more challenging to consider changing healthy habits. In that case, present the same information, but go into more depth in terms of encouraging them to engage in these strategies, build motivation, and problem-solve through potential barriers, or take a slower pace and introduce one healthy habit at a time. We illustrate this through the following dialogue with our patient Ashley, who has cardiac symptoms:

DOCTOR: So those are the healthy habits. Any questions so far?

ASHLEY: Well, I know you said that I need to do all of those things, but my symptoms are too bad to do any of them. Any one of those could make my symptoms worse, and then I won't be able to do anything for the rest of the day. Like drinking water. That makes my stomach feel terrible and makes me dizzy, so then I am probably going to fall down.

DOCTOR: Of course it is difficult to have symptoms in the first place, and to think that doing something like drinking water or eating regular meals could make you feel worse makes it even harder. That's how you got into this pattern of *not* doing these healthy habits in the first place! But noticing your symptoms increasing after doing these healthy habits doesn't mean that you can never make these kinds of changes. We just have to find creative ways for you to take care of yourself. We can do that slowly, one step at a time.

ASHLEY: But my symptoms are signs that I can't handle it!

DOCTOR: Or it means that you are more sensitive to signals in your body than other people. For instance, you may have friends who can stay up all night and skip breakfast and are OK going to school the next day, but that will not work for you. Your body handles physical stressors in a different way than your peers do—not better or worse, just different—so you need different ways to cope with those challenges. Engaging in healthy habits is one way to do that. Which one seems the most possible to you?

ASHLEY: Well, I want to say none of them, but I know you want me to pick one. I guess eating. I don't eat breakfast, but usually I eat lunch and I always eat dinner. I don't want to eat breakfast. I feel too dizzy in the morning to eat.

DOCTOR: I think eating is a good way to start changing healthy habits. Many people who are dizzy in the morning don't want to eat, but your body needs *something* in the morning for energy and salt, which decreases dizziness. Instead of eating a perfectly nutritious breakfast, let's just think about replenishing the salt in your body. When you feel dizzy, what kind of salty snack do you eat?

ASHLEY: Well, usually I have some baked chips. My mom buys small snack bags.

DOCTOR: That's perfect. What if you eat a small bag of baked chips along with some water in the morning? You can keep them on your nightstand by your bed, and when you wake up, sit up in bed, take small sips from the water bottle and eat about half the bag of chips before you get out of bed. Then sit on the edge of the bed with your feet touching the floor, drink more water, and eat some more chips, for a total of about 5 minutes. Once you have had all of the chips and least half of the water, slowly stand up. That way you will do two things at once—we will give your body a little energy in the morning while also targeting your cardiac symptoms by just changing one pattern in the morning.

ASHLEY: I guess I can try that. I'm not sure if it is going to work.

DOCTOR: I am not sure either, Ashley. Just like with all of the healthy habits and the rest of the coping tools we will be working on, I ask that you give each one a try. That's the only way we can see if it will be helpful or not.

SYMPTOM MONITORING

Monitoring symptoms early in treatment allows you to find triggers and identify patterns to symptoms, which can help with treatment, in addition to prompting children to notice times when they feel good or even just OK, thus changing their attention to and awareness of symptoms. Providing children with a good rationale for why they are tracking symptoms helps them understand that while this does call attention to symptoms briefly—which seems like the opposite of taking attention away from symptoms—it is used to better understand their presentation, find the right coping tools, and understand how they can be proactive in preventing symptoms altogether by identifying not only the symptom, but also the context in which the symptom occurs. This enables children to make the connection between symptoms and other experiences in their lives, like difficult activities or emotions.

Many times, just by tracking, children make the connection to symptoms and patterns on their own.

Rather than engage in a long dialogue with children about this strategy, simply present the "Symptom Tracking" worksheet (in the Appendix) at the end of the first level one session and review with them the areas to track, including symptoms, how long they lasted, what the child was doing at the time, and what he or she was thinking. Both "positive" and "negative" symptoms are included on the form. Explain to children that in addition to logging their somatic symptoms, they should also notice as least one time when they felt *good* during the week and treat that the same way as the negative symptom tracking in terms of noting the context. Finally, ask them to write down what they doing before and/or after the symptoms started, and any other details they think are relevant.

The goal is for children to complete the log on a daily basis, with one tracking form per week. If the child is seen weekly, you can provide one form, or more as needed. Unlike healthy habits, which once incorporated we expect children to continue, this is a strategy that we want to use in a time-limited fashion. If you are able to get the information you need after the first week of tracking, then stop this practice and have children report on their function at the beginning of each session, either verbally or through a tracking tool. If children do not bring the symptom monitoring form back or more information is needed to determine the patterns, or if a new symptom pattern that develops, continue using the form until this information is clarified.

DAILY SCHEDULE

Finally, after you have set healthy habit goals and described symptom monitoring, you are ready to put it all together into a daily schedule. In a typical course of treatment delivery, this would be the fourth session, after children have learned healthy habits and symptom monitoring in the previous session. You can incorporate what they successfully implemented in their homework into building the schedule. Introduce this strategy to children by saying "Using a schedule is a way of not letting symptoms choose what you are doing but allowing *you* to choose what you are doing!" It is a concrete way to shift attention and focus away from symptoms—breaking the reactionary cycle of symptoms and disability—and toward completion of the daily tasks that children want and need to do. When setting up a schedule, create a typical day as the standard using the "Daily Schedule Template" (in the Appendix), making mention of how that can be altered on a nonschool day or weekend. Ensure that healthy habits and symptom monitoring are included, as well as standard activities such as school, extracurricular activities, family time, interaction with friends, and pleasant activities. Remember to refer to the assessment session to get some idea of what activities children are missing out on that they want to build back into their daily life or what goals they had for being able to return to activities. Bring back information from the education session to remind children that it is safe and OK to engage in functional daily schedules, and is another way for them to rebalance their system. The overall idea of scheduling is to stop the brain's "bottom-up" processing of attending to symptoms and then deciding what to do based on that information, and instead use a "top-down" model in which the child decides what to do and just tells the body to do it, rather than getting its opinion.

The primary goal of creating the schedule is to increase function. You can sit all day with children in the early stages of treatment debating about thoughts and feelings, but if you are not getting them out there into their lives on a daily basis, you are not giving their bodies a chance to work for them physically, and as a result they may continue to be stuck mentally. Engaging in a functional daily schedule allows children to get endorphins flowing, have positive experiences, and get them on board with making these changes that you are talking about. For all of these reasons, behavioral activation is also a cornerstone of CBT as applied to somatic symptoms, and a functional daily schedule is an excellent way to make this happen. In fact, we often say, "The schedule is the medicine." Increasing function through creation of an actual daily schedule is a great way to make this goal concrete and ensure that children have a balance between time spent on the "need to do" activities (e.g., school, chores, healthy habits, symptom monitoring) and the "want to do" activities (e.g., distraction, fun, friends). There are a lot of popular culture references that children find entertaining that illustrate the importance of function, including Nike's "Just do it" motto, the ancient quote "a journey of a thousand miles begins with one step," or the most popular of all, Yoda's mantra of "Do or do not. There is no try." Children sometimes enjoy putting together an actual or virtual collage of inspirational quotes and pictures as a motivation tool to stay on a functional daily track.

Once a schedule has been established, the best way to increase activity is through pacing. Adults understand this through the idea of "Rome wasn't built in a day," and children resonate with Goldilocks's "too much, too little, and just right" mentality. The main goal of pacing is to avoid the overdo/underdo cycle, or a pattern that cycles between the extremes of overactivity and underactivity and often results in a symptom flare, and strike a moderate balance between activity and rest. For example, many children with somatic symptoms who do not have great body awareness will go full throttle without realizing they are doing it, such as jumping for hours on the new trampoline in the neighbor's backyard. They are surprised that night when they are completely wiped out and sore, and wake up the next day with a dizzy head and difficulty walking. As a result, they miss school and lie in bed all day, which represents the "underdo" part of the cycle. The problem is that for children with somatic symptoms, rest does not solve the problem but instead perpetuates it, and they miss out on more activity until they are sick and tired of missing out and go outside to jump on the trampoline again for 2 hours to make up for lost time ... and the cycle repeats. Instead, recommend that children have a more balanced, moderate level of activity, in which some activity is followed by a rest break *before* they overdo it, followed by more activity, and then rest again. This can be incorporated into the daily schedule by explicitly stating that we want to avoid doing too much of anything back-to-back.

Finally, a functional daily schedule engages children in activities they have avoided because while they know they need to do them, they either do not want to or let the symptoms decide that they cannot. A great example is homework. Most children have homework to do when they come home from school, and they know that if they ask themselves, "Do I want to do homework?" the answer is usually no! This might lead them to put it off until some late hour of the evening, which could result in a fight between children and parents or a stressful time trying to fit it all in at the end of the day, or both. The solution to this dilemma is putting the activity into the functional daily schedule. When children have these activities scheduled, they say, "It's time to do homework" rather than asking themselves if they want to, making it easier to *just do it,* because it is important to do regardless of whether they feel like doing it. Structure the schedule so that mandatory activities come before elective activities to set up a natural reward system. Activities that are a "need to" come before ones that are a "want to." This approach increases active coping and self-efficacy and decreases reliance on a passive or reactionary approach to managing symptoms and stressors. This is how we introduce a functional daily schedule in general:

> "OK, so far we have talked about the healthy habit goals that you are going to work on as well as how to track your symptoms so we can get a better idea of the patterns. Now let's put it all together into a plan that you will follow every day. Using a daily schedule to do these strategies and get you back into all of your activities is a way to regulate and balance your body. We want to do this in a way that we call pacing, meaning that you do not do too much or too little, and that everything is just the right amount, with plenty of time for activity and rest, both for what you need to do and what you want to do."

The schedule is individually created with the child. We typically use a computer program that allows us to build a table, or you could also use a paper copy of a blank table (in the Appendix). An example of a completed home instruction schedule is presented in Figure 6.1. Once the schedule has been created, print it out for the child or send home the paper worksheet and suggest that the schedule be hung on the refrigerator door or on a bulletin board in the bedroom so it is visible and can be used daily. Discuss it as a model for the child to follow in the initial stages of treatment, but just like anything in life, schedules change over time and it should be used as a flexible tool.

THE FAMILY'S ROLE

For level one intervention, the role of the family is to support children's engagement or reengagement in the functional strategies presented in this chapter. The most effective way families can do that is by setting up positive modeling in the home. Some families have done this by adopting a set of "house rules" so that everyone in the family abides by these physical strategies. This way, children do not feel singled out by having to do something different, and families can send the powerful message that everyone in the house stands to benefit from improved healthy habits, regardless of symptoms. House rules can include everyone exercising together, offering a healthy meal daily, turning out lights for all children in the family at the same time, hydration competitions, and so forth. A family approach to increasing function allows the family to engage with the child positively around health instead of around illness, which is a very successful way of reducing the child's attention to symptoms and breaking the cycle of disability. Parents can also pair age-appropriate rewards with completing

DAILY SCHEDULE TEMPLATE

Time	Activity	Did I do it?
7 A.M.		
8 A.M.	Wake up, bathing, dressing, breakfast	
9 A.M.	Schoolwork at the table or a desk	
10 A.M.	Break for relaxing or distracting activity	
11 A.M.	Schoolwork at the table or a desk	
12 P.M.	Lunch	
1 P.M.	Schoolwork at the table or a desk	
2 P.M.	Exercise	
3 P.M.	Schoolwork at the table or a desk	
4 P.M.	Break for relaxing or distracting activity	
5 P.M.	Break for relaxing or distracting activity	
6 P.M.	Dinner	
7 P.M.	Family Activity	
8 P.M.	Quiet Activities	
9 P.M.	Bedtime preparation and relaxation	
10 P.M.	Lights out	

FIGURE 6.1. Example of a completed daily schedule.

tasks on the schedule, like getting to earn an allowance, a fun outing on the weekend, or extra electronics time.

At this stage, families benefit from instruction on how to reduce focus on their children's symptoms, such as asking fewer questions about them. This is an important conversation to have with parents, one that will sound counterintuitive at first but makes sense when you recall the education on attention to symptoms. It is natural caretaking behavior to check on children who are unwell or allow them to rest and disengage from life while they are sick. However, this is the *opposite* of how children recover from somatic symptoms, and just as they are asked to train their brains to focus on function, parents are asked to do the same. We have worked with many children who have asked us, even *begged* us, to tell their parents to stop asking them about how they feel, because just as they have taken their attention off their symptoms, a well-intentioned loved one comes along and refocuses all of their attention back on their struggles with four little words: "How are you feeling?" The children themselves are asking us to teach their families the importance of breaking the cycle of symptoms and attention.

Some parents benefit from hearing children say this themselves, as it gives them direct permission to stop that line of questioning. Or you can instruct parents to stop checking in while providing the rationale (e.g., to decrease attention to symptoms). Make sure to give the parents something else to ask, such as what children learned that day in school, or if they got to see friends at lunch, or what they plan to do for fun, because if you take something away you have to replace it with something else! Because the focus of these initial sessions is on improving function, luckily there will be plenty for parents to focus on in terms of asking children about the activities they have been doing. The other assurance to provide is to let children know that if they are struggling, they can go to their parents for help. It is not that symptoms cannot be discussed at all, it is just that when children are otherwise occupied we do not want to create an opportunity for them to focus on how they feel, and even when they are distressed, it is more helpful to focus on coping efforts. The parenting role in terms of attention to symptoms is discussed in much more detail in Chapter 9, including dialogues to engage in with parents if they are having a difficult time implementing these changes.

TREATMENT PROGRESS

At this point in treatment, children have learned the basic physical strategies that help them remove the focus from their symptoms and readopt normal, basic patterns of function in their lives, with family support. Children and families need to know that after these initial sessions, while some positive patterns are expected to begin, big changes do not happen overnight. New strategies must be practiced on a daily basis over time to become a habit or a routine that ultimately improves function and symptoms. Sometimes, children and families get very excited about engaging in these new strategies and do it all the first 2 days after we discuss it in session, but then something throws them off course and they do nothing for the rest of the week. Other times, children engage in the strategies until they do not feel good, which they may mistakenly believe is an indication that the strategies are not working for them, and then they throw the whole plan out the window. Communicate to families that this is a marathon, not a sprint, and committing to learning coping tools is committing to a *process* of change.

Concrete ways of describing the idea of change as a process include growing hair or increasing in height—children easily relate to the idea that you cannot look in the mirror 10 times a day and expect to see anything different, but that does not mean that they are not growing; after all, when friends haven't seen you in a long time they usually say, "You're so much taller!" "Your hair is so long!" Change is happening all along; it can just be difficult to notice. Also, let children know that it is OK if there is a day where they do something "wrong" or "forget" to engage in one of their strategies; no one is perfect, and each day will have a different challenge. Encourage children to note what was hard about meeting their goal, remember to talk about it at the next session, and try again the next day.

Finally, when evaluating and discussing progress in treatment with children, reflect to them that it is easier for us to see changes on the outside before they feel changes on the inside. For this reason, feed back to them the areas in which you see improvement, making special note of what their friends and family members notice as examples of progress, especially if they have a hard time recognizing progress themselves.

CHAPTER SUMMARY AND TAKE-AWAY POINTS

- Regulating healthy habits, which include exercise, sleep, hydration, and nutrition, promotes overall physical well-being, rebalances an unbalanced body, and helps children feel a sense of accomplishment over something physical that they can control.

- Symptom monitoring is used in a time-limited fashion to improve children's body awareness so they can recognize good signals as well as better understand symptoms when they do occur, incorporating cognitive, emotional, and physical factors into their understanding of symptom patterns.

- The use of a daily schedule helps children and families readopt a typical, functional life regardless of symptoms and incorporate healthy habits and symptom monitoring strategies into a routine.

CHAPTER 7

Level Two: Emotional and Behavioral Factors

Once children have adopted a better physical routine and have begun to normalize basic daily function, they are ready to benefit from the next level of intervention, which focuses on how to understand emotions, help their minds and bodies feel better from a physical standpoint, and gain more control over both emotional and physical symptoms and related impairment. This chapter introduces emotion identification, a precursor to the cognitive work presented in the next level, as well as the behavioral strategies of distraction and relaxation.

This level of intervention takes two sessions to cover the information in a straightforward case: one for emotion identification and distraction, and one for relaxation techniques. This gives enough time for presentation of new material, practice in session, and the child's own practice between sessions at home. For children with more significant symptoms and impairment, it may be beneficial to spread out the relaxation training into multiple sessions (one session for each strategy, even) to ensure they are getting the time and support to learn and practice the skill effectively in session as well as enough time between sessions to incorporate it successfully into their lives.

The emotion identification and behavioral strategies presented in this chapter are designed to teach children about the mind–body connection in a practical, skills-based manner. Emotion identification allows children to gain much-needed practice in recognizing the emotional aspect of what they typically feel in a physical fashion, which builds the connection of emotions to physical symptoms. This is a crucial foundation for children to build at this level of treatment so they are ready to undertake the next level of cognitive strategies, as well as to normalize the experience of emotions and symptoms occurring simultaneously.

Moving into the behavioral strategies, distraction is introduced as a tool that reinforces function and helps to balance the ANS, closes the gate on the pain signal, and redirects attention away from symptoms. When done through engagement in pleasant activities, distraction has the added benefit of getting children active again in meaningful areas of their lives that they may have been neglecting. Reengagement in pleasant activities not only allows children to break the avoidance cycle, it also builds or rebuilds positive experiences and self-efficacy in their abilities by focusing on what they *can* do instead of what they cannot. Finally, relaxation strategies disengage children from the activation cycle (due to symptoms or emotions or both) and lets their bodies rediscover balance and the rest state, which is an essential part of treatment for somatic symptoms. Training on the three major relaxation techniques specifically geared to somatic symptoms is provided, as well as comment on the adjunctive role of biofeedback.

Throughout this level of intervention, ensure that children are blending their newfound emotional understanding and behavioral tools to understand how relaxation and distraction are helpful in terms of managing physical symptoms *and* emotional distress, while improving their identification of when these tools will come in handy. The chapter concludes by reviewing the role of the family in terms of motivational techniques for parents to support their children's engagement in these new skills as they work toward breaking the cycle of symptoms and disability.

EMOTIONAL IDENTIFICATION

Before the introduction of behavioral strategies, teach children the connection between their emotions and how their body feels physically. This is crucial for children with somatic symptoms, as they often struggle to understand their feelings from an emotional standpoint because they are more focused on the physical sensations associated with these feelings. A better understanding of emotions and situations in which they arise enables children to continue building the mind–body connection. The first step in this process is identifying the emotional feelings and understanding the associated body responses. A side benefit of teaching children emotion identification early in coping skills training is that it provides a nonthreatening way of finding out if there are any areas of emotional distress the child has not yet expressed.

Our favorite way of teaching emotion identification is through the use of the "Feelings Identification" worksheet (in the Appendix), or you could accomplish the same idea on a white board on which you have drawn six squares. Ask children to pick six different feelings, putting one in each box (drawing the face or writing the word or both), making sure they have a good variety of both positive and negative emotions. For younger children, you can use feelings flash cards to give them ideas of different feelings, and for older children and adolescents you could use posters or Internet searches to give them ideas. Make sure that a few strong emotions, such as scared, mad, or excited, end up on the worksheet, as that sets you up to talk about the physical connection of "activation" to different emotions. Coach children to include one "good" feeling, such as calm, relaxed, or happy, so you can illustrate that the opposite of activation is relaxation.

Once children identify six emotions or feeling words, the next step is to have them think of two or three situations that might cause them to have each different feeling, and write a brief description of each in the corresponding boxes. Some children notice patterns right away through this process, such as realizing that the same situations cause them to feel mad and sad, or that it is easy to come up with situations where they are nervous or worried but they have a hard time thinking about what will make them feel happy or calm. Notice these patterns as they arise, as those are areas to target for homework and further intervention.

The last step is to ask children how their body feels with each different emotion, and add those physical sensations in the boxes, too. Some children do this well, and others are stumped, having never noticed the signals their body gives them. If they are struggling, make observations to guide them along, such as noticing that every time "worry" or "excited" shows up there is a funny feeling in the stomach. Here is an example of how we engage in this activity with our patient with conversion disorder, Alex, after he has identified his emotions and is connecting them to his physical feelings:

DOCTOR: Nice work identifying these six emotions and when you feel them. Let's look at "mad," and the situations of "when I do not get the grade I want," "when I get in trouble," and "when my brother takes my stuff." How does your body feel when you are mad?

ALEX: Just angry.

DOCTOR: That's the emotion that you are feeling. Let's connect those emotions to the physical sensations, or body responses, which is what happens when your gas pedal goes down and your body is racing. What are your body responses when you are mad?

ALEX: Maybe that I kind of want to punch something, like my muscles feeling tight.

DOCTOR: Good observation! So we can put "muscle tension in hands" in that box. What else? Sometimes kids notice they get sweaty or their stomach feels funny.

ALEX: Yeah, my hands do get a little sweaty now that you mention it.

DOCTOR: Let's write that in the box, too. Now, let's look at "worried." That happens "when I have a big test," "when I have a track meet," and "when my parents are running late." What is your body response for worried?

ALEX: I feel shaky, a little like I want to tap my feet. I also feel like I might throw up.

DOCTOR: We'll add those to the worried box. For excited you said, "when it is my birthday," "when we go to the fair," and "when I win." How does your body feel when excited?"

ALEX: I feel like I can't sit still! And sometimes I get butterflies in my stomach.

DOCTOR: Interesting, let's write that down, too. Do you see how worried and excited have similar body responses? Do you know why that is?

ALEX: No, that's weird. They're opposite feelings.

DOCTOR: They *are* opposite feelings, but our body only has *one* response when it needs to get ready for something: hitting the gas pedal. Below the neck, your body just knows that something is happening—it is up to your brain to decide if it is good or bad. The connection between our mind and body helps us figure out body responses, when they are signaling something helpful and good or when they are alerting us to trouble. When we understand the situations and emotions that lead to body responses, we can figure out how to change the pattern. Did you notice that some of the emotions and situations that you wrote down on your list give you the same physical sensations that your body feels when you are having conversion symptoms?

ALEX: Hmm, yeah, I guess there are some of the same things on here. Like this box for "worried" when I'm at a track meet and I get that funny feeling in my legs.

DOCTOR: Excellent job, Alex. You made a great connection there. The reason we are doing this activity is to understand that the mind and body are connected—so your body responses are affecting your feelings and vice versa. This is an important connection to make; we are working together to help your legs feel better, and now we can also work on making your worries better, since that leads to the same body responses. You can use coping tools *both* for how your body is feeling and how your mind is feeling, too.

ALEX: OK, that sounds good.

DOCTOR: For your homework, keep track of the feelings you notice in different situations. Here is a blank worksheet with six empty boxes, like the one we just did. Keep track of at least one feeling that you have each day, writing down the situations and body responses. Bring it back next time!

For the next part of the emotion identification session, recall the cognitive triad from Chapter 1 that illustrated the interrelationships between thoughts, feelings, and actions that provides the foundation for CBT. We are now going to add "body responses" to this model, as this is pertinent to children with somatic symptoms. Shape wise, think of this as moving from a triangle to a diamond, which is illustrated in a diagram we call "The Roadmap" (in the Appendix). As discussed earlier, launching into a conversation about the role that emotions play in symptoms can be tricky; children are just getting used to the idea that their symptoms might be related to their level of arousal or stress. However, this is more easily done after teaching emotional identification and relating back to the connection of how the body feels in those different emotion states. Then, we can focus on what we can do to change those emotions and physical sensations, which "The Roadmap" allows us to do. Following is a dialogue with Johnny illustrating how to introduce this concept to children:

DOCTOR: Now that you understand the connection between feelings and body responses, let's take a look at this diagram called "The Roadmap" to see how all of these concepts are connected. Just like houses in a neighborhood or cities in a state, each of these places are connected to each other by these lines that are like roads on a map. Each one has a different word—thoughts, feelings, actions, and body responses—and they are all connected together by roads. You can travel in different directions; sometimes your thoughts change feelings, or your feelings change body responses. They're all connected, so, if you feel happy, you tend to have positive thoughts, your body feels pretty good, you are active in whatever you are doing, and that makes you continue to feel happy. This goes around and around like a racetrack, and it is a fun ride. The same thing happens if you something is bothering you, and it doesn't seem fun anymore, but it is hard to exit! Can you think of anything that makes you feel unhappy that would be a good example of this connection?

JOHNNY: Oh, I get really mad when I lose at a video game.

DOCTOR: Good example! So, when people feel mad, they usually have thoughts that are focused on the not-so-good parts of the situation, their bodies feel more tension, and they want to give up. It is like their gas pedal is stuck and they are racing past the exit they want, but they cannot get off the track. Does that happen when you lose at a video game?

JOHNNY: It does! That definitely happens to me. I get so mad I stop playing. Then usually I go back later and sometimes I can beat the level.

DOCTOR: What do you do in that time between when you quit and when you come back?

JOHNNY: I go outside, or play with something else, or do my homework, or have a snack.

DOCTOR: So it sounds like you take the action exit, which gets you off the track of feeling mad, and then because you *do* something else, you *think* about something else, and your *body feels* more relaxed. It is like you are able to slow down long enough to drive your car where you wanted it to go. Then, your feelings change and you can be successful at the game.

JOHNNY: Well, I never thought about like that, but I guess that's what happens.

DOCTOR: Remember, you cannot just change feelings by snapping your fingers and wishing to be happy. Maybe you have tried that! If after you lost, I said, "Alex, just stop feeling so mad, it's just a game!" how would you feel? Would that work?

JOHNNY: Oh my mom says that to me all the time and it just makes me madder.

DOCTOR: Just *saying* you are going to change a feeling doesn't work. If you use this Roadmap as your guide, you can change what you are doing, relax your body, or change your thinking, and because all of the points are connected, your feelings change too. This is what we are going to work on in our upcoming sessions.

Now children are ready for the next set of strategies that direct attention away from symptoms and toward activities they enjoy, and that teach them how to relax their bodies. As you progress through the behavioral strategies, refer back to the educational framework as needed to remind children that the strategies they are learning benefit the nervous system because they "retrain the brain" to attend to other signals, restore autonomic function, and balance the degree to which symptoms receive the spotlight. If children struggle with a behavioral strategy or have trouble making sense of why those strategies are important to learn or practice, that is a good time to refer back to the education concepts presented in Chapters 3 and 5.

DISTRACTION AND PLEASANT ACTIVITIES

The importance of distraction and engagement in pleasant activities as part of typical child development is undeniable, and becomes even more so when working with children who have been struggling with physical or emotional problems. From a mental health perspective, behavioral activation improves depression because it gets people's feet moving, which increases social interaction, releases endorphins, and disengages the mind from a cycle of negative thinking. This concept is no different for children with somatic symptoms. Children have gotten so far away from their usual activities that they are either missing out on them completely, or not able to engage in them as much as they would like. Simply doing something fun has psychosocial benefits, as children's mood and social interaction improves when they normalize activity patterns. Training in distraction through engagement in pleasant activities is the primary way in which we introduce this coping tool. Distracting and pleasant activities work well in children's daily functional schedules when done after "must-do" activities like schoolwork or chores to serve as a motivator/reward.

Distraction can be divided into two parts; active and passive. Active requires more purposeful engagement and can be thought of as something a child *does* (e.g., playing a game with someone, playing music or singing, doing crafts), whereas passive is less purposeful and can be thought of as something a child *receives* (e.g., watching a movie, listening to music). Personality type and preference for activity play a role as well, and children can typically tell you what distractions they find the most fun and engaging. Finally, keep in mind that neurological processing factors, such as attention, factor into the efficacy of this strategy; those who are more "natural" pain or symptom attenders may have a harder time disengaging themselves from the signal. In general, we recommend having a mix of activities for children to choose from so that they have a variety of distractions from which to choose depending on the situation.

When it comes to the reasoning behind introducing distracting activities, "something is better than nothing" also applies to taking attention off of symptoms. Building from the thoughts, feelings, body responses, and actions framework of "The Roadmap," distraction serves as an "action" children can take to change a negative series of events to a positive one. It also represents an opportunity to think about something else, which changes attention to symptoms, relieves pressure on the gas pedal of the ANS, and closes the pain gate. Even if children make a *tiny* change in what they are doing or to what they are paying attention, it introduces new information for the brain to process, different signals to attend to, and a break from whatever stressor was sending them racing down the track. We illustrate the introduction of distraction as a coping skill through a dialogue with Ashley, our patient with cardiac symptoms:

ASHLEY: Why do we have to talk about distractions? I'm really behind on schoolwork so it seems like I should focus on that right now.

DOCTOR: I understand what are you are saying, and you are correct—you do have a lot of schoolwork to complete. But how much of it is actually getting done?

ASHLEY: Well, not very much because every time I try to do homework I have a hard time focusing, get really tired and foggy, and I usually have to take a nap.

DOCTOR: Since your current system is not getting you to your goals, let me propose another idea. In your current situation, dizziness and symptoms are the only thing you are thinking about or focusing on; that takes up all of the space in your brain, and that is all you can think about, even when you are trying to do something else like homework.

ASHLEY: I can't think about anything other than feeling dizzy.

DOCTOR: Remember the "Roadmap" we looked at before that shows the connections between thoughts, feelings, body responses, and actions. Is it fair to say you feel frustrated when you feel dizzy, and that makes you feel like you do not even want to try working because it will probably make you feel worse?

ASHLEY: Yeah, but sometimes I have a good day and then I can get a lot done.

DOCTOR: OK, tell me what is different about those days.

ASHLEY: I usually have something I am looking forward to, like going to the movies with my best friend. I don't have to do a lot of moving around, and if I feel dizzy, I'm already sitting. And it is my best friend, so I don't have to pretend I'm OK if I'm not.

DOCTOR: So during the movie, the dizziness signal gets a little smaller because there are other signals to focus on. Can you tell me about the last movie you saw?

ASHLEY: Oh sure, it was one of the superhero movies. It was really good.

DOCTOR: So that tells me you were able to focus on the movie and not on feeling dizzy.

ASHLEY: Well, I was still dizzy.

DOCTOR: Yes, but you were not 100% focused on feeling dizzy; you were able to direct at least *some* of your attention to something else, which means that you had at least a *little* symptom relief in the sense that your brain was processing those signals a bit less. So even if those physical sensations were still present, the effect of distraction was that you enjoyed the activity more. That's how distraction works. It does not make your symptoms magically disappear. It is a way of shifting your focus, allowing your brain to pay attention to something different than the signal that's playing like a broken record, and giving your brain a chance to form new associations with activities that are safe and enjoyable. When you think of the movies, do you think "dizzy" or do you think "fun"?

ASHLEY: Mostly fun. I see what you are saying.

DOCTOR: Good. This is why distraction is a great daily activity. It is a way of retraining your brain *off* the symptoms and *on* to what you would like to be more focused on, either because you need to do it or you want to do it, or both. When it comes to getting schoolwork done, perhaps distraction could be a useful coping tool to use either right before or right after your school time.

As illustrated above, explain that distraction is used as a symptom management tool because it helps people pay attention to appropriate signals. Many children get stuck in the cycle of thinking they cannot do something fun or distracting due to the constancy of their symptoms. Teach children that the signal is going to be there whether they want it to or not right now; the choices are focusing on that signal, which would make symptoms worse, or having that signal *and* doing something else, which will either keep their symptoms the same or possibly make them better because they are having a fun, or least an interesting, experience as well.

The next dialogue provides a framework for helping children select personalized activities and allows for more discussion of the importance of reinstating pleasant activities into the child's life as a way of practicing distraction. As with most coping skills, some children are really good at generating ideas, and some have a harder time, so be prepared with ideas to suggest to them and refer to the "Distracting and Pleasant Activities" worksheet (in the Appendix) for a list of activities from which children can select. Remind children that no one activity is going to work perfectly all the time, and they may have to try a few different activities until they find something they like that is effective. Luckily, the Internet is also filled with ideas, and just looking up distractions is a distraction in and of itself! Finally, introducing distraction and pleasant activities is a great way for children to continue improving their function by choosing something they have not been able to do in a while or have avoided since having symptoms. Next, our patient Johnny comes up with a list of pleasant activities:

DOCTOR: Let's talk about the "actions" you can do from "The Roadmap" (in the Appendix) that can make your feelings and your body responses more balanced. This one is all about having fun.

JOHNNY: Yeah! There are a lot of things I like to do for fun.

DOCTOR: Why do you think we would use having fun as a coping tool?

JOHNNY: Well, I guess that having fun gets my mind off of pain?

DOCTOR: Yes—remember how that would work in terms of the pain gate?

JOHNNY: Having fun would close it?

DOCTOR: Yes! Having some fun, both on a regular basis *and* as a coping tool, gets your mind off of pain signals and trains your brain to think about something else—like what?

JOHNNY: Well, I like to watch TV, play video games, go outside, ride my bike, see friends.

DOCTOR: Those are all fun distractions! I have a list of activities that includes some of those ideas as well as some others. Let's check off everything that you can think of doing. I want you to challenge yourself to find something you enjoy but haven't been able to do.

JOHNNY: Oh there are lots of fun ideas on here, like learn a new joke, do a magic trick, cook, watch a movie ... go to a restaurant is something I like to do but haven't done lately, since I might get a stomachache if I eat out.

DOCTOR: All of those are good ideas, including eating out at a restaurant to get your body used to doing more of what you like to do. Along with your everyday healthy habits, do at least one thing off this list every day, which we can even include on your schedule. This list is your first official coping tool for something to *do* when you are having symptoms—the goal is to do something, *anything*, when you have symptoms.

RELAXATION

Relaxation is a cornerstone of the behavioral strategies that improve children's control of their bodies and their physical experience of somatic symptoms as well.

Biologically, relaxation both closes the pain gate and puts on the brakes by activating the parasympathetic nervous system. Psychologically, it decreases distress and improves children's perception that there is something they can do to turn symptoms around, which improves self-efficacy and can promote more positive coping actions. There are three main ways to teach relaxation: diaphragmatic breathing, progressive muscle relaxation, and imagery. For each of these relaxation skills, we have included a corresponding worksheet of the same name (in the Appendix) to use in treatment and for the child to take home to support their individual practice. While it is beyond the scope of this book to cover mindfulness techniques (which are a treatment all their own), we have included a "Mindfulness and the Five Senses" worksheet (in Appendix) to offer another form of relaxation that is helpful during acute symptom flares. This section covers how to tailor relaxation strategies specifically for children with somatic symptoms. When introducing these techniques to children, make sure they know that this is not what they might *imagine* relaxation to be like (i.e., just lying down on the couch or bed), but instead is a very purposeful, active, focused effort to get their bodies to quiet down, close the pain gate, and regain a more effective balance of their ANS by manually pushing on the brakes.

The role of relaxation in treatment for somatic symptoms is twofold. First, we are training children to engage in *regular periods* of relaxation during the day to break the cycle of symptom activation and allow their bodies to slow down and rest. Think of this as a *proactive* approach to relaxation, rather than a reactive one. Second, we train children to use these relaxation techniques as a strategy to manage symptoms or emotional distress in the moment to combat the activating response to physical symptoms or fear/anxiety. The key is that they must use *both* types of relaxation practice to be successful. Children have a tendency to save their techniques *only* for when symptoms or distress are high, adopting a reactive rather than proactive approach; without their bodies knowing how to engage in these techniques from routine practice, the strategy simply will not be effective for them in those difficult situations. Children will erroneously conclude that relaxation "doesn't work for me." The research on relaxation training in children with somatic symptoms has mostly focused on functional pain disorders (e.g., abdominal pain) and has found that practice over time improves physiological markers that were poor at baseline, such as heart rate variability, suggesting that one of the mechanisms for improved symptoms is improvement of ANS function (Sowder, Gevirtz, Shapiro, & Ebert, 2010). For older children and adolescents, we share this information about how these strategies can make a lasting physical change to build their confidence that investing in this practice will be worthwhile.

In addition to sharing the rationale for relaxation practice and information about its benefits, draw the analogy that learning relaxation strategies is like learning any new skill, such as playing a musical instrument or playing a sport. If a child knows the rules of playing soccer already, they may go to a soccer clinic to learn a particular move, which will be difficult at first but with practice becomes easier. After some time, the new skill will be so integrated into the way they play the game that they will hardly even need to think about it. The process of learning relaxation skills is similar: children should be able to use these skills without thinking too much about it, so that this response becomes naturally integrated into their daily life. With this approach, they can regain the "automatic" part of their autonomic balance that they have lost.

And when it is time to make the game-winning goal and the pressure is on, they will have all the practice and skill to be able to perform in those acute moments, too. Compare this to what would happen if children only used their new soccer skills in the biggest tournament of the year when it was up to them to score the game-winning shot. Children understand pretty easily that it will not go well for them in that circumstance, because they have not practiced and therefore their bodies do not know what to do. This analogy works well to encourage children to integrate these skills into daily life. Adding one to two daily periods of relaxation to a child's schedule is recommended. Although this section focuses on breathing, active muscle relaxation, and guided imagery, we recommend that you teach children all relaxation techniques (including mindfulness and passive muscle relaxation), and allow the child to choose the strategies they like best. Sometimes children like all of the techniques and rotate between them for their daily relaxation practice, and some prefer one or two strategies over the rest and practice those on a daily basis. Introduce relaxation skills within the ANS and/or pain gate education framework and reinforce the importance of practice when introducing each skill. Review the ANS or pain gate description in Chapter 3 as needed to personalize it for the children with whom you are working. In the following dialogue, relaxation is introduced to Alex, our case example patient with conversion disorder, using the "Learning to Drive the 'AUTO'nomic Nervous System" worksheet (in the Appendix):

DOCTOR: Today we are going to learn strategies to relax your body. First, let's talk about why we do that to understand how relaxation makes your body feel better when you are having symptoms. Remember when we learned about the ANS?

ALEX: Yeah, I think that was the thing that makes our body go fast and slow? Like a car?

DOCTOR: Yes, like a car! There are two parts to the ANS, the "fight-or-flight" response that gives us energy to act and the "rest-and-digest" response that slows us down to relax. When the fight-or-flight response turns on, it is like pushing on the gas pedal in our body ...

ALEX: And you go faster!

DOCTOR: That's right! And then when the rest-and-digest response turns on, it is like pushing on the brakes, which makes you ...

ALEX: Slow down or stop.

DOCTOR: One way our ANS does that is through our heart rate and breathing. Do you notice changes in your heart or breathing when your body is pushing on the gas or brakes?

ALEX: Yeah, before I had trouble walking, my heart used to beat really fast when I ran around outside. But at night then when I'm getting ready to go to sleep, it goes really slow.

DOCTOR: Very good! Those are just the times we would want your heart to go fast and slow. Other times, like when you have symptoms, have you ever noticed that some of the same effects are happening with the gas pedal making your heart and breathing go fast?

ALEX: I have noticed that whenever my legs are shaking my heart starts racing. I don't like it when that happens, it makes me feel worse.

DOCTOR: That makes sense—when you have symptoms, your body responds by pushing on the gas pedal because it knows something is happening, but unfortunately that makes you feel worse. A racing heart beat is a sign that your body is going too fast and it needs to slow down, but sometimes our bodies forget that we have any brakes! Relaxation makes your body slow down when it is going too fast, which makes symptoms feel better.

ALEX: Cool, I never thought about it that way.

DOCTOR: It is like learning how to drive—and you get to be in control of your own car!

ALEX: I'd like to be in control!

In addition to the connection with the ANS, link back to the pain gate for children with painful somatic symptoms to illustrate that activation opens the gate and relaxation closes it. Therefore, relaxation is helpful to both close the pain gate and engage the parasympathetic nervous system.

DIAPHRAGMATIC BREATHING

The most effective way to relax is to slow the heart rate down, and the best way to do that is through diaphragmatic breathing. Some children are already familiar with this type of breathing if they have taken a yoga class or are in the school choir. Some children will say they have already tried that breathing and it did not work, or it sounds like such a simple strategy they cannot possibly imagine that it will help them. The quick answer to give them is that breathing is the most effective way to turn on the parasympathetic nervous system, which is equivalent to "hitting the brakes" because it regulates heart rate. If children have tried this before and it has not worked, it is usually because they have only done it at a time of distress (which will not work if they have not put in the practice) or they were not doing the strategy correctly. Encourage them to try it again and to see if you can find some different ways of doing it that will be more effective for them, providing the rationale for doing it and educating them about why this strategy is beneficial.

Normal breathing (the kind we do not think about) is disrupted by stress and pain, which results in a faster baseline respiration rate. Children who are in a chronic state of tension, which is the case when somatic symptoms are present, get used to this elevated breathing rate and corresponding elevated heart rate over time and begin naturally breathing more from their chests ("thoracic breathing") and less from their diaphragm ("belly breathing"). The diaphragm is a flat, dome-shaped muscle that sits under the lungs. During a deep inhale, it pushes down, allowing the lungs to fully inflate with the maximum amount of oxygen, and the heart rate accelerates to rapidly deliver the oxygenated blood to the muscles, brain, and organs. During a slow exhale, the diaphragm returns upward, the lungs expel carbon dioxide, and there is a corresponding decrease in heart rate. When you think about breathing this way, it makes sense that if you are not using diaphragmatic breathing, your lungs cannot take in the maximum amount of oxygen to efficiently circulate oxygenated blood, and your heart might have to work extra hard to do its job well. Teaching children to engage in deep breathing as a regular practice improves respiratory and cardiovascular function, as well as achieves greater autonomic balance.

In addition to regular practice, diaphragmatic breathing is useful in acute situations of symptoms or distress. An example of this is the efficacy of deep breathing when children are undergoing medical procedures (e.g., getting a shot); the heart stays calm, muscles stay relaxed, and the shot hurts less. It is also useful under conditions of stress or worry, such as a big test at school or a music recital; taking a deep breath calms the body by sending physiological relaxation signals, which allows for better focus and calms shaky muscles and sweaty hands. One of our patients actually used deep breathing as a way to calm down after her family was in a car accident and credited the technique with keeping her from panicking at the scene. Relating these physiological benefits to children provides an additional reason for them to practice and improves buy-in to this skill.

If you are not familiar with how diaphragmatic breathing looks and feels, practice it yourself before teaching it so you can demonstrate the different types of breathing during the session yourself alongside the child, referring to the "Diaphragmatic Breathing" worksheet (in the Appendix). When teaching younger children how to breathe, it is helpful to have them lie down and put a stuffed animal or action figure on their stomach, between their belly button and the bottom of their rib cage, where the diaphragm is located, and use this as a visual cue for them to inhale as they watch the toy rise up, and exhale to watch the toy come back down. Using this process allows them to learn to engage their diaphragm and abdominal muscles rather than their chest. Deep breathing can also be described by imagining that you are filling up a balloon in your stomach with each breath in, and then deflating the balloon as you breathe out. Blowing bubbles or blowing a pinwheel during the exhale is a successful way to aid in children's practice, as both require slow controlled inhales and exhales for big bubbles and long pinwheel twirls. It is helpful to keep bubbles and pinwheels in the office for these occasions and send children home with small bubble bottles for practice. For older children or teens, encourage them to sit up comfortably and put their hands loosely on their stomach to feel the action of the diaphragm. You can use the example of blowing out birthday candles as a good way to remind them of the importance of taking a big breath in and making a slow exhale. Here, we instruct Ashley, our patient with cardiac symptoms, on diaphragmatic breathing:

DOCTOR: The first way we are going to learn how to relax our bodies is through breathing. The reason we learn this one first is because we have to breathe anyway, so you always have the ability to change your breathing no matter where you are. The key is to learn how to take a slow and deep breath, which we call a diaphragmatic breath or a belly breath. The reason we call it this is because you use your diaphragm muscle, which sits at the bottom of your lungs. It acts like a pump to draw air into the lungs and then pushes it out again. To find it, put your hand at the base of your rib cage, right between the bottom of your ribs and your belly button.

ASHLEY: Here?

DOCTOR: Yes, there in the center of your torso. To make sure you have the right spot, a way you can find your diaphragm muscle is to sniff in through your nose quickly, like you have a cold (*have the child sniff quickly several times and see/feel a corresponding quick movement in the diaphragm muscle*).

ASHLEY: (*Sniffs.*) OK, I think I felt it move.

DOCTOR: You got it. Move your hand around if you need to until you have it exactly in the right spot, so that when you sniff with your nose you feel a little push in your diaphragm. That is the spot you want to use to take a big, deep slow breath. Your breathing and heartbeat are connected, so when your breathing goes slower, your heart goes slower too, which will push on your brakes and let you relax. Just like a car, our bodies do not like to step on the gas and the brakes at the same time, so enacting the relaxation response necessarily means that your body will lay off the gas. We use breathing to make our hearts beat slower, which turns on the brakes, which improves your body's response to distress and symptoms.

ASHLEY: OK, I get it now.

DOCTOR: Let's take a few practice breaths. With your hand on your diaphragm, take a slow, deep breath in, feeling your stomach push out against your hand, hold it there for a second or two, and then slowly let that breath out again, feeling your hand fall back in toward your stomach. It is like filling up a balloon with air as you breathe in, and letting it deflate as you breathe out. Good, let's do it again. Nice slow breath in, noticing your hand move away from stomach, filling up your lungs with air like a balloon, and now letting all the air out, watching your hand go back in and your stomach lying flat again. Great job. How did that feel?

ASHLEY: It felt good. But it made me a little bit dizzier than usual.

DOCTOR: I am glad you told me that! Sometimes when people learn how to breathe deeply, they take in too much air or let out too much air, and it disrupts the balance of carbon dioxide and oxygen in your body, and the result is feeling a little dizzy. It is not dangerous, but it might not make you relaxed. Let's try it again, and this time take in a slow breath, but not so much air that you feel like your lungs are bursting. Just enough so that you feel comfortably full, hold your breath for a second, and then let it slowly out. The idea is that you want to breathe in just as slowly, but not take in as much air, so just add a little pause to your breathing pattern. Ready?

ASHLEY: Yes.

DOCTOR: Great. Go ahead and put your hand back on your stomach and slowly breathe in, nice and slow, filling up your lungs just until you are comfortably full of air, hold, and now slowly let out. Excellent! How did it feel that time?

ASHLEY: Better. I didn't feel as light-headed.

DOCTOR: Good. Now let's add some counting to the practice. It turns out that there is an ideal number of seconds to breathe in and out that matches up with the most relaxed heartbeat that humans can have. How long do you think that is?

ASHLEY: I don't know, 2 or 3 seconds?

DOCTOR: It is actually 5! Breathing in for 5 seconds and out for 5 seconds turns out to give us the most relaxed heartbeat pattern. That's only a total of six breaths a minute.

ASHLEY: Wow! That's not a lot.

DOCTOR: I know! Usually people breathe about 12 to 20 times a minute. Slowing down your breathing to six breaths a minute is nice and relaxing compared to what our bodies usually do. I will count up to five and you slowly breathe in. Remember to only breathe in as much air as is comfortable, so that might mean you stop taking in air when I reach 3 or 4 seconds and then just hold it until I say breathe out. Ready?

ASHLEY: Yes.

DOCTOR: OK, get ready, and breathe in for 1, 2, 3, 4, 5, and out, 2, 3, 4, 5. And in, 2, 3, 4, 5, and out 2, 3, 4, 5. One more in, 2, 3, 4 holding, and out 2, 3, 4, 5. Very nice job. How does your body feel now?

ASHLEY: Relaxed, I guess.

DOCTOR: You look relaxed! What do you notice feels relaxed?

ASHLEY: My heart is beating slower and my muscles feel relaxed. And I feel tired.

DOCTOR: That's great. When you push on the brakes in your body, it is like preparing your body for sleep, so yawning is a great sign that your brakes are working! No one yawns when they are activated. Let's talk about when you can use breathing.

ASHLEY: When I'm going to sleep at night.

DOCTOR: Absolutely. It is a great strategy to use at night when you are slowing your body down to sleep. It is actually an ideal time to practice because you are already getting relaxed, and you want to try it at a time that's easy for your body to learn. I recommend practicing 5 or 10 minutes every night when you are going to bed. When is another time you could use this breathing?

ASHLEY: When I am stressed or having symptoms.

DOCTOR: Absolutely. It might be a bit harder than when you are going to bed, because your body is not relaxed already and you might have some other distractions, depending on the situation. It is useful to practice breathing for 2 to 5 minutes during those times of distress, and you can even combine it with another strategy like distraction. Practice at *both* of these times, when you are relaxed already at night *and* when you are having some difficulties. If you just save it for the hardest times, your body will not be familiar with the skill and it will be less likely to work. You can also relax your body throughout the day by taking just one deep breath at different times, such as every time you sit down, before meals, or whenever you feel that your body needs a little tap on the brakes.

There are several ways we encourage children to practice breathing at home. Simply setting aside a regular time on their schedule and engaging in slow breathing by counting works, as well as listening to a favorite slow piece of music, or looking at a timer counting seconds. There are a number of free apps that are available on phones and tablets that regulate breathing and have either a visual cue (e.g., lungs inflating and deflating) as well as an audio cue (e.g., a high tone indicating inhale and a low tone indicating exhale). Many allow for adjustment of time of practice and length of time for inhale and exhale; the recommended setting is six breaths per minute, which is 5 seconds in and 5 seconds out. Children can also use it to track their progress, which you can review in session for homework. Reminders can even be set to notify children of when they need to practice.

PROGRESSIVE MUSCLE RELAXATION

If a person's body is in pain, has physically distressing symptoms, or is under any kind of stress, the natural response is to tighten the muscles in accordance with sympathetic activation. Over time, that leads to a lot of muscle tension, which children end up getting used to as part of their chronic symptom experience. Many children with somatic symptoms say, "I am not tense, I don't know what you are talking about," and benefit from signs of tension being pointed out, such as tightened shoulders that are closer to their ears than they should be, jittery feet, or clenched hands or jaws. Often, children are either so used to this that it just does not register as tension, or their body awareness is so poor that they have not noticed. One patient that we have worked with had a panic episode in session and was startled and confused to find her hands shaking; she was so focused on the emotional experience that she had not noticed what was happening in her body at the same time. When children recognize these physical representations of tension, it improves their body awareness. Children with somatic symptoms tend to avoid thinking about their body because it does not feel good; learning to relieve tension gives them a positive experience with their body, which is something they are not used to having.

Progressive muscle relaxation (PMR) is a technique to increase awareness of the areas of the body that feel tense and provide a way to relieve that feeling; it is like learning how to give yourself a massage! It is called "progressive" because it moves through all the muscle groups in the body, starting in the feet and then working up to the head, having children tense and then release each muscle group, noticing how the muscle feels when tightened and then switching the focus to how it feels when released and relaxed. As with many of these strategies, it is best for children to practice and become familiar with it before the skill is needed in an acute moment. As with diaphragmatic breathing, PMR can be practiced at bedtime, or placed at another convenient time on the child's daily schedule. Again, if this is not something with which you are already familiar, practice first so you can teach and describe it effectively. Both active (tensing and releasing) and passive (imagining tension release) PMR scripts are included in the Appendix; these can be read to children and recorded or given to them as a guide to use at home. The dialogue below with our patient Alex, who has conversion disorder, illustrates the descriptions and questions that may arise during teaching of active PMR:

DOCTOR: We are going to talk about a new strategy called progressive muscle relaxation, which is a way to tense and release all the muscles in your body. After practicing, you will get better at figuring out when your muscles are tight and how to make them loose and relaxed. Can you think of any reasons why a strategy like this would be helpful?

ALEX: Well, you have been talking a lot about how muscles are tight when your gas pedal is down and it doesn't make my legs feel better, so I guess if I can figure out when they are tight I'll be able to slow my body down by relaxing them?

DOCTOR: That's the idea. Let's get some good feelings going on in your muscles that have been bothering you so much. Let's start with a pretty easy one. Have you ever made lemonade before?

ALEX: Sure, we make it with a mix at home.

DOCTOR: Well, we are going to pretend we are making lemonade the old-fashioned way with real lemons. Imagine you have a lemon in each hand, make a fist, and now squeeze all the juice out by making a tight fist, as hard as you can. That's it, keep squeezing, and get your arm muscles involved, we have a lot of lemonade to make! OK, now relax your arms and let your hands be loose, shake out your fingers.

ALEX: Wow, that kind of hurt! I was holding my hands really tight. But now my hands feel kind of warm and tingly.

DOCTOR: Holding our muscles really tight lets us know what muscle tension feels like, and then when we relax the muscle we pay attention to what it feels like when they loosen. That loose, relaxed feeling is what we want to focus on. Let's try another one—this time, get your muscles to the point where they are tight but not to the point that they are hurting you. I call this one stretching like a cat. Lift your arms as high as you can above your head. Stretch each one a little higher, spread your "claws" out—Good! Now hold it for 1 more second really high, and now release and let your arms slowly come down and rest back on the arms of the chair. What did you notice?

ALEX: Oh, it feels like kind of flowy into my arms and in my back. It feels really nice to relax my arms and shoulders after they were so tight.

DOCTOR: That's great. Now let's try this out in your legs, as that's a spot where we really want you to feel more relaxed. Slowly lift up your legs and hold them straight out in front of you.

ALEX: I'll push my chair back a little.

DOCTOR: OK, slowly breathe in while you lift those legs up, make them straight in front of you, pulling your toes toward you to feel the stretch in your calves and using your quad muscles in the top of your thighs to lift your legs up even higher, hold that inhale and notice the tension that is building in all of those muscles— now, slowly exhale and let those legs go back down to the ground, notice the muscles slowly release and feel the sense of relaxation going through your legs from the toes up to your waist.

ALEX: I think my heart is beating slower and my legs feel, they feel good, actually!

DOCTOR: Great work! It is nice to slow down our breathing at the same time we are relaxing our muscles. Now we are going to practice a few more areas.

This is an excellent strategy for children to practice at night before bed, as we mentioned, and when they are sitting at their desks for a long time at school or after coming home from a high-energy activity, such as sports. It is great if they can match their deep breathing practice, breathing in when they tighten, and breathing out when they release; that way, they can practice two relaxation techniques at once. Children can follow along with the script provided in the Appendix. There are also several good videos and audio tracks available online that offer guided practice, or you can make an audio recording of yourself reading through the script on the child's phone or a CD/MP3 track that the child can listen to in order to facilitate practice as well.

IMAGERY

The third and final relaxation technique that is beneficial to children with somatic symptoms is imagery, which is the practice of conjuring up a peaceful, calming image in the mind either individually or as led by someone else (guided). Imagery is a useful strategy because it serves as *both* a distraction and a relaxation, taking away attention to the signal while producing physiologically beneficial effects in the body. Something we like to share with children as we introduce this strategy is that while this relaxation doesn't directly ask their bodies to slow down breathing/heart rate or reduce muscle tension, which the other two strategies target directly, the body shows those positive physical benefits anyway. This is a great example of the power of the brain to relax the body simply by thinking peacefully. Similar to the other relaxation techniques, thinking about a positive image is beneficial in terms of providing distraction, hitting the brakes on the ANS, as well as closing the pain gate.

Regarding content of the image, the only real "rules" are that it has to be pleasant, relaxing, comforting, or restorative. It can be something real that children have previously experienced (e.g., a past vacation) or something entirely imaginary (e.g., flying), or a combination of both (e.g., flying over their past vacation destination). Reinforce the notion that children are totally in charge of this experience, and the goal is that it is something they can do for themselves to feel good. A neat, specific application of imagery for use by children with somatic symptoms is to have them purposefully either choose to remember a time or imagine a future time in which they are functioning without symptoms, perhaps doing something they love to do that is difficult for them now with ease and confidence in the future. Children also enjoy creating images that relieve symptoms, such as imagining swimming in a pool filled with a special liquid that takes all negative sensations away or a magic wand that they wave over themselves to alleviate symptoms. It is easy to carry this idea over to distress relief as well; for a child worried about an upcoming test, we might suggest an image of the child sitting at his or her desk in that class, doing well on the test and knowing the answers.

The other guideline is for children to use all of their senses while picturing their scene. Typically, children enjoy beginning with the sense of sight and can easily picture everything they would see in their scene. In order to make the image more realistic and engaging, and therefore more effective for distraction and relaxation, ask the child to expand on that sense to incorporate what he or she would also hear, taste, smell, and feel. Again, remind children that all of these additional details should also be pleasant; for example, if they choose to go to the beach, they can choose for the temperature of the sand to be just right and no pesky seagulls to be squawking. End on the sense of feeling, and not just in terms of imagining what they would or did feel in their image, but also how they feel in their body *right now*. Help them carry over the sense of relaxation they have created from imagining their scene into their bodies to feel that way in the moment.

Of all the relaxation strategies, this one is a favorite; children are natural imagery users. They do this all the time. It is fun to hear the scenes they come up with—some of our favorites include Candyland (complete with lollipop trees!), inside a cookie jar (why not?), and orbiting Saturn in a high-tech spaceship. It also provides a nice opportunity to put children in charge—they are the only ones who can choose the most relaxing image for themselves, after all—and you can reinforce their independent efforts by telling them, "You know just what to do to help your body and mind feel good." We have included an imagery handout in the Appendix that children can use to create both pleasant and restorative images. There are also many videos and audio tracks available online that children can explore if they prefer a guided experience. In session, depending on how much time you have and how important it is for the child you are working with, you can either just describe the technique as we have done here and have the child practice it at home, or you could fully immerse the child in a guided imagery experience in session that you could record and send the child home with to practice. Either way, ensure that the child picks a time to practice this skill each day routinely.

BIOFEEDBACK

Biofeedback is a therapeutic modality that goes hand-in-hand with CBT. While a full description or training of biofeedback techniques is beyond the scope of this book, biofeedback can be a valuable way of engaging children in relaxation training, and it is particularly beneficial for children with somatic symptoms who benefit from increased awareness of their bodies that biofeedback shows them. When describing biofeedback to children, break it down into two parts, because the word sounds technical or medical and we want to reduce fear and increase understanding. We say that the "bio" stands for biology, or physical sensations, and the "feedback" stands for information. In those terms, biofeedback is simply a tool we use to teach children about their body by looking at information from their own physical sensations. Biofeedback can be very low tech; having children simply make a fist with their hands to check their skin temperature and sweatiness or manually check their heart rate are both ways to get information about how their body is reacting in any given situation is biofeedback. Biofeedback can be very high tech, especially now that there are widely available computer programs with associated hardware that can detect a variety of physical sensations, display them on a computer screen, and teach children about how to change their body responses through interactive games.

Biofeedback is useful in practice as an adjunctive way to train relaxation for two reasons. One, it gives children objective feedback on how activation and relaxation work in their bodies while giving visual and physical reinforcement of relaxation training. It makes the mental health provider's job easier when they do not have to convince children that their bodies calm down as they relax; they can see it with their own eyes! And two, children get really excited about the prospect of using a fun computer game to learn coping strategies, which improves buy-in to treatment. Biofeedback is recommended to be used as part of treatment, but not as somatic symptom treatment alone; CBT is still the most effective treatment modality and biofeedback is a part of that. If you are interested in becoming more familiar with these techniques, we recommend consulting the Biofeedback Certification International Alliance, which is the professional certification body for the clinical practice of biofeedback recognized across the globe.

TREATMENT PROGRESS

At this point in treatment, children have learned a number of strategies to cope with somatic symptoms and improve function, including healthy habits, daily scheduling, emotion identification, distraction, and relaxation, which are all coping tools that children should now be using for managing symptoms and building up their coping repertoire. Use the "Coping Skills Toolkit" (in the Appendix) to summarize and personalize children's favorite coping tools, which can be used and added to throughout treatment. For most children, progress up to this point represents an increase in function (e.g., improved participation in school, daily activities, restoration of daily schedule). That is great—they are on track and ready to engage in the next and last level of treatment, cognitive strategies, during which the stage will be set for children to maintain these gains into the future. Other children may not have yet achieved a significant functional gain. That is OK—continue to the next level while problem solving any barriers keeping them from engaging in the skills they are learning. Also, keep an eye out for systemic issues affecting the child, including family factors, school factors, or ongoing medical concerns. Family, parental, and school factors are addressed specifically in the last section of the book, but if a child's progress in treatment is stymied by any one of these factors, it may be beneficial to look ahead to those chapters now to incorporate those aspects of treatment before moving on to level three intervention.

THE FAMILY'S ROLE

Include parents in the emotional identification and behavioral intervention sessions at the end of each of those sessions so that they can see the progress the child is making and help make system-level changes that enable the child to engage in his or her newfound coping skills outside of session. When teaching the behavioral strategies in particular, this is a good time to be aware of the role of reinforcement the family provides for the child's behavior, which can be a very positive influence in terms of providing motivation for increased function and use of coping skills, or an unintentionally negative one, so that the child is accidentally reinforced for illness behavior that may perpetuate a cycle of symptoms and disability; reinforcement cycles are addressed further in Chapter 9. The goal for parents at this level of intervention is to help children get motivated to engage in their coping skills and reinforce their positive function, while addressing any family patterns that are keeping them stuck.

To help families break out of a cycle of symptoms and disability and return to more normative patterns of positive reinforcement, instruct parents to start by simply "catching them being good." Encourage parents to notice and reinforce even basic behaviors and actions that their children are doing positively, such as helping to set the dinner table or interacting nicely with a sibling, with a simple "I am proud of you" or "Great work" or "Thank you." This is also a good time to encourage parents to reinforce the coping skills children are learning in the same way. Parents also can help with adherence and motivation to practice new coping skills by creating a reward chart with their child; this is a concrete way for the child to get more attention for behaviors associated with function than for behaviors associated with somatic symptoms. Parents and children can do this as a way to engage together about treatment and check in about the positive use of coping skills.

Overall, the message to families is that ultimately, through whatever factors are motivating to children, they should encourage children to try these strategies out. Not attempting something new means not actually getting better, and if children do not at least try these strategies, they do not get back to function or effectively manage symptoms. Children (and adults) are sometimes inclined to approach something new with avoidance, because they want to prevent something bad from happening from a new approach or that while negative, the old pattern is at least familiar. A way to help children and families buy in to the need to at least try these new skills is to remind them that something bad is *already* happening; what have they got to lose by trying out something different? The worst that could happen is that the bad thing still happens, but the best thing that could happen is that their body is given a new opportunity to feel different or even better.

If children are reluctant to try something new, have parents challenge the symptom with behavioral experiments, not arguments (i.e., "let's try it and see what happens). Remind children that when we are doing something new, we are telling our body that although symptoms feel bad or uncomfortable, they are not dangerous, and the way our body learns that is by actually doing the new thing until we realize it is safe. When children stop responding to symptoms with avoidance, the signals become quieter and quieter, and repeated exposure over time leads to habituation. It is helpful to have the parent in the room for these discussions, as parents can often be very supportive of children trying new things and it also gives parents some positive behavioral tips.

CHAPTER SUMMARY AND TAKE-AWAY POINTS

- Emotion identification helps children figure out the feelings behind their physical sensations, enabling them to make the mind–body connection and setting the stage for the next level of intervention with cognitive techniques.

- Distraction is an effective symptom management tool that decreases attention to the symptom signal, and doing so through pleasant activities reinstates normal function that improves children's mood and social interaction.

- Relaxation improves children's ability to regulate their bodies and their physical experience of somatic symptoms by turning on the parasympathetic nervous system through diaphragmatic breathing, progressive muscle relaxation, and imagery strategies. Biofeedback can be used as an adjunctive treatment to enhance relaxation training.

CHAPTER 8

Level Three: Cognitive Strategies

Now that children have learned to use healthy habits on a daily basis, identify emotions, and engage in distraction and relaxation, it is time to focus on the cognitive part of the intervention. At this point in treatment, children should be adept at identifying their emotions and can now consider the role of their thoughts to fully develop their understanding of the cognitive-behavioral process. For many children, particularly younger ones, this can be the hardest part. Our brains are really good at generating thoughts, analyzing information, and solving problems. But as good as they are at generating helpful thoughts, they are even better at unhelpful thoughts. And of course it is easy to think that because the brain is thinking it, it must be true, right? This is exactly the struggle for children with somatic symptoms—thoughts that are actually far from plausible *seem* like they are true.

Because of the relationship between thoughts, feelings, and actions, negative thoughts set children up to have negative emotions, poor coping responses, and ultimately, increases in somatic symptoms. Worse yet, many children worry about the somatic symptom experience itself, which unfortunately, through the same processes, becomes a self-fulfilling prophecy: worry about the symptoms and they will appear. A simple way to phrase the message of this chapter is: "You will learn to manage your thoughts about how you are feeling!" We will examine this relationship in detail through the course of this chapter, while focusing on how children can break out of this difficult negative thought/feeling cycle to adopt more realistic, positive thought patterns in a logical, problem-solving fashion that reaps physical benefits as well.

It is generally best for cognitive strategies to be the last set of skills learned rather than the first. Sometimes, but not all of the time, children have gotten the message they have some level of control over their symptoms or that they are causing their symptoms on purpose. To dive in with "this is how anxious thinking produces symptoms" often reinforces that notion that children are controlling this experience and can lead to distrust of the process, with yet another provider sending the message that they are making up their symptoms, or worse, insinuating that symptoms are "all in their head." However, cognitive strategies are an important part of the treatment and fit in very well at the most advanced level once children have gained back some degree of functioning. It can be hard, or threatening, for children to recognize how their cognitions relate to their symptoms, but it is an essential connection for them to understand, and one that has a big impact on their treatment. In addition to improving symptom presentation, cognitive strategies are useful in terms of maintaining progress and preventing relapse. Even if children know that thoughts are related to emotional feelings, most do not recognize at first that thoughts are also directly related to physical feelings.

Incorporating the "C" of CBT into treatment for somatic symptoms makes sense when we consider the physiological and theoretical background of CBT. Understanding the influence of cognition on emotion and behavior enables the translation of that information into interventions for children with somatic symptoms. Physiologically, consider the role that thinking plays in activating the sympathetic nervous system, and the cascade of physiological changes that occurs as a result. In other words, simply *thinking* about a potential stressor can automatically elicit a series of physical responses consistent with the fight-or-flight response *without even experiencing the actual stressor.* Even the quickest recognition of a threat will elicit feelings of anxiety and the body "stepping on the gas pedal"; as a result, symptoms increase and avoidant actions are more likely to follow. We worked with a child who feared bugs, and even the mere *mention* of looking at a picture of a firefly led to accelerated breathing, sweaty hands, and shaky muscles. In this chapter we present a number of cognitive strategies that teach children about the connection of negative thinking to physiological arousal. Once children have developed an understanding of that connection, work with them to challenge those automatic thoughts or come up with more helpful ways to think about situations to change emotions, body responses, and behavior.

There are a few additional ideas to keep in mind. Consider the developmental level of the child when working on cognitive strategies and related coping skills. For younger children it can be helpful to use visual cues when illustrating the concepts and employ a "multiple-choice" approach with a few descriptions from which to choose. From a motivational perspective, it is advantageous to let them choose *from* a number of possibilities rather than choosing *for* them, and from a cognitive perspective, the task becomes less overwhelming when you provide some choices to work from. For older children and teens, see what they like best; some are more easily engaged with worksheets and concrete exercises, while some prefer a more natural, conversational format. For children of all ages, it can be helpful to add some separation when talking about what they think. Instead of asking, "What are you thinking about?" you can ask, "What did you notice your brain thinking about?" This allows for depersonalization and provides some perspective to better teach children about these connections between their thoughts and body responses. And one really neat thing about the cognitive coping strategies that we like to remind children of is that they can use them *all the time*—they always have their brains with them! They do not require leaving the room, changing an activity, or missing class. When introducing cognitive strategies and the connection of thinking to symptoms, normalize the experience of feeling anxious or apprehensive about having symptoms. The term "anticipatory anxiety" works well for this purpose. For instance, if every time you walked into a certain room in your house you began feeling sharp pains in your stomach, you would begin to worry about walking into that room because you would know that you would soon be in pain. Communicate the message that anticipatory anxiety is *normal* from the beginning when introducing cognitive strategies, or it might accidentally sound like *all* symptoms are due to anxiety, and for whatever reason, people tend to believe anxiety is more under conscious control than other biological protection mechanisms, like pain, although both of those processes have strong biological ties. As touched on in earlier chapters, this is a good place to remind children about the biopsychosocial model, as this chapter illustrates the connection between the mind and body in a way that normalizes the connection between thoughts, feelings, and symptoms.

If you are familiar with CBT already, this level of intervention should fit into your existing framework and will be a new application of the same model, with physical symptoms swapped out for other childhood and adolescent adjustment problems. Overall, this chapter focuses on cognitive strategies including identifying automatic negative thoughts, information processing, cognitive distortions, reframing, problem solving, and goal setting. Regarding progression of cognitive skills by session, in the first session we typically begin with the first two concepts described in this chapter—identifying thoughts and information processing—and end with a homework activity that asks children to track their automatic negative thoughts. In the second session, we introduce cognitive distortions and reframing, using the examples that they tracked from their homework or examples that are generated in session. We often finish treatment and transition into a maintenance phase with goal setting and problem solving. As in previous intervention chapters, the speed with which you progress through sessions can be modified based on the needs of the child you are working with. Finally, include children's families into this aspect of treatment as well, so the whole system can learn to adopt a more balanced and realistic cognitive framework.

IDENTIFYING THOUGHTS

The first step in introducing cognitive strategies is increasing awareness of thoughts, which we begin with in this chapter. As people go about everyday life, thoughts pop into their heads; after all, the brain's purpose (in addition to keeping the body running) is to generate thoughts and solve problems. Beck et al. (1979) called these thoughts "automatic," and believed a person's reaction to negative automatic thoughts contributed to depression or negative mood. The goal of this step is to identify automatic negative thoughts, which are associated with negative mood states. But first, in the treatment of somatic symptoms, children must recognize that thoughts impact their physical experience as well as be able to distinguish between a thought and a feeling, something that can be difficult for children to do. This level of intervention teaches children to recognize negative and unhelpful thoughts or patterns of thinking that are associated with negative mood or body responses, and ultimately, trains them to change those thoughts and patterns.

This first section in this chapter covers ways to teach children about the cognitive factors that affect symptoms, including identifying the situation, the amount of concern about symptoms, the perception of how much the symptoms can be controlled, and how thoughts can affect emotional states and impairment related to symptoms. This introduction sets the stage for then teaching children how thoughts work in their brains, the types of thinking traps that result from that, and how they can take charge of their thoughts by changing them for the better. We introduce the role of thinking in coping with symptoms with the "What Affects Somatic Symptoms?" worksheet (in the Appendix), whose use is illustrated here with our patient Johnny, who has abdominal pain:

DOCTOR: Today we are going to talk about the kinds of thoughts and feelings kids have in different situations and how that affects their experience and the way they cope with their symptoms. Let's take a look at this worksheet; it describes four major experiences that affect the symptoms you feel, including what you are doing in the situation, what feelings you have, how much worry you have about your symptoms, and how much you feel you can cope with the symptoms. A few of these ideas will be familiar to you, like distraction.

JOHNNY: Yeah, that definitely is true, distraction helps me more than anything.

DOCTOR: Yes, it does! Let's take a look at the other parts. We know that if a person has pain and symptoms, they naturally feel more worried, which is like having an increase of negative emotions, which results in noticing the symptoms even more. The degree of concern you have for symptoms is also important, because if you think that what you have is really dangerous, that's also going to make your symptoms stronger because worry makes the gas pedal goes down and speeds everything up. How much you believe you can manage the symptoms is also important, because if you feel totally out of control, what happens?

JOHNNY: I feel worse. It doesn't feel good to be out of control of my own body.

DOCTOR: Exactly. But if you can learn to cope with the symptoms, that allows your body to be less affected by them. You've done nothing wrong to think those thoughts or feel those feelings; those are expected responses to symptoms. But the trouble is that none of that thinking or feeling helps you out, and in fact it makes you feel worse. Your body naturally focuses on pain, with increased worry, concern for danger, and feelings of being out of control when somatic symptoms happen. So our goal will be to change your thoughts in the opposite direction, so you can turn symptoms down or even better, turn them off. That means you will learn to think about what distracts you from symptoms, to have feelings that are calm or neutral, have an explanation for your symptoms that can reduce your worries, and remind yourself of your coping skills.

JOHNNY: OK, that sounds like a good plan.

With the rationale in place for the importance of thinking strategies, there is a natural transition to the connection between thoughts, feelings, and actions, which we continue illustrating with Johnny with the aid of the "Thinking, Feeling, and Doing" worksheet (in the Appendix):

DOCTOR: Let's talk more specifically about how thinking works. Thoughts are related to the feelings we have and the actions we do, like in our Roadmap. Let's understand that more by working through a few examples. Take a look at this child who just won a trophy. What is she thinking?

JOHNNY: She looks really happy!

DOCTOR: Yes, it seems like a good situation to be in and that smile on her face is telling us she is happy, but that is her *feeling*, not her thought. I like to say that feelings do not usually come from nowhere—they usually come from somewhere, and that place is your mind! Feelings come from the thought, message, or idea your mind is having about a particular situation. So if we look at the picture again with that definition in mind, what would you say she is thinking? What is on her mind that is making her feel so happy?

JOHNNY: Oh! That she just won and got a trophy, so she is really proud of herself.

DOCTOR: Good! So she is thinking, "I just won a trophy!" and she is feeling happy and proud as a result. Now let's do the next one. What do you think this girl is thinking?

JOHNNY: She looks really nervous! That's the feeling—so she is probably thinking, "I wonder if I should jump off this diving board."

DOCTOR: Nice work! You did a great job figuring out the difference between the thought and the feeling for that one. How is her body feeling?

JOHNNY: I'd guess butterflies in her stomach, and she probably wants to run back down the ladder.

DOCTOR: Yes! Now, those were two different kids in two different situations. Let's look at an example of two people in the *same* situation, but with very different thoughts. How do their thoughts lead to different feelings, body responses, and actions?

JOHNNY: This girl is imagining getting to the top of the mountain, so she is probably feeling excited and motivated to go hiking. The boy is imagining getting bitten by a snake, so he is feeling nervous and like he does not want to go.

DOCTOR: So two kids can be in the same situation but one is imagining fun and the other is imagining danger, and they have different thoughts and different feelings as a result. Now, let's take it one step further and imagine what they might *do* in the situation.

JOHNNY: Well, I think the girl who is excited will probably go on the hike and get to see cool stuff. But the kid who is nervous might tell his parents he does not want to go, but if they still make him he might miss out on seeing cool stuff because he's keeping an eye out for snakes.

DOCTOR: Absolutely! If these kids have equal chances to have stomachaches, which one do you think is more likely to feel bad?

JOHNNY: Oh, definitely the boy who is worrying about the rattlesnake. He probably has his gas pedal pushed all the way down, so he would not feel great at all.

DOCTOR: Yes, and it all started with the way he was *thinking*. Here is the last one. This is just one person in the situation, but he could be having two very different thoughts. How would those thoughts affect his feelings, body responses, and actions differently?

JOHNNY: Oh, he's standing on the free-throw line and the score is tied!

DOCTOR: Yes. We can't really tell whether the situation is going well or going badly, so let's see if you can come up with an example of a negative thought, then a positive one.

JOHNNY: Oh no! The whole gym is watching me make this basket; if I miss we could lose.

DOCTOR: That's a great example. And how does that thought make him feel?

JOHNNY: Nervous! Look at the scoreboard!

DOCTOR: With that thought and feeling pattern, what would happen in his body?

JOHNNY: Well, since he is nervous and thinking about losing the game, he might tense up his muscles too much or he might be shaky, and that might make him miss the basket!

DOCTOR: I agree with you—those negative thoughts and feelings make him pay attention to the threatening parts of the situation, which pushes his gas pedal down. But that thought and feeling pattern is not so helpful, because the outcome is that he doesn't make a good shot! Look at that—the thing that he was worried about might actually happen!

JOHNNY: Oh yeah! That's so weird.

DOCTOR: If he can think about the situation in a positive way, it could change his emotions and actions. What's a positive or realistic thought he might have?

JOHNNY: He could think about all the times he's made the shot no problem.

DOCTOR: Yes! And how would he feel?

JOHNNY: Well, it would make him feel better—less scared and calmer—so then he could make the shot and probably have a better chance of winning.

DOCTOR: I agree. Much better chances for winning! What we learned through these worksheets is that we can have different thoughts that are related to different feelings. Some of the thoughts might be true, like "if I miss the basket we could lose the game," but do not necessarily help us out if we focus on them too much and might lead to more chances that the bad thing will happen, since thoughts change your feelings and actions. You did a great job understanding those connections, Johnny. Just as we learned about today, our goal is to focus on coping tools that keep you distracted, calm, and prepared to handle challenges. The way to do all of that is through our thoughts, and we are going to work a lot more on understanding how thoughts work, what negative thoughts or thinking traps are, and most importantly, how we can use realistic thoughts as coping tools.

This example illustrated how to teach children the difference between thoughts and feelings, how two thoughts can lead to two different emotional and behavioral responses, and the impact it all has on physical experience. At this point, children should be able to identify the connection between thoughts and feelings, know whether thoughts are helpful or not helpful, relate the connection of thoughts, feelings, symptoms, and actions, and have at least an initial understanding of the idea that thoughts can be changed to lead them in a more positive direction. The next cognitive strategy involves information processing and the influence of one's emotional state.

INFORMATION PROCESSING

Information processing is guided by cognitive schemas that determine how we pay attention to, interpret, and remember information (Beck et al., 1979). In any situation, a stimulus gets interpreted as positive, dangerous, or irrelevant, with attentional bias toward threat-related information (Lazarus & Folkman, 1984). For example, if a person is getting ready to cross the street, that person is more likely to attend to the dangerous aspects of that action rather than the safe ones, which is a normal survival mechanism. This works well in acutely dangerous situations; however, it can backfire in situations that are difficult but not life-threatening, such as having somatic symptoms.

Recall the example from the "Thinking, Feeling, and Doing" worksheet of the child shooting the basketball for the game-winning shot; he is more likely to attend to the negative aspects of that situation, thinking he might miss the shot and lose the game, and feel the associated negative emotional and physical responses. However, it would be more productive for him to take in that information in a positive or neutral manner by thinking that he has practiced these types of shots a thousand times before and is likely to do well based on past experience, which would generate calmness and allow him to be more fluid in his actions. He will be more likely to make the shot processing information the second way rather than the first. Discussion of these skills assumes a foundation of emotion identification skills and awareness of body cues in different emotional states, as presented in Chapter 7. The following dialogue with our patient Alex illustrates the role of information processing and attentional bias in coping with somatic symptoms, using the "Information Processing" worksheet (in the Appendix):

DOCTOR: Let's talk about the role our thoughts play in managing different situations. Can you think of any situations in which you were feeling nervous about something or really did not want to do it? I can think of a few we have talked about.

ALEX: Oh, well probably the first day I went back to school! Before I went back, I spent all night thinking about whether kids would ask me where I had been or make fun of me for using a wheelchair, and if my teachers would let me use my coping plan. I had a really hard time going to sleep, and when I woke up I had a flip-floppy feeling in my stomach.

DOCTOR: Let's talk about how your brain was doing all that thinking. Our brain is like a computer. When information comes in, we analyze it and make decisions, depending on what information we paid attention to. Our brains are designed to pay more attention to danger than safety, which is something we call an "attention bias." It is like wearing glasses that change the way the world looks, or block your ability to see out of one eye. When we see something that we are even a little anxious about or are anticipating might have some negative effect on us, we are more likely to pay attention to the scary or threatening information than we are to the positive information. For example, you were thinking about whether kids would tease you because of the wheelchair, but you probably were not thinking about all of the kids who would offer to help you out.

ALEX: That's true. I just thought about the ones that would probably make fun of me.

DOCTOR: Let's look at this worksheet. Here is a child who is having a lot of different thoughts about going to school, too. There are a few examples of what he is paying attention to in these thought bubbles, and we can add a few more of your own.

ALEX: He is thinking about a test, playing sports in gym, and the other kids.

DOCTOR: Yes, and this is just neutral information coming in, but how do you imagine he is thinking about it? How would that make him feel emotionally and in his body?

ALEX: Well, he probably is thinking about all of the negative parts of school, like failing a test, or getting teased by those kids, or not getting to play soccer during gym. If he is like me, his legs probably feel wobbly or maybe his stomach hurts. He is probably feeling nervous and maybe kind of mad at his mom for making him go.

DOCTOR: I think that's a pretty good description. What else would you add to this example that you were thinking about when you went back to school that was negative?

ALEX: I was worried that I might not get to sit with my friends at lunch because I have to sit in a special spot in the lunchroom because of my wheelchair, and whether my teachers would be annoyed at me for being late to class, since it takes longer to use the elevator.

DOCTOR: Let's add "teachers" and "lunch" to the thought bubbles. Just as you noticed, both you and this kid were more likely to take in that information about school and think of the negatives first. Is there another way to think about these same aspects of school?

ALEX: I guess so. I mean, he could think that he might do OK on the test and play soccer just fine and hang out with his friends. For me, I did get to sit with my friends at lunch, and the teachers all seemed to understand that it was OK for me to be late.

DOCTOR: And if you had those thoughts, how would feelings and body responses be different?

ALEX: Better. If I thought about how all of those same parts could be good parts of school instead of bad, I would not be so nervous and my body would feel calmer, too.

DOCTOR: That's right. So what do you think we learned about how someone like you can learn to "process" a tough or new experience like going to school?

ALEX: I guess that there's more than one way to think about the information that comes into our brains. We might think about it as bad at first, but it could be OK or even good, and thinking that way makes feelings and body responses better.

This description of information processing applies to all children, not just children who come to see mental health providers or have somatic symptoms. However, part of the challenge for children with somatic symptoms is that their bodies end up being more physically sensitive to perceived threat and therefore make them more likely to negatively process information, which increases impairment. In other words, they might feel dizzier, notice their pain more, or have more disability related to motor symptoms in a potentially challenging situation as a result of bias toward the negative cognitive information. The solution is to teach children that even if they cannot directly change the threatening situation (e.g., attending school), they can modify their thinking to pay more attention to its positive aspects, which will make them better able to cope with symptoms in any situation. To help them start to work on this skill, ask them to complete the "Thought Record" worksheet (in the Appendix) which will serve two purposes; (1) increase awareness of thought patterns, and (2) provide examples of automatic negative thoughts to discuss in the next session when introducing cognitive distortions.

COGNITIVE DISTORTIONS

A key part of the cognitive processing system is cognitive schemas, "structures" that act as organizers to store meaning and experience, that affects attention, memory, and recall (Beck et al., 1979). Essentially, cognitive schemas are the lenses through which we see the world, our fundamental beliefs developed over time based on experiences, emotions, and perceptions. A child might have a schema that all dogs are scary, and upon seeing a dog will filter information about the dog through this lens and perceive the dog as threatening (paying less attention to clues that suggest otherwise). The stress response will be triggered, leading to negative emotions and reinforcing the idea that dogs are scary. Another child, who has grown up around dogs, may have the schema that most dogs are pretty friendly and will filter information about this very same dog through his or her own lens, assess the dog as positive, walk up to the owner, ask if it is OK to pet the dog, and have a good experience, reinforcing the idea that most dogs are pretty friendly. Same dog, but the two children have very different cognitive, emotional, and physiological responses based on their cognitive schemas. This process is applied to the treatment of somatic symptoms by addressing the ways that cognitive schemas and accompanying thinking styles, called cognitive distortions, affect the way thoughts and feelings interact and how incoming information is processed. Through this process, children are taught to retrain their brain so that previously threatening situations (e.g., having symptoms at school) end up being less threatening than predicted.

Cognitive distortions are exaggerated thought patterns that reinforce and categorize negative thoughts. Beck et al. (1979) identified cognitive distortions in people's information processing, including all-or-nothing thinking, overgeneralization, mental filter, disqualifying the positive, jumping to conclusions, magnification/catastrophizing or minimization, emotional reasoning, "should" statements, labeling/mislabeling, and personalizing. Some people are more affected by cognitive distortions than others, and there are certainly more prevalent styles of thinking among individuals with anxiety and depression. But everyone has them, and teaching children to identify when their thoughts are getting stuck in a negative thinking trap is a great coping tool to move them forward in their treatment. This information may feel familiar if you are already working within a CBT framework, but instead of predicting negative outcomes on something like a test, children predict negative outcomes for their physical symptoms. Show children the "Cognitive Distortions" worksheet (in the Appendix), and have them go through each one, asking them to identify which types of thinking happen to them most often. You can also call them "thinking traps," "unhelpful thinking styles," or "sticky thoughts." In our experience, the most common are all-or-nothing thinking, overgeneralization, catastrophizing, mental filter, and jumping to conclusions. Once the patterns are noted, work with children to identify helpful thoughts and differentiate them from unhelpful ones. In the following dialogue, we introduce the concept of cognitive distortions to our patient Ashley and help her work through the effect of those types of thoughts on her overall thinking pattern:

DOCTOR: Let's talk about what affects how we make decisions about information. We have reviewed the "Cognitive Distortions" worksheet, and you identified that you tend to have pretty black-and-white thoughts, and also jump to conclusions a lot.

ASHLEY: I was just noticing that today. I've been thinking that if I don't get back to school soon, I won't be able to go to college and then everyone will think I dropped out.

DOCTOR: What happens if we examine that negative thought? Is it true? Is it helpful?

ASHLEY: It is true. My grades are not where they should be, so I don't want to tell myself not to be nervous. I don't know how I will graduate from high school.

DOCTOR: It's understandable that this is on your mind—school is important to you. Let's focus on those thoughts to see if we can find some patterns. Worries can be tricky, because they have a way of growing. Have you ever planted flowers or vegetables?

ASHLEY: No. I live in the city.

DOCTOR: Well, do you know how flowers grow?

ASHLEY: Sure, you plant a seed, water it, hope it is sunny, and then you have a flower.

DOCTOR: Absolutely. Worries are the same, but maybe more like big trees than pretty flowers. A "seed" gets planted—let's say our seed is "I do not know if I can pass this test." We give it lots of sun and water by paying attention to it, and voilá! A little worry sapling is growing. It is quite small at first, so we work around it. We can still pay enough attention to schoolwork, and we can still easily pull the sapling out of the ground by thinking, "I did fine on that test, I do not need to worry about whether I will get into college, everyone gets in somewhere." But let's say we do not do that, we let it keep growing by paying attention to the negative thoughts, and our little worry sapling grows and gets branches. One branch is "I am going to fail the test," another is "I won't get into college," one is "My family will be so disappointed," and one is "I will never get better." Now the tree is getting big and hard to ignore; it starts to block out all the positive or realistic thoughts. Even the branches grow their own little branches. The "I won't get into college" branch also grows "All my friends will go," "I will be embarrassed," and "I will have to live at home forever." Soon, you have got a giant tree of worry that is hard to cut down or see around, and everything is in the shade because the worry tree is blocking the sun and all the nice flowers. And how did it all start?

ASHLEY: A tiny thought.

DOCTOR: Yes, a tiny thought that's part of a larger pattern. Turns out that it is hard to change your thinking when the tree is full grown, but it is not quite as hard as when it is still a tiny sapling. It is just like not waiting until your dizziness is the worst, but taking a break earlier on so you can manage it.

ASHLEY: When I first started coming in I did not think I was worried, but now I can see how this process works. Of course I would feel nervous with all of these symptoms.

DOCTOR: You have made great progress in seeing how all of these factors are connected. Now, let's talk about ways to change your thinking so you can keep the worry tree from growing by recognizing the patterns that worries and negative thoughts can have. Next time we will talk about what you can do to change these types of thoughts and talk about any goals you might want to set regarding school attendance, and how these strategies can help you achieve that.

When children are learning about cognitive distortions, have them do some tracking at home. You can again utilize the "Thought Record" worksheet (in the Appendix) that allows the child to fill in situations, thoughts, feelings, body responses, and actions to do initial tracking of negative thinking patterns. Children can also keep a tally on the "Cognitive Distortions" worksheet, or electronically via a note-taking or memo application. The importance of tracking is twofold: it increases children's awareness of thoughts and helps them carry over the skills learned in session into their daily lives.

REFRAMING

Once cognitive distortions have been introduced, the next step is to teach children how to manage them. Some children and adolescents find that once they are aware of their thought patterns, and aware that they are just *thoughts*, not truths, that having that awareness alone is the only tool they need to pay less attention to negative thoughts and pay more attention to active coping behaviors instead, which allows them to successfully move forward. However, children who have more difficulty managing symptoms, waited longer before coming into therapy, or have comorbid anxiety and depression often have a harder time managing these types of thoughts and benefit from learning an additional skill to address negative thinking, called reframing. Once children have identified their own negative thought patterns and corresponding negative emotional, physical, and behavioral consequences, reframing is the tool that gives them the opportunity to change those patterns for the better. Reframing or restructuring is the approach of challenging cognitive distortions and changing your thoughts and beliefs to a more neutral, balanced, or positive outlook. A mantra we often say to introduce this idea is "You're not responsible for automatic negative thoughts happening in the first place, but you are responsible for what you choose to do with them."

The process of reframing can be compared to hypothesis testing. We teach children first that thoughts are not facts, which can be surprising to them! Thoughts come from all over the place; they could be weird, true, untrue, or silly. But they are not necessarily facts. Children have to learn to evaluate the accuracy of their thoughts, particularly as they relate to their symptoms. If a child gets to school and automatically thinks, "I'm going to have a terrible stomachache today," he does not actually *know* that is true because the day is just starting, but simply because he believes he will not do well, his fight-or-flight response activates and actually makes him *more* vulnerable to having a stomachache. To improve this pattern, it is crucial to teach children to examine their thoughts and determine whether there is evidence for their beliefs; if evidence is lacking, this is a perfect place to engage in reframing for emotional and physical benefit.

Reframing is based on the knowledge that negative thoughts lead to negative feelings and actions, and it allows for neutral, balanced, or positive thoughts that lead to positive actions, feelings, and outcomes. This is a technique that consists of disputing and then changing any thoughts that are irrational, such as cognitive distortions, whether they are maladaptive and making the situation worse, or maybe true but just not very helpful. It is not advantageous to send the message to children that they can or should think perfectly positively all the time. In fact, a child we worked with commented that when someone tells her to "think positive," she stops listening to them, particularly if the person is encouraging her to be more active, because she knows she will have symptoms with activity and the idea that she will be symptom-free is not realistic to her. But when she was encouraged to "think neutral," she was better able to make use of reframing techniques and went into the situation thinking, "I might have symptoms, but I will be able to cope with it," which positively affected her mood and motivation. Teach children to aim for neutral or realistic thoughts, neither overly positive nor overly negative. For example, if a child worrying about failing a test thinks, "I am definitely going to get 100%," they may be disappointed with anything less, but if they think, "I will probably do fine," their anxiety is reduced and success is more likely to be achieved. The goal of reframing is to reduce symptom impairment.

When teaching reframing, always reinforce the notion: Is there another way to think of this situation? One that is more positive, realistic, balanced, or more valid, or that will help you reach your goals? Henry Ford once said something along the lines of "If you think can or you think you can't, you're right." Thomas Edison said, "I haven't failed, I've just found 10,000 ways that did not work." Those are reframes; it is easy to look at both men, who made very important discoveries, and think that they were successes. But imagine how many times they were *not* successful prior to those discoveries, and where the world would be had they stopped working on their inventions. We illustrate the introduction of reframing with our patient Johnny, using the "Reframing Thoughts" worksheet (in the Appendix):

DOCTOR: OK, Johnny. We are going to pull together all of these ideas—the connections between thoughts, feelings, body responses, actions, and negative thinking patterns—into a helpful thinking strategy called reframing using this worksheet. As you can see, the first thing we do in a situation is come up with the negative thoughts, feelings, and actions that happen because that is how our minds do it! Then we will figure out how to think about the situation differently, and see if we can come up with more helpful thoughts, feelings, and actions. What situation would you like do?

JOHNNY: Well, when I have a stomachache, of course!

DOCTOR: OK, so let's fill in "having a stomachache" as the situation. When that happens, what are some of the automatic negative thoughts that your mind thinks about?

JOHNNY: "The pain is never going to go away" and "Pain will keep me from having fun."

DOCTOR: How do you feel after thinking those thoughts? What do you do?

JOHNNY: I feel sad, sometimes mad if it interrupts me. And worried that it is going to get worse, so I don't really do anything about it except feel bored and rest.

DOCTOR: That's a tough situation to be in, and those thoughts and feelings do not seem to lead to any of the good coping actions that you have been working on. Reframing is a way of looking at these negative thoughts to see if they are true or helpful and coming up with realistic ways to think about the situation that lead to more balanced feelings and helpful actions. The way we do that is by looking at your thoughts, one by one, which lead to new feelings and actions that can come from them. Let's take the first thought here that we wrote down: "The pain is never going to go away." Is that what happens for you?

JOHNNY: Well no, I guess not. Usually, the pain gets better after a little while.

DOCTOR: Let's put that down as one of our realistic thoughts over here in this section of the worksheet: "Usually the pain will get better in a little while." The next thought says, "Pain will keep me from having fun." Is that one true?

JOHNNY: Yes, definitely. When I have pain, I can't have fun at all.

DOCTOR: Well, OK, but does that mean you can *never* have fun again in your whole life?

JOHNNY: No, I guess that doesn't mean I can never have fun, just not at that minute.

DOCTOR: OK, so maybe another way of saying it is that pain might keep me from having fun *right now*, but it is not going to keep me from having fun forever. If you were thinking those two realistic thoughts you just came up with, then how would you feel?

JOHNNY: A little better. It seems like those thoughts are more hopeful. Maybe I'd feel more motivated to use one of my coping tools.

DOCTOR: I agree, let's put all of those feelings down here as positive feelings. So, then what do you think you might do once you are thinking and feeling better?

JOHNNY: Well, I might take a short rest, but then I might start doing my other activities probably, because my pain only lasts a little while, usually. Or maybe I could do a distraction for a coping tool or at least think about something fun to do later.

DOCTOR: Let's finish off the reframing worksheet by writing those down as your positive actions. Look at that—just *thinking* about the situation differently led to *feeling* differently which led to *doing* something differently, and what do you think that will lead to?

JOHNNY: My body feeling better.

DOCTOR: I agree. And all because you changed your thinking! Reframing is a pretty powerful tool. I will send you home today with some blank reframing worksheets that you can use to record your thoughts when you find yourself in a tough situation and thinking negatively. Pick three different examples of changing negative thoughts to realistic thoughts for next time.

Some children are able to engage in reframing relatively easily once the patterns are identified, but others may need to be taught a step-by-step process. In order to be successful at using reframing strategies, children should first identify which parts of the situation they can control, and which parts they cannot. While focusing on the parts they can change, children can determine the realistically positive aspects of the situation in order to take a more balanced or neutral approach and increase their belief in their ability to cope with the situation. The key is teaching children to determine the *realistic* possibility of their negative expectations and figure out the outcomes that are more likely, which are usually less negative and more neutral/ positive. Reframing ideas are listed in the "Ways to Challenge Thoughts" worksheet (in the Appendix). Once children get comfortable with the self-questioning process, they can use the information they have discovered to change their negative thoughts to neutral or positive ones, reduce emotional and physical distress from a situation, and have a more balanced outlook. Let's revisit the conversation with Ashley using the "Ways to Challenge Thoughts" worksheet in order to engage in reframing as she plans to return to school:

ASHLEY: I know that last time we talked about one of my goals as getting back to school. But I don't think I can change what I'm thinking about school. My brain thought it, so how can I make my brain unthink it?

DOCTOR: The good news is that this strategy is not about unthinking anything. Our brain's entire job is to have thoughts. But should you pay attention to every single one of them?

ASHLEY: No, I guess not. Sometimes I think about whether people will like my outfit, but then I remember that I like it and it doesn't really matter what other people think.

DOCTOR: And that's a realistic thought! It will feel harder to think this way about school, but we will practice it together. Once you have identified the thinking traps that we worked on before, you can figure out how to make changes in your thinking. You noticed a lot of fortune-telling, like "I will be too tired to make it through the day." Let's see if there is anything we can do to change that thought, either by thinking of parts of the situation that you can change or finding different ways of thinking about the situation.

ASHLEY: Well, I guess I could get enough sleep the night before and use my healthy habits like staying hydrated and getting exercise. But I cannot control what time school starts or how much the teachers are going to ask me to do there. That's what got me into trouble before.

DOCTOR: You have control over your schedule, but you cannot predict what demands school will place on you. However, you can control how you manage them. Let's try some reframing questions. What evidence goes against this thought? Can I predict the future?

ASHLEY: Ha, not really. I guess the evidence for being too tired is that I have felt really tired all day before, but since I have been coming here, I have had more energy. I hung out with my friend for 5 hours, so that's evidence I could be at school for 5 hours.

DOCTOR: Good work. And what is the worst thing that might happen? Is there anything good that could happen? Is there a middle ground?

ASHLEY: The worst thing that will happen is I'll feel sleepy, my body might feel weird, I'll have a hard time concentrating, and I might nod off in class. Best-case scenario, I get to see friends and I get to get back to actually learning and doing my work like a normal student. Realistically, I think it will probably be somewhere in the middle. It is going to be a big adjustment. I'm just really worried about it not going well. So I guess I could remind myself I don't know what the day will be like, and if I don't know, I could predict it will be at least OK ... like, maybe I'll feel tired but I'll still be able to get to school.

DOCTOR: Great. And you might have noticed something; like we talked about, black-and-white thinking often comes with extremes of language (like "always/never") and does not use "maybe," "probably," or "sometimes."

ASHLEY: Oh, I said maybe! I see how that makes it feel less hard to do something. It also helps me to think about the ways something could work out instead of all the ways it is going to go wrong. But then I'm not prepared for the bad things that might happen.

DOCTOR: I think a lot of people feel that way. Like we have talked about before, negative thoughts are not necessarily untrue, they are just unhelpful because they usually have a small chance of happening. Even if they do happen, people usually find they are able to handle them better than they thought they would be able to. You do not have to be positive all the time; aim for "thinking neutral," which will help you take a balanced approach. You may find that activities go well when you have realistic expectations.

GOAL SETTING

For children who are successful at this point in treatment, goal setting is a nice way for them to plan for functioning into the future or as a motivational strategy that will keep them engaged in positive coping as you wind down treatment. For children who feel stuck or unable to use coping skills, take some time to review their goals in order to address motivational factors that may underlie those challenges. Children might have a hard time motivating themselves to get back to school and might therefore not practice coping skills as readily, but they might be more motivated to go to a friend's house to play. Both of these goals require the same basic level of function; to be able to get out of bed and use coping strategies to manage either anticipation of symptoms or the symptoms themselves in situations outside of the home. If a child understands that using coping skills improves function, and improved function means children can reach their goals, this enables them to engage in different and sometimes difficult new patterns. One way to say this to a child is "If you are doing something hard, remember the reason that you are doing it." In addition, setting their own goals gives children something concrete to look forward to.

There are many ways to set goals with children. Ask them to think about where they would like to be or what they would like to be doing in a week, a month, and a year, and then work backward to ensure they have all the skills needed to reach those goals. Let's imagine a child's goal is to be able to play in the championship soccer game at the end of the season. This goal can seem unreachable to a child who has been missing school and spending more time in bed. The first step is just to get back on the soccer field, either to watch a practice or to start working out with the team, and to do this she would need to have a good plan for healthy habits management, a note for the coach on how to support her with symptoms should they arise, and a plan for managing negative expectations by using reframing techniques and setting reasonable expectations for the practice. For a long-term goal, like attending college in the future, the conversation can turn toward how daily use of coping skills leads to improved school attendance, focus, and educational engagement, which then leads to improved academic performance, ability to participate in activities, and a better chance of success in meeting the college goal. Overall, allow children to see that using their coping skills and setting goals are both related to their overall value system, or what matters to them in their lives; if they find themselves working toward something they are truly passionate and excited about, children might be surprised to find out just how much they can do even in the face of symptoms. The next strategy is problem solving, which can be a good way to continue the goal-setting conversation and useful in generating strategies for other areas in which children are struggling.

PROBLEM SOLVING

The final cognitive strategy that we cover in this chapter is problem solving. To some degree, you already have been working on problem solving along the way in your discussion of symptoms from a biopsychosocial framework; you have likely worked with children and their families to determine what they can do to manage the aspects of situations that they do have control over, which are usually the factors that pertain directly to their own thoughts and actions as opposed to direct symptom resolution. This is the crux of problem solving: to identify the problem, identify the desired outcome (what is controllable), think of a number of ways to get the desired outcome by using the coping skills they have learned, choose the best one, and try it out. Problem solving is an excellent skill for children to end on in treatment, as it provides them with a framework for deciding which coping skills to use in which situations, connecting that process to how it can benefit their physical function (and thus symptoms), and makes a nice transition to the maintenance phase of treatment.

Consider children's ability to influence the outcome of situations when teaching problem solving, as well as their thinking and communication skills. Younger children may need a more concrete approach. Children with negative mood or depression may need more help developing strategies depending on how successful they view their efforts to be. Use clinical judgment in determining how much facilitation to provide when having them choose coping skills in a problem-solving framework. For younger children, or children struggling to come up with ideas, try giving them a few options and letting them pick. Be careful not to choose for them; part of the goal of problem solving is changing children's thinking and their approach to difficult situations, as well as encouraging advocacy and self-efficacy, rather than just providing them with a solution.

The "Problem Solving" worksheet (in the Appendix) includes the steps outlined above and can be used in session or given to the child for use at home. The first step is to identify the problem in a detailed and concrete way. The second step is for children to decide not how to solve the problem, but rather what their goal is or what they would like to have happen. The next step involves generating possible solutions, before going back to decide whether each situation is likely to be successful, paying attention to not only whether the solution would work, but also whether it would create unintended consequences. Children should consider benefits and drawbacks of each solution in their rating. One solution might work well in isolation, but would cause other consequences that make it not such a great solution. Finally, the child chooses a strategy to try, evaluates its success, and either celebrates the success or goes back to the list as needed. We illustrate problem solving with our patient Alex:

DOCTOR: Today we are going to talk about a coping skill we call problem solving. How do you usually solve problems?

ALEX: Well, if it's math I try to write down the steps, unless I can solve it in my head.

DOCTOR: What about if it is something a little more complicated? Like putting together a project for your robotics club?

ALEX: We usually work together on a team, so I would ask for help from my teammates if I was stuck, but that kind of stuff is pretty easy for me.

DOCTOR: You just identified some good strategies without even realizing it! Following the steps and asking for help. Do you feel like you can use those same strategies when you are having a hard time managing a problem related to your symptoms?

ALEX: I never tried. I didn't think I could solve my walking problem in the same way I solve a math problem.

DOCTOR: Let's look at this worksheet together, which has some steps for solving problems, even ones that seem really hard to solve. The first step is to identify the problem, because if we do not know what the problem is, we cannot figure out how to fix it. Then, we identify what you want to happen, think of ideas for how to make that happen, rate the ideas, decide on the best, and then try it out. So, what is a problem you have been having that we could use as an example?

ALEX: Oh, definitely getting my homework done. I'm so behind and it makes me mad. And feeling mad makes my legs feel worse.

DOCTOR: That is a good example of how negative thoughts and feeling make symptoms feel more intense. Let's see if we can use problem solving as a strategy that will keep that from happening for you. We'll put "Feeling mad about homework" for number one. What do you want to happen?

ALEX: Well, I want to feel calm and get my homework done so I don't feel like I have so much to do and have more time for fun. And not have my legs feel worse.

DOCTOR: So when you sit down to do homework, you sometimes feel really overwhelmed, which makes you want to procrastinate and not do your homework, which makes you feel worse. Is there anything you can do to look at the situation differently?

ALEX: I could make a list so I know what I have to do, I could ask my teachers if I could get excused from it, I could ask my friends for the answers, and I could do some and then take a break.

DOCTOR: Those are great ideas! I like how you just listed them off and didn't try to decide if they would work right away. Let's see if you can think of a few more.

ALEX: Maybe I could try some relaxation while I'm doing my homework. I can't think of any more.

DOCTOR: OK, what do you think one of your friends would do?

ALEX: Oh, two of my friends live next door to each other so sometimes they do their homework together.

DOCTOR: Let's write that down, do homework with a friend. Any other possibilities?

ALEX: No.

DOCTOR: OK, that's a good list. Let's go through and rate them from one to 10. One is going to be not so likely to work, and 10 is going to be very likely to work. Are there any drawbacks to the first one, making a list?

ALEX: No, I think that is a pretty good one, so I would rate it 10. My mom already told me my teachers won't excuse any more assignments, so that's maybe a 2 since I could try to convince them, but it would probably take a long time. Asking my friends is a 4, they might not know the answers and it might be cheating. Doing some and taking a break is a 10, and trying relaxation is an 8. Doing homework with a friend is a 7, I guess.

DOCTOR: Good work. Now we have to decide which one to start with. Usually it works best to start with one of the top-rated ones. Which one would you like to pick?

ALEX: I guess sort of a combination of two, making a list and taking breaks.

DOCTOR: OK, and how long do you want to try that before you decide if it is a good way to solve your problem?

ALEX: Well, I guess maybe a few days.

DOCTOR: OK, so today is Monday, so you can reassess on Wednesday to see how you are doing. Can you guess what you would do if it was not working?

ALEX: Probably pick another thing from this list. A 7 or an 8?

DOCTOR: Good work! So, let's do a quick review. First, we figure out what the problem is, we think about what we want to happen, we come up with a bunch of possible solutions, then we rate our solutions, thinking of the benefits and the drawbacks of each solution, we pick one and decide how long we will try it for, and then give it a try. If it works, great, if not, back to the list, and pick another one if needed. Remember, what you are trying to do is use the factors that are in your direct control, like how you think about something and the actions you take, to help the factors that are a bit out of your direct control, like how your legs are feeling. That is how problem solving can be an effective symptom coping strategy.

This problem-solving approach can be used to solve an acute problem and as a guide for approaching difficult situations in the future, such as finals time at school, or when children have to go back to the sports field where symptoms occurred, when they get sick with a virus, when school is back in session in the fall, or when they have a symptom flare. Children do not have to go back to square one if their symptoms pop back up again; just because they fall off the bike, they do not have to roll all the way back down the hill. They have to step to the side, hop back on, exert a little extra effort to get going again, and keep riding. Getting started is sometimes the hardest part; once a child gets going, momentum does the rest!

Problem solving should feel very familiar to children at this point in treatment, as you have modeled it all along: identifying what one can or cannot control and figuring out different strategies to adapt to the situation at hand. Assess children's expectations as this framework is introduced; if they think, "OK, if I do this thing, it better work!" they may be disappointed, as rarely does a single solution work perfectly. But if taught to use the more adaptive approach of "I will try it, and if it doesn't work I have lots of other ideas" they show more flexible coping, which is typically more effective. In addition, children should be able to identify when they need help and how to ask for it. Sometimes being ready to move on to the next stage is not knowing or having all the answers, it is just using the knowledge you do have and knowing when to ask for help.

THE FAMILY'S ROLE

There are several ways that parents can support and model these skills for their children at home. First, parents can structure thought tracking, as well as observing and identifying times their children get stuck in negative thinking patterns. For younger children, we encourage parents to use a short phrase to catch children when their thinking is "stuck." Parents may say something like "Those are your worries talking," or "that sounds like the worry bully." As the child progresses in therapy, parents can challenge cognitive distortions and engage with the child in problem solving. This support also helps the child to verbally express the worries, rather than allowing them to remain internalized and affect physical symptoms. For adolescents, talk with them about what role they want their parents to have in supporting coping strategies at home. Some teens feel that once they learn the skills they are able to use them inde-pendently, and some find that they still need or want parent support.

It is important to address the fact that parents sometimes model maladaptive cognitive coping too, such as taking a black-and-white approach themselves. As we teach children coping tools, parents also need to be made aware of the ways they can model positive and adaptive coping for their children. Just as we train children to be flexible and adaptive, parents also need reminders that they sometimes need to alter their expectations for success and failure.

TREATMENT PROGRESS

This chapter concludes the intervention portion of the book; upcoming chapters cover working with parents, schools, and health care colleagues. At this point in treatment, a majority of children will have reached their functional goals and may experience diminished frequency or intensity of symptoms. It is then pertinent to discuss with children and families bringing the active treatment phase to a close and shifting the focus to maintaining gains into the future. It can be difficult to know when to shift from intervention to maintenance. The most important factor is an indicator that function has been regained. If you administered assessment tools at the start of treatment, it is wise to readminister the same measures at the conclusion of level three intervention, paying attention to recommended cutoff scores for each tool and comparing current scores to the baseline. Alternately, use the child's and family's self-reports as a guide: Are children attending school? Are they socializing with friends and participating in activities? Has there been a reduction in distress or impairment related to symptoms? Have they been able to recover when they have had a symptom flare? Are they getting closer to their developmental and/or treatment goals? This is a good time to refer back to the initial assessment as a guide; if children are participating in activities they were too impaired to participate in prior to treat-ment, this is a good indication of return to function. If the answer to many of these questions is "yes," it is appropriate to meet less frequently. This provides more time for the child to utilize his or her skills outside of your office, which is the ultimate goal of treatment.

Prior to discharge from treatment, spend at least one session summarizing prog-ress and problem-solving future areas of concern, while reviewing or role-playing how children can maintain healthy lifestyles, and use behavioral or cognitive coping strategies as needed. Either review the "Coping Skills Toolkit" and/or use the "Cop-ing Plan" worksheets (in the Appendix) to provide children with an overview of the skills that work best for them with personalized instruction on when and how to use them. Summarizing progress gives an opportunity to celebrate the successes, while emphasizing and reinforcing all of the positive changes children have made. It also provides time to talk about how children's perspectives and awareness have changed over the course of treatment. It may be that children are more aware of the role of physical health needs like staying hydrated, the importance of behavioral changes like engaging in relaxation, or how thinking patterns can affect the way the body feels. A foundation is then provided to talk with children about times they perceive to be high stress, ranging anywhere from the good (a fun vacation, making a new friend) to the expected (a new school year, a musical performance) to the dreaded (semester exams, soccer tryouts), so they can have a plan of action ready for those events based on what strategies they feel have been most helpful. The "Take a Break" worksheet (in the Appendix) provides a visual reminder of how to cope with challenges for future reference. If children are functioning well when they return for a maintenance session, they are released from treatment with an instruction to call should symptoms reappear or if a booster session is needed to deal with a particularly challenging stressor. If children are not functioning well, reassess for the source of the difficulty, and either provide further intervention for ongoing somatic symptom challenges, change the course of treatment, or make a referral for other presenting concerns.

CHAPTER SUMMARY AND TAKE-AWAY POINTS

- Cognitive intervention includes teaching children to recognize the link between their thoughts, feelings, and actions, and how their feelings relate to their symptoms based on the situation or on more global emotional functioning.

- Thoughts can lead to different emotional and physiological experiences; some thoughts can be "helpful," while others are "unhelpful."

- Cognitive strategies to manage unhelpful thoughts and maladaptive thinking patterns include identifying automatic negative thoughts, information processing, cognitive distortions, reframing, goal setting, and problem solving.

PART IV

Collaboration

INTRODUCTION

Children do not live in a bubble—they come with parents, siblings, extended family, friends, neighbors, teachers, coaches, doctors, nurses, therapists, and other community members who all influence them. Attending to factors within children's larger social structure *must* be part of the intervention to make treatment for somatic symptoms truly successful and enable children to transition coping skills into the rest of their lives. The degree to which children are able to utilize the strategies presented in this book meaningfully and effectively out in the world is truly the ultimate test of whether the treatment goals have been met. It would be a mistake to deliver treatment to children but then overlook the importance of intervening with the larger system. CBT is not a success if children use coping strategies perfectly in the office but fall apart when they leave the session. In order for that translation of skills to occur, it is critical to include the influences within their system as a part of treatment. In this final section, we address these larger contexts and relationships, with a focus on how to work within this system to support the functional changes children are working hard to make. Specifically, we review three main areas in which children with somatic symptoms need support: parents, school, and health care. In the final chapter, we wrap up with a few thoughts about successes and challenges in working with children with somatic symptoms.

The ecological systems theory provides a framework for considering contextual factors based on the idea that child development is a product of the interaction between children and their environment (Bronfenbrenner, 1979). The theory posits that children interact with the environment at four levels: children themselves are at the center, their immediate caretakers are at the next level, the community after that, and finally the culture in which they live. Children with somatic symptoms are affected by the environment at every level.

Starting at the center, children's own experience is significantly influenced by somatic symptoms in that they are directly challenged by their physical experiences and related impairment, often on a daily basis. In their immediate context, such as at home with their families, at school with peers and teachers, and at the doctor's office, they are influenced by others' responses to their symptoms, which can either support function through a focus on positive coping efforts, or keep them in the sick role through attention to symptoms, promotion of a "symptoms are dangerous" mentality, or secondary gain/reinforcement of avoidance. Children and their families can be affected by the community around them in terms of how well acquaintances, neighbors, and social services understand and work with children with somatic symptoms. After all, there is no neighborhood fundraiser or casserole delivery for a family caring for a child with somatic symptoms, whereas communities often rally around families of children with other chronic conditions, and these types of interactions have an effect on families in both scenarios. Finally, the culture in which children live plays a role, particularly in how somatic symptoms are viewed or understood. Whether illness is seen through a biopsychosocial lens or a more dichotomous mind–body framework is often culturally dictated.

For all of these reasons, consider the role of the environment when treating children with somatic symptoms, so that children are not held back in using their newfound coping strategies by a system that is struggling to understand or support them. Truly successful treatment of children with somatic symptoms requires a reboot of children's own management of their symptoms *and* a simultaneous reboot of the environment around them, particularly among their immediate influences of family, teachers, and health care providers. Attending to these environmental factors is particularly unique to pediatric treatment. Working with children necessitates working with adults. It is one thing to work with an adult and teach him or her to become adept at engaging in effective coping; in contrast, children don't control their environment like adults do. Children look to adults for validation and assistance at every turn, and when they do, adults need to acknowledge children's symptom experiences while providing supportive messages about function.

Throughout this section, as we address ways to work with the adults in children's lives, the major theme we will return to is how to ensure that parents, teachers, and medical providers understand that somatic symptoms are just as real as organic symptoms; it just requires a different approach to manage them. If adults are supportive of this message, then it is quite likely that children will be able to use their newfound coping skills successfully in the environment, and true treatment success will be reached in improved function and effective symptom management.

CHAPTER 9

Parents and Community

It might be the case that parents have the hardest job when it comes to managing somatic symptoms in children. Above all, it is the parents' job to keep their children healthy. As such, when children are sick, parents dutifully get them checked out by the doctor, make sure they take their medicine, and provide them with a comforting environment in which to heal. Most parents are naturally quite good at this, and usually the approach is effective—except, as was the case with Johnny at the very beginning of the book, when that approach does not work and symptoms get worse instead of better despite parents' care and devotion. Again, quite naturally, parents' anxiety increases because the usual plan did not work as expected, so they visit more specialists, and more school and work get missed; yet the child still does not get better. Anxiety shifts to fear, and all of a sudden parents find themselves quite helpless in a situation in which they desire to be the most helpful; they cannot make the symptoms go away, when it is all they want to do.

In this highly challenging, abnormal circumstance, it seems entirely reasonable for parents to say, "Well, keeping the child home will at least give him some rest even though he has missed a lot of school," or "Sleeping in the child's bed ensures safety at night even though I haven't done that since he was little," or "I'll just let him eat in front of the TV since he has so much trouble with his stomach, even though it's a family rule to have dinner together at the table," or to make any number of statements that parents would never otherwise say. This is the beginning of the slippery slope that parents find themselves on when trying to find the right strategies to manage their child's somatic symptoms. In no time at all, parents find themselves living a life at home that is quite different from what they envisioned for their family, and worse yet, the new routine may accidentally perpetuate their child's cycle of symptoms and disability. No matter in what maladaptive patterns children and families end up, it usually comes from a normal and reasonable response to a really abnormal and confusing situation.

So far, the focus of this book has been the challenge that *children* face when managing somatic symptoms. In this chapter, we turn to the *parents'* experience, as they are faced with the equally challenging task of caring for a child who is sick with symptoms that are entirely different from the usual course of illness. While you may be surprised to find parents engaging in what seem to be very obvious maladaptive strategies, remember that they have arrived there out of sheer desperation and desire to help their child, and unfortunately their efforts have backfired. We say to parents all the time that children don't come with instructions in the first place, and there certainly are no rules about how to help them when they have a challenging problem like somatic symptoms. As you embark on your work with parents, it is important to send the message that no one has done anything wrong; everything that has been tried to this point was in a genuine effort to help the child; those efforts were unsuccessful due to the tricky nature of these types of health challenges; and it's simply time for a new approach. Keep this perspective in mind while reviewing the factors that affect parents' responses to children's somatic symptoms and the strategies that can help them break out of unhelpful cycles.

In addition to the role of parenting behavior and responses to symptoms, parental modeling of illness behavior may play an even larger role in the cycle of symptoms and disability in their children. Levy and colleagues (2004) found that children of parents with IBS went to the doctor for general health concerns and GI-specific concerns more often than their peers whose parents did not have IBS. A similar pattern was identified in adolescents with FAP whose parents also had pain, and the more in tune adolescents were with parents' pain behaviors, the more disabled they were with regard to their own pain (Stone & Walker, 2016). Further, the Levy study found that the effect of parents' attention to children's symptom complaints was independent from parents' own illness status, indicating that both nature *and* nurture play a role in this relationship. Parents who model more illness behavior have children who notice more symptoms in themselves as well as their family members.

Mental health providers can help parents navigate these challenges and encourage the whole family to adopt a functional routine. Our message from the beginning of treatment to children and parents may sound harsh at first as we exclaim, "Stop! Stop missing school, stop lying on the couch, stop sleeping and eating somewhere different, stop focusing on the symptoms." However, we make those exclamations while providing a rationale for why these normal protective mechanisms make symptoms and impairment worse instead of better. While we expect parents and children to change directions, it can be challenging. Consider, too, how parents' own mental health and medical status as well as the experience of going through unpredictable medical encounters influence parents' response to children's symptoms. As mentioned earlier, parents feel anxious in uncertain situations such as receiving few medical answers for children's symptoms, and their own medical experiences and mental health status influences the care they seek for their children. It is essential to be aware of these factors when incorporating parents into children's treatment.

Parents have a variety of responses to engaging in CBT for somatic symptoms with their children. Some are on board; maybe they share our biopsychosocial approach and easily recognize that somatic symptoms are worse or better in different contexts, they believe in the power of the mind and body working together to overcome symptoms, and they see the overall utility of returning a child to function. There are also parents who are adamant that there are no psychosocial triggers or patterns to symptoms and it must be an organic problem, because the idea that stress or anxiety could trigger a physical symptom might sound to them like "the child is making this up."

And then there are parents in the middle, who just want their children to get better and are willing to try just about anything to get there. It is important to understand where parents are on this spectrum. Some parents need more reassurance, and some need less; some are more frustrated, and some understand that the health care world is not perfect and even the very best medical assessments do not tell the whole story.

In this chapter, we present tips for parents to use as they function in three main roles in their children's symptom experience: structuring the environment, interacting around symptoms, and managing their own coping and emotional functioning. Of course, there is overlap between all of these roles that play into parents' behaviors toward their children, but thinking about parental roles in these three main ways works well when considering how to provide support to parents in the context of delivering CBT. For example, you may find that many parents need more help with structuring the environment, while some need more individual support of their own, and others need help with the dyadic interaction—some may need all three. Throughout the intervention chapters, we recommended bringing the parent in at the end of each session to summarize the information learned, as well as instructing the parent on how to support the child in coping with symptoms. Without parent support and understanding, the child is less likely to successfully make changes.

As we discuss working with parents, we also have to address the most significant connection between children's behavior and symptoms that is often most evident in the parent–child interaction, mentioned briefly in Part I, which is unintentional secondary gain. As it relates to illness, secondary gain is the side advantage or reward that comes from having symptoms, such as successfully avoiding something that was going to be difficult anyway or receiving a benefit because of the symptoms, and "unintentional" refers to the process in which this happens by association and *not* by design. To be clear, we do not think children with somatic symptoms are intentionally plotting to stay up late with a stomachache so their parents will allow them to stay home from school the next day to play video games instead of taking a math test. However, it is certainly the case that maladaptive associations can be made between symptoms and situations that become reinforced over time, often by parents, which makes them more likely to reoccur.

For example, imagine that a child with nonepileptic seizures tries to go back to school but has an episode upon stepping into the classroom. The child naturally thinks, "Oh, last time I did that, something bad happened, so I'd best not try it again because it's dangerous." That is an association, and the "gain" comes in if that child goes home and does a special activity for the rest of the day with a parent who suddenly takes off work to be with the child because of the difficult morning. The next time the child even *thinks* about going back to school, that association will be automatically conjured up, and another day will be spent at home because having an episode at school is scary *and* having a special day at home with a parent is comforting. It is easy to see how parents become embroiled in this process—after all, what parent would not want his or her child to do something pleasant and relaxing after going through such a difficult and scary experience? But if we take a step back and look at the overall pattern that is created, it is clear that this parent and child will have an even harder time getting back to the regular routine now that this unintentional secondary gain pattern has been established.

The same process can happen for children with dizziness or pain, particularly during physical exertion or times of higher anxiety (e.g., sports practices, games, presenting in front of the class), who stop the activity in favor of something better. Most children and parents have the best of intentions about getting back to school or activities, but each time the children try, the symptoms get worse, the activity gets associated with discomfort, and the parents pick them up to take them back to the safety of home. The first step, which is often part of what you are doing through education about the cycle of pain and disability, is to help parents and children see these patterns and understand that they come from a normal place but have abnormal and detrimental consequences in terms of the child missing out on important life events. The parents' role is to be the enforcer and the cycle breaker, and in essence what we are asking them to do is tolerate the child's distress and their own distress to promote improved function, which is really, really hard to do. This might be why parents have the hardest job of all when managing children's somatic symptoms. All the strategies and tips we review in this chapter are designed to empower parents to do one of the hardest jobs they will have to do as parents: watch their children struggle while trusting in the knowledge that the struggle will lead to success. These tips and strategies can be incorporated into treatment when the parent joins in at the end of child intervention sessions or in the context of a parent-only session to focus solely on parenting factors if needed.

First, we review how to provide in-session modeling of the types of skills parents can use to support children when they have symptoms. Second, we review five important concepts that parents, or other adults, should be aware of when supporting children with somatic symptoms. These ideas line up with our "Providing Support to Children with Somatic Symptoms" handout (in the Appendix), which we give to parents either at the end of the education session or during one of the first intervention sessions when the focus is on improving function in the home setting. Finally, we cover the importance of being mindful of parents' own emotional regulation, as well as provide a guideline for use of strategies to handle symptoms in the community.

MODELING COPING

If we have one rule for our intervention sessions, it is to remain calm at all times, even when children and/or their parents are highly distressed. The best examples of this are times when children had somatic symptoms in our offices, including passing out, nonepileptic seizures, or throwing up. Parents look scared and go straight into protection mode, and we just keep going. Although we are certainly thinking that this situation is not ideal, we see it as an opportunity to model effective coping, and part of that is to register no external distress. As such, we successfully model to parents and children the practical approach required for teaching children to effectively cope with their symptoms. The father of a child we worked with once told us that he learned so much from just watching the way we interacted with his son, who was having an active symptom flare in our office during the assessment, and how we showed that it was OK to keep talking even when he had symptoms, which led the father to change his behavior with his son at home. This was valuable feedback to hear from a parent—in the first 5 minutes of the first session we had with that child and family, an important lesson had taken place that had a lasting and positive effect on the parent–child interaction.

Many children have told us they do not worry about having symptoms in our office because they know they will be safe: the ambulance will not be called, they will not ruin their relationship with us, they will not distress their classmates, teachers, or family, and best of all, they may be able to work on a technique with us that will help them feel better. As a result, we can confidently estimate that the likelihood of somatic symptoms happening inside our office is *lower* than it is outside of our office. We believe this is because children perceive their work with us as helpful and therefore do not anticipate negative outcomes, so their systems are not activated and symptoms remain at bay. We can truly count on our fingers the number of times we have seen significant symptoms in session, although the majority of our treatment population is comprised of children with somatic symptoms. Although we ask children to confront challenging problems, we provide a safe environment in which to try out new approaches and skills.

Overall, our goal is to use the safety of our environment to model the skills that we train children to do in treatment, and this carries over to parents as well. Basically, we tell parents to carry out the same strategies we tell you as therapists to do in terms of interacting with children. And it can be hard, for you *and* for parents, because it means that you also have to keep talking when a child has a symptom during a session, just as you expect the parent to keep taking the child to school if he or she is having symptoms in the car. It is something that gets easier and feels more natural over time, which both therapists and parents need to know.

PARENT TIP ONE: ENCOURAGE NORMAL ACTIVITY

There are two ways we encourage normal activity: the first is to ask parents to enforce the schedule created during the first intervention session; the second is to ask them to choose the activities in which their children should participate. Often, when a child with somatic symptoms arrives in our office, the demand at home has been reduced (e.g., fewer chores, lower self-care expectations), and the daily schedule has changed quite a bit: later wake times, less participation in family activities, and a less structured day overall (more time in front of the television, napping, etc.). Just as one of the first parts of the intervention with children is healthy habits, one of the first interventions with parents is asking them to provide the structure and support for the child to successfully do that. For this to happen, there have to be rules in the house, and parents have to enforce them on a daily basis and understand the rationale for *why* they need to do that. Some parents just need someone to say, "It's OK to get Johnny out of bed when he has a stomachache, it's OK to have him do chores, and it's OK to say no to video games if it's not time for video games." Sometimes, parents *have* conveyed those messages to their children, and is helpful for the children to hear someone else say it as well.

If children have symptoms, parents need to stay on message on those days, too: business as usual, with no special treatment. A symptom flare does not equal staying in bed all day playing video games, as we don't want to reinforce the symptom pattern both physically (i.e., the body gets the message that symptoms must be really serious if all activity stops) or psychologically (i.e., children feel relief that something potentially anxiety provoking was avoided). Sometimes parents need direct instruction and reassurance to make these changes at home, and for those families, you want to be certain to spend extra time at the end of the session to relay these tips or consider scheduling a parent-only session.

Parents are a big part of a child's motivational structure. For example, a child is unlikely to go to bed earlier just because the therapist said so, and is much more likely to go to bed earlier if *parents* are the ones making the rule. If parents have a hard time tolerating the child's emotional distress (or sleeplessness) when trying to change the bedtime routine, parents may come back and say that they tried to make the child go to bed earlier but the child refused. This is a good example of when to do additional education and problem solving around bedtime (or any other healthy habits) with parents, as we model through the following dialogue with our patient Johnny, who has developed some trouble going to sleep:

DOCTOR: Susan, thanks for joining us at the end of the session today! How has Johnny been doing with his healthy habits? It sounded like you had some concerns about his sleep.

MOTHER: Yes, he is usually such a good sleeper, but lately he's been having a hard going to sleep. It can take him hours, his pain just keeps him awake.

DOCTOR: When Johnny and I first talked about his sleep, we learned that he has a great bedtime routine. Johnny, has anything changed that has made it hard to go to sleep lately?

JOHNNY: I don't know. My pain is just higher at night and it keeps me up.

MOTHER: That's true, he gets into bed on time, he just has a hard time falling asleep. Last night he kept getting up to tell us that he was still awake and was hurting, so I finally just went in there and slept next to him. It seemed to calm him down so he could get some sleep. I know we talked about the importance of Johnny sleeping on his own, but he needed his sleep and that was the only way to help him rest.

DOCTOR: Many parents have a hard time making changes in sleep routines or handling pain at bedtime because at first these changes seem to cause *extra* disruption in sleep. We have to help kids endure those difficulties to succeed in changing the pattern. Tell me a little more about how the evening and bedtime went last night.

MOTHER: Well, we got home from his brother's baseball practice at about 7:30 P.M., and the kids still had to do their homework, so I bet it was about 8:45 P.M. by the time they got ready for bed, and Johnny's stomach already was hurting. We did take a minute to review his coping tools; he had his books and we put some ice water on his bedside table. We let him try to manage it on his own until about 9:45, but then I finally went in because he kept calling for me. He had his math test today, and I did not want him to be too tired.

DOCTOR: Sounds like you guys did a great job of remembering to practice the coping skills and setting the situation up for success, but it didn't work out as you had hoped. What do you think worked well about that plan and what did not work as well?

MOTHER: Well, we definitely should have started earlier and had more time to relax before bed, but that just is not possible with his brother's baseball schedule. So we are just going to have to figure out a way to work around that. And then I think that the reading probably distracted him for a little while, but Johnny could read all night so that does not usually make him feel tired. And I'm sure I probably should not have gone in there. It's like what you were saying last time about trying not to rescue him too much.

DOCTOR: This is all a learning process; we have to be flexible problem solvers—there's never just one answer, and as long as we are trying to learn and evolve our problem-solving skills we are making progress. So what do you think would be a good next step?

MOTHER: Well, my husband is much better at dealing with this than I am. So I think maybe what we can try tonight, especially since his brother does not have baseball, is to have more quiet time before bed, and then if Johnny has a hard time falling asleep, I am going to ask my husband to help him relax and stay in his room.

DOCTOR: Great idea, sometimes one parent has a different approach than the other, and that can make it a little easier. Just remind his dad to stay calm, pop his head in quickly, help with self-calming, and step back out again. Would you be open to trying a reward for Johnny if he is able to stay in bed and use his coping skills, even if it takes him a really long time to fall asleep? He could earn a prize in the morning—it can be something small he earns every day, like extra electronics time, or something bigger he can work up to.

JOHNNY: Like getting a new video game!

MOTHER: We can try it! I guess the worst-case scenario is that he is tired in the morning, and then maybe he'll have an easier time going to bed the next night. Maybe we can practice it first on a weekend so we don't have to worry about school the next morning.

DOCTOR: That would be perfect. Reward his *effort* in terms of staying in his room and using his coping skills, and not necessarily whether or not he falls asleep exactly on time. As he keeps practicing, it will get easier and easier for him to fall asleep.

Similar to the challenges associated with establishing healthy habit routines and independent coping skills, parents also have questions about how to make decisions about whether or not children should participate in an otherwise normal activity they have been struggling with since having the symptoms. For example, we worked with a parent who was deciding on whether to allow her daughter to go back to a regular school setting after she had several blackout episodes associated with cardiac symptoms that caused her to pass out and fall down in school. To address these questions on how to reinstate normal function, we use a rule of thumb that we call "Consult the List" when choosing whether the child should do an activity. We tell the family:

> "When your child first had symptoms, and you had to choose whether or not you were going to do something, the symptoms were always at the top of that list when it came to deciding what they could and couldn't do. And that made sense because you didn't have a full understanding of what the symptoms meant to your child's health or if it was safe to do that activity. Now we know that the symptoms are somatic symptoms, which are real symptoms but they are not dangerous, and that children actually *benefit* from getting back to regular activity as a way to break the cycle of symptoms and disability. Now we have to go back to the 'normal' list of rules of choosing an activity, the ones you consulted before your child ever had these symptoms, which are:
>
> 1. Does the child want to or need do it (based on likes, interests, age)?
> 2. Does the family want the child to do it (consistent with family values)?
> 3. Is it logistically possible (time, money, availability)?
>
> "Then, after asking those three questions, you should have a yes or no answer. Now there is a fourth item, which is the symptoms. They are still on this list, but now they are in the fourth position instead of the first position, so they aren't determining *if* the activity should be done or not—that has already been decided based on the first three factors, which are the most important. Symptoms are now simply informing you about *how* the activity can be done."

In order to re-create a normal routine in the family so children aren't missing school and parents aren't missing work, you can ask parents what their expectations would be for the child's function if there were no symptoms, as this can give you a good baseline to work from. If they want the child sleeping independently, attending school daily with good grades, doing one or two chores, and sitting with the family for dinner, then that is a good place to start. Some families are off and running after hearing these guidelines—they just needed someone to say it was OK—and easily get back to typical expectations and household rules. For other parents, this is a really hard sell because with enforcing rules comes an increase in child distress, which comes with an increase in parental distress. This leads us to the second tip.

PARENT TIP TWO: TOLERATE DISTRESS

Allowing children to experience distress is exactly what they need to develop problem-solving skills and resiliency. The goal of helping parents tolerate children's distress is to send the message that it is a normal developmental process for children to undergo distress as a way to learn resiliency skills. In this way, parental tolerance of child distress plays a role in a larger context than just the symptoms. If a child has a problem with a teacher and expresses worry or frustration about it to the parent, and the parent jumps in to solve the problem, the child does not learn to manage distress and come up with a solution. This process, although very well intentioned, sets up children to have underdeveloped problem-solving skills because they never have to resolve challenges since someone else has done it for them. Many parents look at this as a natural, positive parenting response; of course they want to help their children, and they do not think about their actions robbing the children of their ability to learn to deal with distress. Unfortunately, the result is that children learn to avoid problems rather than cope with them. Teach parents that the benefit of allowing children opportunities to cope with distress is building resiliency, which includes coping with somatic symptoms.

Parents must learn to cope with their own distress as well. Distress is easily visible on a person's face or evident in what is said; if a parent is distressed, a child is likely to notice, which results in the child getting biologically activated, psychologically upset, and socially communicated that there is a problem. The consequence of parental distress is child distress and less adaptive coping with symptoms. Parents must work to break this cycle by taking the lead in managing their own reactions to children's symptoms.

The parent of one of our patients shared that one of the most important lessons she learned through her son's treatment was "not to show my worries" in front of her child. She gave a specific example of watching her son play on the playground at school with his friends and worrying about whether he would hurt himself. She noticed her mind considering all of the terrible things that could happen to her son, who was just getting back on track physically, and she had every reason to shout "Stop!" or "Be careful!" However, she chose to keep these worries to herself while presenting a neutral and supportive face and *not* calling out in fear, but instead cheering on her son. Afterward, she recognized that showing her son those worried feelings would have resulted in higher anxiety and tension for him, maybe more symptoms, and definitely more difficulty with the activity because now *he* would be thinking of the ways it could go wrong. The result was that her son had a great time and so did she.

In asking parents to tolerate distress, we are not asking them to be void of emotion; we are asking them to manage their emotions. Here is how we discuss this concept with the family of Alex, our patient with conversion disorder:

DOCTOR: When I walked with Alex down the hallway for the first time without him using his wheelchair, I thought, "This is scary, there's a chance he could fall!" but I said, "Great work!" and "Look how far you've walked," and then we talked about what we were going to have for lunch. Before you knew it, we had a very calm, safe walk down the hallway. How do you think that Alex would have felt if I told him that I was really scared that he might fall or showed that worry on my face?

MOTHER: Well, I imagine that it wouldn't have made him feel very confident. He probably would have worried because you were worried!

DOCTOR: That's right! And how would that have affected his walking?

FATHER: Well, I imagine he would not have done as well. He might have actually fallen.

DOCTOR: Yes, and it would have happened because he saw the worry on my face, interpreted that as him not doing very well or being unsafe, and that would have made him focus on his symptoms. As we know, those thinking patterns make symptoms worse. This is why we have to tolerate our distress as caregivers so children can improve their function.

Although it is normal for adults to feel apprehensive when asking children to cope with their somatic symptoms, it is crucial for them to project confidence. It is easier for a professional to do this since it is not their child and they have the training to know that they are helping, not harming, the child by reengagement in normal activities. It is more difficult for parents to do this for their own children and without the professional background. Ask parents to put on their most neutral, relaxed face when their children are improving function, followed by a healthy dose of positive verbal reinforcement for children's attempts, whether successful or not.

PARENT TIP THREE: BALANCE ATTENTION TO SYMPTOMS

When we think about children with somatic symptoms and their parents, the first parents we think about are the ones who are overattentive and protective, who might not be on board at first in terms of promoting children's function or distracting them from symptoms because it feels dangerous. Parents in this situation may prevent children from participating in activities due to concern about symptoms, ask children constant questions about symptoms, and have a protective, sometimes defensive attitude when asked to increase children's function. These may also be the parents who provide a lot of reassurance, which is a natural tendency with a child who is ill but in the context of somatic symptoms only promotes further avoidance of situations in which children may experience symptoms and perpetuates the cycle of disability.

Research on parenting interactions is very supportive of the positive role of distraction and engagement in normal activity for improving children's symptoms. In one study, parents of children with FAP anticipated that distraction would lead to more negative outcomes in comparison to reassuring their child; however, results indicated that parents who reassured and attended to children's symptoms had children with *more* symptom complaints than children of parents who distracted them from symptoms (Walker et al., 2006). Reassurance communicates that there is something wrong—saying "You'll be OK" indicates that you are not OK right now. These illness interaction patterns are common in children with somatic symptoms, who perceive their parents as providing more encouragement for illness behaviors than healthy children or even children with emotional problems (Walker et al., 1993; Walker & Zeman, 1992).

At the other end are parents who pay too little attention, so that the children are in situations with high distress and no guidance on how to manage symptoms. These are the parents who send the message "Suck it up" or "Deal with it," which at first glance may look like a functional message but actually is not helpful, because it gives the impression that the child just has to suffer through it without any guidance on what to do about the challenge. What we prefer is for children to participate in different situations *and* cope with them effectively. In the intervention sessions, we work on teaching the children tools to cope with the symptoms instead of just throwing them in a situation and hoping that they will float. Ensure that parents understand this subtle but important difference. The message that gets sent with "Suck it up" is that there must be something wrong with the child if he or she cannot engage in the situation without difficulty or symptoms. Everyone has a hard time in one way or another when they are in situations that cause them distress, particularly when they do not have a plan to deal with those challenges.

In either case, you as the therapist are a powerful model for how much attention to pay to the symptoms, which is a balance between asking too much and paying no attention at all. It takes a combination of acknowledgment, validation, and distraction, which we handle like this with our patient Johnny, who has abdominal pain:

> "Hi, Johnny. I hear from your mom that your stomach is hurting today. I'm glad you still came to the session, because this is exactly what we are working on, after all! First, let's try some of those coping skills we have been working on to see if we can change something about the situation or your body's responses. Then we'll keep going in treatment by learning some new skills today. Which strategy would you like to use?"

In this response, we are acknowledging symptoms—we are not just ignoring him—but doing so in a manner that does not reassure him, and we don't ask questions either. Note that we did not pull our emotions into it and say, "I'm sorry your stomach is hurting," or "It's sad that your stomach is hurting." Acknowledge the symptom and move along by providing a functional message and rationale for coping. As mentioned earlier, we have told parents on many occasions that we are prepared to give the trash can to a nauseated child as needed in the session. We have kept calm while patients had nonepileptic seizures as parents looked on fearfully, and when the child roused we all took a deep breath and continued our work. Although this was challenging for us, too, we succeeded in being a positive model of nonanxious coping. Through this process, you can teach a new way of coping adaptively with somatic symptoms for children and parents alike.

Another comment we make to parents around the idea of attention is that if they find themselves inclined to ask children how they are feeling, chances are they have observed something on children's faces or in their behavior that has led them to want to ask this question. Because parents are the ultimate experts in their children, we tell parents that if they are motivated to ask the question, then they already know the answer! So we suggest skipping the question and going to the solution, which is to offer a coping strategy. Asking children about symptoms only increases attention to negative cues, which activates all of the biopsychosocial factors that make the symptoms worse. Starting with the physical strategies, we instruct parents to cue children to engage in a healthy behavior, monitor/track what they are feeling, and move on with their daily schedule. As children move through treatment, parents can cue them on their other emotional, behavioral, and cognitive strategies as well.

One of the best ways we have found to help parents understand that attention to symptoms often worsens them is by using an example from early social development that everyone can remember and relate to:

DOCTOR: Children are social creatures. They look to parents for how to react in unfamiliar or scary situations. Remember when your child was a 1-year-old learning how to walk? All children in that situation toddle a few steps and at some point, they fall down. And what's the first thing they do? They look at you! They look right at your face to see your expression. And what you do with your face in that split second determines their reaction. Children are hardwired to get information about their surroundings by detecting their parents' emotions. If your face is full of concern and upset, what are they going to do?

MOTHER: Cry!

DOCTOR: Correct! Because your expression has communicated fear, they take away the message that something bad has happened to them and react accordingly. Now, what if you had a totally calm face? What are they going to do then?

MOTHER: Well, probably get up and keep walking.

DOCTOR: Yes! Because you have told them through your expression that this is a normal part of learning to walk and it is not dangerous. So when thinking about how to interact with children who have somatic symptoms, it is the very same dynamic that plays out. If a child grimaces in pain or stumbles and parents display fear or worry in their expressions or words, then that danger has been communicated, and the child will react like that 1-year-old who cries after falling down. Although it's really hard to do, we have to give them that "OK" look, because we know that falling down is part of learning how to walk. It's the same mentality with somatic symptoms, and it holds not only for making the "right" responses in the moment when children have symptoms, but also in avoiding asking children about how they feel.

The key to reassuring parents that it is safe and OK to do this for their own children with somatic symptoms is to tell them that in this situation, children are hurting but are not injured. When parents understand that somatic symptoms are real physical symptoms but not dangerous, they will be more ready to adopt this approach. Instead of symptoms, we ask parents to pay attention to the coping behaviors, as illustrated in the fourth tip.

PARENT TIP FOUR: PROMOTE POSITIVE COPING

By the time children and families seek treatment, there usually has been a lot of focus on and reinforcement, often unintentional, of illness behavior and minimal attention to times when the child has coped or functioned well. If children hear parents say, "School is really tough because of the symptoms," then the child is primed to pay attention to that pattern. The goal is for parents to focus on what children *can* do to shift the pattern of reinforcement to function and coping behaviors, and away from illness and disability. Then, if children hear parents say, "Symptoms are still there, but school is going well" those coping behaviors are more likely to continue.

Parents are typically very motivating influences in children's lives. Children have a desire to engage in behavior that they have been taught is positive from the time they were little and everyone in the room clapped when they sat up or crawled for the first time. When children have somatic symptoms and disengage from activities, the opportunities for positive reinforcement from family members also decline. When there are not as many events happening, it is hard to find things to give children credit for, and a lot of focus and concern is placed on symptoms and disability in the absence of anything else to discuss. For this parent tip to succeed, parents need to reinstate previous patterns of activity and reinforcement.

For anyone familiar with parent training for preschool behavior problems or parent–child interaction therapy, the gist of this recommendation is similar to those approaches in that we want parents to pay more attention to the positive behaviors (coping) than the negative ones (symptoms). In addition, parents need to praise the *effort*, not the outcome: "You used your relaxation—that's great!" instead of "You used your relaxation—did it make your symptoms go away?" We do not want children to think they "failed" if their chosen strategy does not work in the sense that symptoms did not disappear; many times, they will not. The important thing is that they tried it, they are functioning, and they can try a different strategy if symptoms are still a challenge. Teach parents to avoid questions that undermine the child's ability to function or are not things that children should have a choice about, such as "Do you want to go to school today?" The answer to that question for any child struggling with symptoms is almost always going to be "no." Instead, suggest that parents reinforce function by stating what children need to do, and then provide choices around how they can cope by saying, "*When* you go to school today, *which* coping skills would you like to use?" or remind them of rewards for positive functioning by saying, "When you come home from school today, what would you like to do to reward yourself for staying all day?" That way, parents maintain confidence in the child's ability and provide coping encouragement and support. Changing the focus to positive aspects of treatment and recovery prevents an overfocus on illness behavior or functional deficits.

One of the most challenging situations in treatment is when families have subscribed to an illness identity, as they tend to have a very hard time focusing on positive coping behaviors because it takes them away from the illness focus that has come to mean something important to them. Families can easily become overly invested in the label or diagnosis of the symptoms, which seems positive at first because it finally explains the symptoms that have been so hard to understand; however, this identification can backfire because it brings additional attention to the symptoms and provides justification for the lack of function. Think, "He cannot do that, he has chronic pain," or "She has conversion disorder, so she does not handle stress well." Neither statement is really true or helpful; an overinvestment in the diagnosis can spell disaster for a return to functioning. One of the reasons for this is that instead of the child being a son/daughter, athlete, musician, friend, sibling, scout, or artist who *happens* to have pain, dizziness, or neurological symptoms, he or she becomes a syncope, or pain, or conversion disorder child. The diagnosis and associated deficits become the child's whole life, and therefore the primary factor in all decision making. This is a difficult situation for the child to be in because somatic symptoms are always going to make the child decide to stay home when given the option, and there will be few opportunities for positive, functional coping to reinforce. We want to support the more flexible, accepting, sometimes harder approach of "I have this, but it does not have me. It does not make my choices," which requires the support of the parents. If you notice this pattern of illness identification in children or their parents, address it to ensure you are working toward similar goals to live a life outside of symptoms.

The other side of the equation is when parents get so invested in treatment and the idea of a return to function that they encourage children to engage in *more* function than is recommended, especially at first. Inadvertently, this sends the message to children that if they struggle (as most would), they are not working hard enough to use their skills, and it also runs the risk of having the child *overdo* activity, which can increase symptoms. If indicated, it can be worthwhile to have a conversation with parents about patience as they support their children in rebuilding normal functional routines, which happens best over time.

PARENT TIP FIVE: RESPOND FLEXIBLY

No parent wants his or her child to suffer. However, when children learn new skills to manage symptoms, they will not be able to cure themselves overnight, so some challenges are expected as children go through treatment and practice their skills outside of session. Parents are children's primary supports at home, and teaching parents to adopt a flexible style will enable them to best assist their children in coping engagement on the home front.

Parents often ask, "What is the one strategy that will help my child the most?" Our answer to that is "Flexibility." There simply is not one best way to manage somatic symptoms. There is not one perfect strategy, or one perfect sentence, or one perfect word of love or support. But there is one concept: *flexibility*. Parents have to be able to look at the circumstances, figure out what children are going through, and help them choose from their toolbox of strategies; the most effective strategy will be different based on those factors. As long as parents keep the overall focus on function, how they get there might look quite different from moment to moment or day to day. This is in effect what we do as mental health providers—when a child walks into the office with a symptom complaint, there is no big book of perfect solutions to consult. It takes flexibility in all settings to best help children cope. Upon hearing this, many parents express relief that there is not a grand solution that has been eluding them. Research has also supported the positive benefits of flexibility in coping style among parents of children with chronic pain (McCracken & Gauntlett-Gilbert, 2011).

It can be challenging to work with parents on developing a flexible style, especially if parents are focused on a "cure" or still searching for an organic cause for the symptoms. In that case, they may not be focused on helping the child cope with the symptoms because they are waiting to see if the next medical opinion might yield a quick fix. Parents in this position often take a black-and-white approach to managing children's symptom complaints, such as either saying, "If you have symptoms, stay home from school," or "If you don't have symptoms, go to school." For successful treatment of somatic symptoms, parents have to be less rigid, gauge the context of the situation, and approach it from a flexible standpoint. In this case, that might be saying instead "What are some strategies you can use if you have symptoms while you are at school?" The way to communicate this message to families in this situation is to go back to the basis of treatment for somatic symptoms, which relies on the understanding that the child has already undergone a medical evaluation that has ruled out dangerous causes for symptoms. Treating somatic symptoms can feel like a leap of faith, and parents and children have to trust you and the team to guide them along this path. It is reasonable to tell the family that regardless of the origin of symptoms, this flexible approach to coping with symptoms will be helpful. We tell parents whether the cause of the symptoms is organic, such as seizures stemming from electrical discharges in the brain, or somatic, such as seizures stemming from difficulty coping with stress and autonomic arousal, the child still has the symptoms and still needs to figure out ways to minimize their impact and impairment by coping with them flexibly. We do not usually stop families from seeking other medical evaluations; however, if parents are working up to a sixth or seventh opinion, it may be appropriate to have a conversation about the effect that continued medical evaluations are having on the child from the standpoint of fear or anxiety, and determine whether each visit is adding information or a repetition of similar information.

If families are concerned about how to handle a new symptom or a symptom that seems different than usual, it can be helpful to have a plan in place for the child and parent to deal with that situation.

First, identify the symptom, then ask the following questions:

- Is it happening in a different location?
- Does it feel different than usual (sensation, intensity)?
- Did something happen to cause it (injury, food, exercise, heat)?
- Does the place where the symptom is look different (color, swelling, position)?
- Are the usual coping strategies failing to help?
- Is the child unable to do the activities he or she usually does, even when symptoms are present?

If the answer to some or most of these questions is yes, it is reasonable to have that symptom evaluated by the child's medical provider. If not, the child and family are encouraged to use their somatic symptom coping tools. Chapter 11 covers collaboration with health care colleagues; these are the types of questions to review with the child's medical provider to ensure all members of the team are giving the same message about symptoms and agree with the medical aspects of the treatment plan.

All families just want the symptoms to go away. That's how the medical model usually works: symptoms, treatment, cure. As we have discussed, that is not the story for somatic symptoms; instead, we have to approach somatic symptoms flexibly, which also means being flexible in our expectations for how we define a "cure." For us, that is when children are back to their normal lives, participating in their activities, and managing symptoms effectively if they arise.

PARENTS' OWN EMOTIONAL DISTRESS

Sometimes parents' own emotional distress gets in the way of children's treatment. Parents worry about children's medical problems, particularly when the diagnosis is uncertain, as is the case with somatic symptoms (Jessop & Stein, 1985). Parents who are anxious are more likely to take their children to the doctor and think their symptoms are more severe compared to nonanxious parents (Hatcher, Powers, & Richtsmeier, 1993), and parents of children with somatic symptoms are more likely to be anxious compared to parents of healthy children (Walker & Greene, 1989). With parents' primary role in managing illness in children, it is essential to understand the influence of parental emotional distress in response to children's symptoms to move forward in treatment.

If you are finding that progress is hampered not because of the child's symptoms and impairment, but because parents are struggling with their own anxiety about the child's symptoms and it is preventing progress in therapy, it is appropriate to discuss the impact of parental anxiety on the child. Here, we address anxiety in the parent–child interaction around increasing function in Ashley, our patient with cardiac symptoms:

DOCTOR: I just wanted to check in to see how you feel it's been going now that Ashley is working on improving her function using her coping skills.

MOTHER: Well, I've done what you told me to, like not asking too many questions and not doing everything for her anymore, which I think is going well for her, but it still feels like a really big change for me. I liked being more involved.

DOCTOR: Well, you do not have to stop asking questions altogether! We just want to try to focus more on function than on symptoms, and one of the ways to do that is to reduce questions about symptoms. I know that's still a really big change for you to make.

MOTHER: I am still convinced there is something else wrong with Ashley. There must be a medical explanation for her problems. Do you think it might be a significant problem we should get checked out? What if she has cancer?

DOCTOR: Well, you've had her medical specialists agree that there is nothing dangerous happening in Ashley's body, so for now we are just focusing on her coping with the symptoms and getting back to her usual schedule.

MOTHER: OK. I just really worry a lot.

ASHLEY: My mom worries more than I do and thinks of things I don't, like what if I fall and hurt myself when I pass out. Or what if my heart stops in the middle of the night.

MOTHER: I do. I just do not want anything to happen. I know she's almost an adult and she can probably do a lot on her own now, but I am just so scared something will happen and I won't be there to be able to help her.

DOCTOR: That's an example of what Ashley has been working on to manage negative thoughts, all those "what if" type of thoughts that are often worst-case scenario types of thoughts, because we know those only increase attention to symptoms and challenges.

MOTHER: Oh, I have some of those too. I'd really rather always be prepared. Is it my fault she is having such a hard time? Did I not do something right?

DOCTOR: Not at all! Ashley's symptoms are no one's fault, least of all hers or yours, but there are definitely times when parents' thoughts can lead to more anxiety in children, which can activate Ashley's sympathetic nervous system and make her symptoms more impairing. What you think about her is pretty important and she pays attention to it! Ashley has mentioned that she worries about increasing your stress.

MOTHER: Oh, she does, she's my good kid. Always makes sure she follows the rules. But I don't need her to be worrying about me. I just need her to get better.

DOCTOR: Yes, and one of the ways she is learning to cope with her symptoms is to manage her negative thoughts about success or failure and use more neutral thoughts that, regardless of the outcome, she will be able to handle it. So instead of having her stay home because you are worried she will hurt herself, what would you think about letting the worry take a back seat and choosing to do something based on whether or not you two would actually like to do it? You could go out to lunch, somewhere close by and familiar that does not involve a lot of walking, and see how it goes. The worst thing that would happen is that Ashley would pass out, and you've already handled that situation, so while it's not ideal, it wouldn't be a disaster, and the best-case scenario is that you have a great lunch.

ASHLEY: And the neutral is that we get out of the house and the lunch is just OK!

DOCTOR: Exactly.

MOTHER: I don't know, if you think that is OK we could try it. I understand what you are saying about reducing my worries and how that will help Ashley, but that is really hard!

DOCTOR: Ashley has really done a great job with this, so it is OK to follow her lead. This is a way you can support her efforts to be more active and confront her own worries about negative outcomes, even if you're not sure yourself!

Addressing parent mood concerns is outside the scope of this book and of treatment of the child for somatic symptoms, but it is appropriate to refer parents for their own mental health support if indicated.

In addition to anxiety in the parent, somatic symptoms can also be influenced by the larger family system. Some children may notice that their symptoms play a larger role in the family dynamic, such as a child who recognizes that his symptoms keep his parents from fighting and is afraid that if he gets better, his parents will go back to a conflictual communication style. Children of divorced parents may notice that they see their noncustodial parent more often when they are in the hospital or when they have to stay home from school. More commonly, family sleeping arrangements change when children have somatic symptoms. This often involves one parent sleeping with the child while the other parent remains in the parents' bedroom, or one parent is ousted from his or her own bed to the couch so the child can sleep in the parents' bed. If sleeping arrangements are not easily returned to normal through healthy habit intervention, it is worth it to have a conversation with the parent regarding what other barriers exist to getting the child back to sleeping independently, and if there are relationship factors between the parents that are perpetuating the sleeping arrangement. While it is beyond the scope of treating the child with somatic symptoms to address parent relationship issues, it is helpful to at least clarify the other sources of the problem to effectively change the behavior you are targeting. Additionally, sometimes parents have changed their work schedule or quit their job altogether to provide round-the-clock care for their child with somatic symptoms, and it is important to address these factors with parents as well as ensure that the parents' role in caring for the child is not a barrier to improved function.

Finally, some parents struggle with guilt that they did not seek out this type of intervention sooner, that there is not an easy fix for the symptoms, that the child is suffering at all, or that they cannot find the "answer." Address this and normalize it. First, parents did not know the first time the child had the symptoms that they might end up being chronic and require a different treatment approach than anticipated, and second, their reactions were normal. After all, if the small child learning to walk in the earlier example falls down and scrapes up both knees, it is normal and appropriate to look and act concerned. Overall, the treatment of somatic symptoms is a big adjustment for the whole family, and it is important to support them in treatment as well.

COMMUNITY INTERACTIONS

Outside of communicating with schools, which we address in the next chapter, parents frequently ask how to explain or talk about symptoms with siblings, extended family, babysitters, and other community members (e.g., sports teams, scouts, religious organizations). We encourage you to provide families with the specific symptom "Fact Sheets" (in the Appendix) as a way to provide information to community members.

For parents who are concerned about play dates with peers, and how friends' parents can manage symptoms, think about it from a graded exposure perspective. Start small and work up to the end goal. If a parent has a concern about whether the child can handle a sleepover at a friend's house, start with an afternoon play date first. Encourage the parent to have a conversation with the peer's parent about what to expect and how to manage symptoms if they arise. This is a great way to practice managing somatic symptoms outside of the home; most children enjoy playing with their friends and often name seeing friends as a good distracting or pleasant activity. Plan on an hour at first, then build up to two. After the child has conquered that, come up with a plan for sleepovers, such as having one at the child's home first before going over to a friend's home, then have one at the home of a good friend whose parent will be around for help. This is a great exercise for the parent and child to engage in together in session while modeling problem solving for how they can take their coping plan into the community.

The process is similar for adolescents spending more time away from home. Encourage the teen and parent to pick a peer with whom they feel close, explain the symptoms and the coping plan, and choose a mildly challenging activity (e.g., seeing a movie rather than walking around the mall). Sometimes this kind of community engagement planning can be more anxiety provoking for the parent than for the adolescent: What if he passes out and hits his head? What if she has an episode in public? Many teens have actually already experienced their symptoms in public; remind them they've already gotten through an episode in public and lived to tell about it. Next time, they'll have more skills to use!

When parents ask, "But what if it happens in the community?" we are honest in saying that there is always a chance a symptom flare could happen anywhere. The message is that children have to live their lives *anyway*; everyone has the chance of something negative happening, whether we know about it or not, and worse yet, there are so many positive experiences that are missed by staying home! Children with epilepsy go to school, participate in sleepovers, and play sports, all situations in which they might have a seizure. Children with diabetes go on field trips, to musical performances, and competitions, and any of those situations may lead to a low blood sugar. The way to manage these situations effectively is to plan ahead; know the situations in which the symptoms might be more likely to happen, be prepared with coping tools, use them, know who is there for support, and continue participating. The coping tools might be fast-acting carbohydrates to increase blood sugar for diabetes or diaphragmatic breathing to hit the brakes on a racing nervous system for somatic symptoms, but they are all coping tools nonetheless. As therapists, parents, coaches, and teachers, we cannot limit children with somatic symptoms from normal activities; it will reduce function and prolong symptom impairment. If parents are worried about whether helpers will understand what to do if symptoms do happen outside the home, there is no harm in putting parent contact information and a brief description of symptoms in the child's phone, on a piece of paper to be kept in the wallet or backpack, or on an ID bracelet.

CHAPTER SUMMARY AND TAKE-AWAY POINTS

- Parents are a child's main support in using coping skills to manage somatic symptoms. Parents structure the child's environment, interact with him or her around symptoms, and have their own emotional response to the child's symptoms. Address parents' functioning with their child in all of these roles to promote the most effective coping in the home setting.

- The role of the therapist in working with parents is to model calm coping with somatic symptoms, as well as help parents encourage normal activity, tolerate distress and remain calm, balance attention to symptoms, promote positive coping, and respond flexibly to challenges.

- Pay close attention to parental anxiety or mood concerns, as well as larger family systems issues and whether they are creating obstacles for the child in treatment. Help children and parents create successful community communication and coping plans.

CHAPTER 10

School

The school environment is arguably the most important context in which children function outside of their family environment. Going to school for a child is like going to a job for an adult—it represents the most basic aspect of a child's function. It would be very concerning if an adult was unable to work due to his or her health status, and the same is true of children when it comes to school. In some sense, it is even *more* concerning when a child misses school than when an adult misses work because of the disruption to developmental milestones and achievements that can have repercussions in future years. Children with somatic symptoms should attend school in the most typical setting possible. Participating in daily, developmentally appropriate activities, *school included,* is not only critical for educational development, but also teaches children's bodies to effectively cope with symptoms by engaging in regular function. However, as indicated throughout the book, children with somatic symptoms often demonstrate significant problems with school. For these reasons, it is essential to address children's school functioning as part of their somatic symptom treatment.

There are many obstacles during the school day that pose significant challenges to children with somatic symptoms. First is school attendance; just successfully attending school and staying for the full day can be a challenge for children who are struggling to make it out of bed in the morning when they are not feeling well. Second, school performance factors, including academic abilities as well as social and physical functioning, are challenging for children with somatic symptoms. Finally, children struggle with their ability to cope with symptoms in the school setting. Attending school requires children to be more independent in their coping abilities and to use their skills without family support in a setting that is more rigid, often with rules and restrictions that may make it even harder for them to cope with symptoms, and around peers who may also negatively impact their perceived ability to cope. Taken together, challenges in all three of these areas can conspire against children to make getting to school, staying in school, or being successful there a near impossible task. Even if children report that they are attending school, be sure to follow up on whether they are staying there for the full day, succeeding in their work, and coping with symptoms. Even when children are physically in the building, most children with somatic symptoms tell us that they aren't really "there" in terms of their attentional capacity to learn, emotional capacity to interact with their peers and teachers, or their ability to effectively cope with their symptoms in that setting.

While it is widely accepted that children with somatic symptoms have significant difficulty when it comes to functioning in school, there is little research on the topic. The few studies that have been conducted demonstrate that school impairment goes beyond the struggle with somatic symptoms and represents a true biopsychosocial challenge of physical symptoms, emotional functioning, and social participation (Chan, Piira, & Betts, 2005). Among children with chronic pain syndromes, those with high levels of impairment related to their symptoms have frequent school absences and poor academic performance, more so among older children with multiple symptoms and those with comorbid depression (Zernikow et al., 2012). In addition, teens with chronic pain who have poor social functioning have more school impairment than children with good social functioning (Simons, Logan, Chastain, & Stein, 2010). In a study of children with chronic abdominal pain, children had lower expectations of their own performance on an academic task, more sympathetic nervous system arousal in response to success, and more symptoms in response to failure on academic tasks compared to healthy children (Puzanovova et al., 2009). Recall from Chapter 2, the study of children with conversion disorder that showed deficits in attention, executive function, and memory, but similar intelligence and overall cognitive function compared to healthy children, suggesting that specific learning deficits impeded their educational performance beyond the negative impact of the symptoms (Kozlowska et al., 2015). In all, these research findings suggest that the impairment that children with somatic symptoms experience in the school setting interacts strongly with biological, psychological, and social factors. Thus, providing support for children in the school setting at all of these levels is essential to creating a positive learning environment in which children can engage.

In this chapter, we'll address how to help children manage these challenges in several ways, including helping them succeed in school based on their level of impairment, advantages and disadvantages of different school environments, facilitating communication with school staff about somatic symptoms and children's needs, and understanding the resources that are available in schools. In terms of how to incorporate this information into your treatment, while we address these school challenges in the final section of the book, they should be attended to throughout treatment, including assessment and intervention. There are different avenues for working with schools to help children be more successful in that setting. We recommend you use these ideas with the children you are treating as needed.

SCHOOL IMPAIRMENT

When discussing children's school function, first get a good understanding of their level of impairment in school due to symptoms, as well as the reasons that school is challenging. This provides a good basis from which to create and enact a successful school plan and is typically done during the assessment process. In addition to the questions listed in Chapter 4, specific school assessment questions include:

- *Attendance*: Are they attending school? What is the setting? Are they missing partial days or full days? Are absences excused/is there a problem with truancy?
- *Performance*: Are grades declining? Are they passing or failing? Are they missing assignments?
- *Challenges*: Do they struggle with academics (e.g., concentration, memory), physical challenges (e.g., stairs, gym class), peers (e.g., bullying, teasing about symptoms)?
- *Accommodations*: What does the school know about the symptoms? Has the school done anything to help? What do the children and families think would help?

This information provides a better understanding of children's overall experience in school and is a basis from which to formulate ideas about specific school interventions that will improve function. To aid in the process, school impairment can be conceptualized in three levels with associated school recommendations; low, moderate, and high.

In a low school impairment situation, children are attending school and keeping up with work overall, but some factors in the school setting could be improved to help them cope better with symptoms. In that case, the goals of treatment are to help children apply coping strategies in the school setting and check in about school engagement as treatment progresses. A school letter would generally not need to be written.

Children with low to moderate school impairment, like our patient Johnny, are enrolled in school but have some absences or are unable to stay for a full day. Children with a moderate to high level of school impairment, like our patient Alex, have a significant number of absences, and are experiencing a decline in their usual grades or ability to keep up with schoolwork. In both of these cases, address school impairment at the beginning of treatment, such as in the first intervention session when addressing establishment of a normal routine. A school letter would need to be written to communicate about the child's symptoms and recommended accommodations for children with these levels of impairment.

Children with a high level of school impairment, like our patient Ashley, are either out of school entirely, enrolled in homebound or online school due to absences from illness, or are failing their classes. In this case, there is benefit to first getting the child engaged in CBT to learn coping strategies, working with the family to at least stabilize the school situation for the time being, and then addressing a more formal school reentry plan once the child has established more basic patterns of function, improved emotional coping, and better symptom management. It is helpful to communicate with the school briefly at the beginning of treatment so they know the child's status and that he or she will be working up to returning to school. Then, you will need to work closely with the school to create a reentry plan once the child has progressed in treatment.

Overall, when discussing school impairment, these guidelines can be useful for case conceptualization and for formulating an initial treatment plan; however, this is an area of intervention that is highly individual in terms of what will be successful for helping the child address educational challenges. Perhaps more than any other aspect of treatment for somatic symptoms, school plans are not one size fits all, and flexibility is key in terms of making educational recommendations. What *is* the same for all children is that education is nonnegotiable; therefore, it is not a choice whether or not a child will pursue education (at least until he or she is old enough to choose otherwise!), but there are many choices about *how* a child does that, and that is exactly the place for creative intervention. More and more, there are many educational supports that can be implemented in a child's current school setting that are beneficial in addressing challenging schooling situations. Specific examples of accommodations are covered later in the chapter; here are a few innovative examples of creative educational accommodations that have worked well for children with somatic symptoms:

- Late start/study hall first thing in the morning to warm up to the school day.
- Structuring a well-balanced schedule so that the first class of the day isn't the hardest and the morning and afternoon are equally weighted in terms of class difficulty.
- Including electives to look forward to during the day.
- Adding a guided study hall to the schedule for instructional support.
- Setting a goal that children will get to school in some capacity every day, even if they have to go in a class period late or go to the nurse's office first thing upon arriving.
- Taking one class online to minimize in-school time and concentration demand.
- Making sure a friend is in lunch or in difficult classes for support.
- Providing alternate activities for gym class (e.g., do own exercises, permission to pace activity).
- Educating other children in the grade about the condition so there is a shared understanding of how to provide support and interact in the school setting (e.g., have the child or teacher present to class, hold a small assembly).
- Identifying a point person (e.g., teacher, nurse, coach) so there is someone to check in with who is up to date about the condition and can provide support in the school setting.
- Dropping down a level from advanced placement to honors or from honors to regular education classes in subjects that are very challenging or stressful.

Through implementation of these supports, children are still able to work toward their educational goals, but in flexible ways that alleviate specific difficulties, thereby keeping them more engaged in the overall academic environment. The more successful they are in school, the more stress will be alleviated, impairment will improve, and even the symptoms themselves may get better or will be more easily managed. It is truly a win–win situation when creative solutions such as these provide so much benefit to children's everyday lives.

One of the hardest conversations to have with children and families related to school impairment is whether children should change school situations entirely rather than have accommodations made in their current school situations. There are two different school settings to be aware of that families may consider as alternate schooling choices for a child who is experiencing school impairment due to somatic symptoms. One is homebound instruction, in which the child remains enrolled in his or her regular school but completes the curriculum at home with the aid of a teacher who comes to the home at least 1 hour a week. This schooling arrangement usually requires the signature of a physician (typically we work with the child's primary care physician for this) and is time limited, as it is designed as a short-term solution for providing children with education while they are recovering from an illness that keeps them from attending school. The other is taking children out of the school system entirely, essentially withdrawing them, and completing a homeschool program either online (many states have free online educational programs) or through a private homeschool program that provides a curriculum that the family follows with the child.

When you are asked whether a child should change his or her school setting, which you *will* be asked at some point in your treatment of children with somatic symptoms, first ask to the child and family: "Imagine that you didn't have these symptoms. What kind of school setup do you think would be best in that case? Would you stay with what you have now or would you want something different?" Posing these questions helps children and families get to the core of what type of educational environment is best for the *child*. In our experience, sticking to the school setting that children and families feel is best based on children's personality and educational characteristics—and not symptoms—is the course that is the most effective. When children and families make schooling decisions based solely or primarily on symptoms, they get away from placing the focus on the child, and as a result, too much emphasis is placed on symptoms. This reactive rather than proactive decision reinforces the cycle of symptoms and disability, which is the opposite of what children are being encouraged to do in treatment: to break out of a disabled pattern into a functional one.

Now, if a child and family asked whether a child should be homeschooled because of symptoms and shared that they had long thought about homeschooling, other children in the family are homeschooled, and this is an education style that the family values, then those would be good reasons to pursue homeschooling—*but for those reasons and not in response to the symptoms*. If the answer is no, the family never would have considered homeschooling if these symptoms had not caused so many problems, the recommendation would be to advocate more strongly for making accommodations within the existing school setting.

There are few situations that we can recall from our clinical practice in which a child changed from a regular school setting to a homeschool setting due to somatic symptoms and the change was successful in the long term; however, we can recall more children we have worked with who have been unhappy with homeschooling and realized that they would be better off in a regular school setting. We also have worked with some families who have found educational settings that are still regular school settings but are more suited to the child's overall personality and have provided successful changes for the child. For example, a shy and anxious child with chronic headaches changed from a large school setting that was stressful and increased symptoms, to a smaller school setting that was better suited to his personality where he had improved symptom management and better grades. We have also worked with children who have engaged in homebound instruction effectively on a short-term basis with a successful transition back to a traditional brick-and-mortar school. Again, these decisions should be informed by getting to the core of *why* a family wants to change a school setting, which should be more about the child and less about the symptoms.

Finally, especially for older children and adolescents, a motivational interviewing style of conversation can be useful when discussing educational goals and creating an effective school plan. Making the connection between where they are now and their future can be very motivating for teens, helping them gain the momentum to improve current school dysfunction, especially when they feel that nothing about 10th-grade history will matter in their futures. We illustrate this with Ashley, our patient with cardiac symptoms, who has a high level of school impairment, and to whom we introduce school reentry after completing all levels of intervention:

DOCTOR: Now that you have been learning the coping tools to manage symptoms, let's talk about one of the functional goals that we haven't worked on yet: getting back to school.

ASHLEY: Yeah, I'm not sure about that one. I mean, homeschool isn't ideal, I miss my friends, and the program I'm doing at home is boring, but there were so many problems when I was in school that I just don't know if I could ever be successful there.

DOCTOR: You had a tough time when you were in school, from what you have told me. It sounds like the school didn't have a good understanding of your symptoms or what you needed for support.

ASHLEY: Yeah, you could say that again.

DOCTOR: When we talk about setting educational goals, it can help to think about future goals. What would you like to do for a career?

ASHLEY: Well, definitely something in the medical field. I'd like to be a doctor, or maybe a physician's assistant, or a nurse practitioner.

DOCTOR: Those are awesome career goals! I could see you doing really well in any of those roles. I bet you could help others understand difficult medical situations like yours.

ASHLEY: Yeah, I will know what to do for other people like me, based on my experience!

DOCTOR: So, thinking about that future goal of working in health care, what do you need to do to get from this point today to that point in the future?

ASHLEY: Truthfully? I'd just like to fast-forward from this point to that point. I just feel really stuck at the moment. I know that this homeschool program is not the best education to prepare me for college, but I just can't imagine going back to school.

DOCTOR: Fast-forwarding would be a good option in the sense that you'd be able to get to that exciting point of doing what you want to do very quickly, but you'd be missing some pretty important steps along the way, wouldn't you?

ASHLEY: Well, I suppose college and medical school are pretty important!

DOCTOR: I would say so! It can be really hard to see yourself getting from point A to point Z when you've had so many challenges, but as you pointed out, there are a lot of experiences that will matter between A and Z ... like all of the other letters! Let's focus on taking small steps to move your education along right now, like telling the school about your condition, coming up with an accommodation plan, and making a slow transition back, all the while remembering the reason *why* you are doing it: for your future! Although it may not seem like it, every step of your education leads you to that job you want to have in health care. Focusing on how these are positive steps toward your future goals is a way of feeling less stuck and more confident.

ASHLEY: I never thought about it like that. I like that way of thinking.

In addition to motivational strategies, never underestimate the power of the coping tools that children learn through the intervention as applied to improving school attendance and performance. A good example of this comes from one of our patients who was approaching a stressful week of testing in school and feeling an increase in stress and symptoms as the deadlines loomed. Positively, she noticed that when she engaged in healthy habits (especially keeping to a good sleep schedule), took study breaks by engaging in pleasant activities, and told herself exams were "no big deal," she not only got all A's on her exams but succeeded in keeping worry and somatic symptoms at bay for the duration of the week. Remind children that while there are some special considerations to be made when it comes to ensuring a good school environment, they have also learned a lot of coping tools that are highly effective for handling school stress and reducing disability. This sends the message that it is a two-way street when it comes to improving school functioning—not only focusing on what the child can do but also what the school can do, which we now address.

SCHOOL COMMUNICATION

When working with children with any level of school impairment, but particularly for moderate and high levels of impairment, facilitating communication with school staff about somatic symptoms and what children need in terms of accommodations to be successful in the school setting is an essential part of treatment. If you haven't had a lot of experience working with schools, it is difficult to know which staff to work with or even what to ask for in terms of what schools are willing and able to do for students. Even if you have experience interacting with schools and advocating for students, it can be challenging to know exactly how to communicate with schools regarding somatic symptoms, in particular. In this section, we address these challenges as well as walk you through the way we communicate with schools in our school letter template.

In terms of staff, there are many people in a school setting who could potentially be great partners to work with to improve a child's school functioning. Some key school personnel include principals, vice principals, guidance counselors, school psychologists, teachers, nurses, secretaries, and aides. Sometimes families already have been working with someone, and it can be helpful to talk to that person to get a sense of who the key players are in that school setting. If children or families do not have a good sense of who to work with, it is good to start with the guidance counselor. Schools have very good resources online, so it is quite easy to find names and contact information if families do not have them readily available. Families often need to sign a release to facilitate school communication, per the guidelines of your institution or practice. It is helpful to keep a copy of the release handy, as sometimes schools request a copy.

When beginning communication with the school, first, educate school staff about the somatic symptom condition. Similar to how treatment is structured with education provided prior to teaching coping skills, it is most successful to first educate the school about the child's condition before launching into the recommendations for school support. Schools are much more willing to make accommodations when they understand where they come from and why they will help children improve school function. Without that explanation, it can sound like a lot of requests for a child whom the school may not see as needing extra help. For example, a study of teachers' understanding of chronic pain syndromes reflected a poor understanding of the biopsychosocial nature of the condition, with a preference for a medical explanation of the condition and more favorable responses to students when they had a physiological understanding of the condition (Logan, Simons, Stein, & Chastain, 2008). This study underscores the importance not only of educating school staff about the psychosocial nature of all chronic conditions, but also reinforcing the medical nature of the symptoms that children experience to promote the best understanding.

With these ideas in mind, we are going to walk you through using the template of our standard school letter, which we view as the first step in communicating with the school. After the school receives the letter, a follow-up phone call may be warranted to further expand on these points. The letter is the best way to start communication, as it allows for full explanation of the condition and suggested accommodations that can easily be shared among school personnel (vs. a phone conversation that may be relayed with less accuracy). We address each paragraph individually to explain the rationale and discuss communication tips. The "General School Letter Template" is provided in the Appendix. As you read the template, remember that you can tailor it to add details about the specific symptom presentation and choose accommodations depending on the child's needs. While we have distilled the template down to the most common recommendations that we make for children to succeed in the school setting, there are some factors that may or may not be required in certain situations. Our general rule is that if it is not a problem, then we do not address it in the letter. Only focus on what the school needs to understand about the child's condition or do for him or her; otherwise the letter will become unwieldy, or it will seem that you don't have an appreciation for what they have already done to help the child. Sometimes we need an additional recommendation beyond the general template, and we will address several common additions that you can incorporate in the letter as needed. We think it is safe to say that no two school letters are alike!

To begin the letter, we describe the details pertinent to the child, including an explanation of the diagnosis and introduction to the treatment the child is receiving. Remember that you are communicating with non–health care professionals, so use as many lay terms as possible. We like to strike a balance, providing enough information to effectively communicate about the condition while not giving so much information that it becomes overwhelming or that the person receiving the letter stops reading. We will begin by presenting an example of the letter we would send to the school attended by our patient Johnny, who has low to moderate school impairment from his abdominal pain condition:

```
Dear Administration:

This letter is to confirm that fourth-grade student Johnny
is receiving cognitive-behavioral therapy (CBT) in our
Psychology Clinic. Specifically, Johnny is receiving
treatment for functional gastrointestinal disorders (FGIDs),
specifically abdominal pain and irritable bowel syndrome,
which are chronic medical conditions characterized by
abdominal pain and diarrhea/constipation caused by a
disorder in the brain-gut interaction. The symptoms are
real, but are not dangerous in the sense that they are
not caused by acute illness, injury, or disease. These
challenging problems have interfered with Johnny's ability
to attend a regular school day and keep up with his work
this academic year. We appreciate all you have done to
support him in school. As a child psychologist specializing
in somatic symptoms, I am working with Johnny, his family,
and his medical team to help manage his symptoms and
increase his ability to function.
```

For children with neurological, cardiac, or pain symptoms, revise the text to reflect those symptom descriptions from the symptom "Fact Sheets" and consider providing a copy of that handout to the school along with the school letter.

Once we have introduced the name of the problem and the specific symptoms the child experiences, we then like to emphasize how the mind and the body both contribute to the condition to best represent the equally important roles of physical and psychological health. We also address the "realness" of the condition:

```
Somatic symptoms have both physical and psychosocial
components. Physically, it's difficult for children with
somatic symptoms to remain in school for a full day. For
Johnny, being dehydrated and having limited bathroom
breaks make stomach symptoms hard to manage. Waking up
early in the morning and the demand on concentration are
additional physical challenges. Like any medical condition,
somatic symptoms are made worse by emotional and social
stress, so it is typical for Johnny's symptoms to increase
on school days when he encounters worry or frustration
with academic work and difficulty coping with symptoms.
Our recommendations include a variety of strategies aimed
at improving attendance and school performance as well as
managing stressful situations that may worsen the cycle
```

of symptoms and disability. Please keep in mind that while stress and symptoms are closely related, this does *not* mean that Johnny's symptoms are made up or that psychosocial challenges alone cause the symptoms.

On occasion, we have had to engage in further conversation with schools around the nature of somatic symptoms, particularly if school personnel questions the reality of a child's symptoms or feel that the child is fabricating symptoms for secondary gain. This seems to occur more in situations when school staff feel they have observed the child looking "perfectly well" during preferred activities, such as lunch or extracurriculars, and having symptoms only when asked to do something that is disliked, such as a test or a difficult class. In these cases, it is helpful to further educate the school regarding the nature of somatic symptoms, adding information such as this:

Somatic symptom intensity fluctuates. Children often ignore or distract themselves from symptoms by functioning in positive activities and then experience more symptoms during times of stress, leading to varying levels of observable symptoms and distress. In a school setting, this can result in Johnny appearing to be quite "well" at times and in significant pain at other times, which can be misleading and cause confusion about the nature of symptoms, particularly when Johnny appears well during fun activities and distressed during a math test. However, when this presentation leads to Johnny being questioned about how "real" the condition is, or to asking him to wait before using a coping skill (e.g., getting water or taking a break), this only adds stress and frustration for him. Eliminating questions about the validity of his condition is the most helpful approach for promoting Johnny's ability to positively manage symptoms.

Next, we introduce the recommendations by assuring the school that despite the condition, it is safe and OK for the child to attend school. If the school is uncertain about a child's condition or there has been confusion on their part as to whether (or how) the child should attend school, they will look to you, in consultation with the medical team, to ensure that the child can return to or remain in his or her educational setting. We also like to indicate that these accommodations should be in place for the length of time that they will be helpful for the child as opposed to a specific time frame:

We strongly encourage children like Johnny with this condition to engage in as much normal functioning as possible, including attending school. This condition is not associated with any specific timeline in terms of recovery, which varies greatly by individual. It would be helpful for Johnny to have a *flexible* school plan that meets his

educational needs while he engages in treatment by allowing
the following accommodations:

Sometimes, families explicitly ask for past or future illness-related absences to
be excused, particularly if they live in a state or district that pursues truancy charges
against families with children who have missed more days of school than are allowed.
In our experience, school absence issues are one of the trickiest balances to strike with
families. On the one hand, excusing any absences, past or future, goes against every
one of our treatment recommendations, which are all focused on improving function and attending school. On the other hand, families are understandably stressed
by the prospect of truancy charges, and stress exacerbates the challenges of getting
the child back to regular school attendance if it is perceived that the family is "fighting" against the school. Therefore, starting with a "blank slate" when getting back
to school can be beneficial to achieve improved school function. For those reasons,
we will excuse past absences when needed, making it clear to the child, family, and
school that going forward, the expectation is for positive school attendance and no
more absence forgiveness for not managing symptoms in a functional manner. To do
this, we would add a sentence like this:

Please excuse Johnny's absences up to this point in the
school year for medical reasons; going forward, we expect
Johnny to attend school daily and the family will need
to provide medical documentation for any future absences
related to acute illness.

Then, we address the specific recommendations that we make for children to
be successful in school. When deciding on the accommodations that are appropriate for the child, it is challenging to know where to draw the line between providing
appropriate accommodations to help a child cope with the demands of a stressful setting and unintentionally rewarding or reinforcing poor coping by excusing the child
from activities that reinforce the avoidance cycle. For each recommendation, we try
to address this challenge by asking for the accommodation and explaining why it is
helpful to the child in the school context. We have heard time and time again from
schools we have worked with that this information is actually very helpful to them,
because they not only know *what* to do for children, but also *why* they should do it,
which helps children, families, and schools be on the same page about the educational
and attendance goals. We have organized our recommendations into three categories:
school setting, coping strategies, and information sharing.

School Setting

For school-specific requests, there are two main areas of support that are helpful
to children to ensure a safe and productive learning environment; academic and
physical accommodations. The goal for this section is to think about the aspects
of the school environment that will need to be different for children to remain in
school—physically and mentally—and be successful there for the full day. Physically,

depending on mobility and symptom impairment, many children with somatic symptoms require help or additional time getting to or from class or in and out of the building (e.g., use of elevator instead of stairs). Sometimes they benefit from a lighter load of books to carry by keeping books in classrooms and/or having a second set at home. Academically, accommodations for assignments and testing are helpful when children have missed a lot of school and are at risk of getting unusually poor grades or not passing. Simple changes to grading practices, such as asking teachers to base the "current" grades on the work that children have turned in give children a better sense of their performance versus just seeing a "0" in the online grading system because of missing work that increases children's anxiety about school performance and decreases motivation to keep up with work. When asking for academic support for older adolescents, some high schools are limited in the amount of work that can be changed, especially for advanced placement or honors classes, or requests for schedule changes due to state requirements for core courses that may be taught only at certain time. We typically make school setting recommendations into two separate paragraphs, one addressing the physical needs and academic needs in the other, as illustrated for our patient Johnny:

> From a physical standpoint, Johnny would benefit from additional time to transfer between classes and not be counted as tardy, not only so he can pace his physical exertion, but also so he has a chance to use the restroom if needed.
>
> If Johnny has periods of substantially increased work to either make up or complete, it would be useful to reduce the assignments in the short term so that he is at less risk of falling behind in the long term. Having less work to make up will limit the stress that accompanies and worsens chronic conditions, making it easier for him to stay engaged in his classes. Having teachers grade work that has been completed instead of giving zeros for missing assignments would also help him keep up his usual level of performance.

These are our standard recommendations for children who have still been attending school in some form or another. If you are working with a child who has been completely out of school for a period of time, we recommend that the very first paragraph of the letter be devoted specifically to the school return, before you even mention physical or academic accommodations. When structuring a return to school, we usually plan a partial return for a few days to a favorite class period or for a half day, working up to a full day of attendance. You can recommend whatever time frame makes sense for the child you are working with. It can be beneficial to have the first few days of the week be partial days (i.e., Monday, Tuesday, Wednesday, alternating which half of the day children attend or adding one class period/lunch each day), working up to full days by the end of the week (i.e., Thursday, Friday) and then giving the child the reward of the weekend after reaching full attendance. This works well for children who have been out of school for weeks, but for children who have been out for months, a longer ramp-up to achieving full attendance may be required, as demonstrated by this recommendation for our patient Alex, with conversion disorder. A statement like this may be helpful in those circumstances:

> Though Alex is encouraged to return to school at this time, he continues to struggle with symptoms and is working on building his endurance and coping strategies. We suggest that he be permitted to attend shortened days (alternating between morning and afternoon schedules) and have reduced academic expectations during the next several weeks as he transitions back to school. This schedule will allow him to get caught up on assignments and reintegrate into the school setting without feeling too overwhelmed.

Physically, an additional recommendation that we include when needed has to do with physical education class expectations, especially if exercise or movement is a specific area of impairment or challenge. Here is an example of how we would ask for that type of accommodation:

> As stated, Alex is experiencing ongoing symptoms and it may be difficult for him to engage in Physical Education class on a daily basis. Please communicate this information to Alex's PE teacher specifically and allow him to participate in class as tolerated. Ideally, Alex should participate to the fullest extent possible, either engaging in the regular activity or engaging in a lower-impact form of the activity or doing an alternative activity, such as stretching or walking. If he is unable to do anything active, please involve him in nonphysical ways such as keeping score or acting as a coach.

Other ideas for academic support include working with a tutor, testing accommodations, a guided study hall, or further testing if a learning disability is suspected. Adding a specific request to this effect is helpful in that circumstance. Note that when recommending additional testing, parents need to follow through on this request in particular, as that will trigger a formal school psychology intervention that parents or the school need to initiate.

> Although Alex is able to attend class much of the time, his ongoing symptoms make concentration and absorption of material more challenging. Therefore, he should be considered for adjunctive tutoring services, extra time on tests, or other supportive services that may increase his academic success. These services should continue until the end of the year or until Alex feels he no longer requires them to stay on track.
>
> Alex would benefit from additional academic and educational testing to determine his learning style and

whether any underlying attention or processing disorders
are interfering with his ability to learn in the classroom.
These challenges appear to be separate from his medical
condition; however, learning difficulties may be adding
to Alex's stress about school, which in turn can worsen
symptoms. Therefore, attending to these concerns has the
potential to improve his functioning with his condition.

Finally we have developed schoolwork-related tracking forms to use on some occasions that help children and teachers measure how children are doing in each subject in an objective fashion while reinforcing effort (see the "School Subject Tracking Form" in the Appendix). We do this as a separate worksheet and send it as supplemental material to the teacher and home with the child. When children are struggling in a class and do not know why, this can be a successful way to both track work and figure out where there are problems. These types of tracking tables can also be useful to help children and teachers improve their communication about work and class performance. To reinforce the importance of communication, include a line for teachers and parents to comment or to sign the form to indicate it has been reviewed. Families can also use it as an incentive program in which children earn a reward based on daily or weekly total goals.

Coping Strategies

The next section of the school letter addresses the coping strategies that children are learning in treatment that we want them to do in the school setting. Children learn a host of coping strategies through CBT; the idea in communicating about that to school is not to provide them with a comprehensive list—children should be independently engaging in their strategies, after all—but rather to focus on the strategies that children will need special permission to do in a school setting. These are typically the strategies that require children to move around the room or leave class, such as standing, stretching, or taking a break, or to have something with them that most students are not allowed, such as electronics for using relaxation apps or water bottles and snacks. As with all of our accommodations, we want the school to understand why we are asking for these special privileges, which at first glance may seem distracting to children's school experience when in fact they are designed to keep them engaged in the educational environment. We would rather have children miss class for 10 minutes to proactively cope with a symptom flare so they can recover and go back to class, rather than suffer through a whole class period with poor concentration and then leave school early because symptoms become too intense to manage. Here is how we ask permission for coping accommodations in school with the corresponding rationale for our patient Johnny:

Johnny is being taught to use breaks and relaxation
strategies to cope with symptoms right there in the school
setting rather than being sent home. Please allow Johnny
to spend 5-10 minutes in the bathroom, nurse's office, or

> another quiet place as needed to cope with symptom flares. He
> should also be allowed to stand up, stretch, and move around
> in the classroom as needed to manage discomfort that comes
> with sitting for long periods of time; a seat in the back of
> the classroom would help him to do this without feeling out
> of place or being disruptive to the class.
>
> Please allow Johnny to carry a water bottle in school.
> Dehydration is a trigger for symptoms, and the length of the
> school day does not allow for adequate hydration to achieve
> his daily fluid intake goal. It would be helpful if Johnny
> could have a permanent pass to allow for bathroom breaks,
> which will be more frequent.

If you have recorded relaxation tracks or introduced the use of apps for aid in relaxation practice, you may need to ask the child whether he or she is allowed to have a phone, tablet, or MP3 player in school. If not, discuss whether the child would like to have it available to engage in relaxation, and if so you will need to ask special permission for that. If you are working with children with any type of orthostatic intolerance, such as POTS or dysautonomia, or chronic headaches, when asking for permission for them to carry a water bottle you should also mention that they also are allowed to have a small, packaged salty snack with them to aid in symptom management.

Sometimes, school staff struggle with how to cope with children's symptoms and support function while watching children go through obvious distress. The "Specific School Symptom Plan Template" (in the Appendix) is a supplemental letter that can be sent along with the general template, or at a later time as needed, to aid schools in responding to symptoms that children are having in the school setting. For instance, it is helpful for school staff to know when children should go to the nurse's office for medication or symptom management, and how that should be handled. Here is an example of how we would provide the school with information about our patient Johnny:

> Please allow Johnny to visit the nurse's office as needed for
> medication that has been prescribed by his doctor. After
> taking his medicine, he may either take a short break to
> cope with symptoms or return to class. We do not recommend
> that he call home or expect to go home when experiencing
> typical symptoms at school. Under extreme conditions or in
> the face of unusual symptoms, such as a fever, the school
> nurse should use discretion with this guideline.

It is particularly important to include specific symptom coping guidelines for school staff when the child has significantly physically impairing symptoms in the school setting, such as gait dysfunction, nonepileptic seizures, or any type of syncope or passing-out episodes. Schools are understandably concerned about students with these types of somatic symptoms, as it is very scary to watch a child go through such an episode, especially if there is question about the cause; a school's typical response would be to call an ambulance or alert the family to come and get the child. For a child with somatic symptoms, these symptom episodes are real, but they are not dangerous or indicative of an acute cause, and therefore need to be handled differently. Specifically communicate about these situations to the school so the staff can develop an appropriate response plan, similar to the tips provided to parents for supporting children with symptoms. In general, schools need to know that although the symptoms are real, they are not dangerous, and if the child has an episode in school, staff should interact with the child in ways that will promote a focus on function, break the cycle of symptoms and disability, reward the child for positive independent coping, and keep a normal schedule going as much as possible.

As mentioned in the research review, social problems can be a significantly limiting factor in children's school success, and unfortunately, negative peer interactions in school are a challenges for many students regardless of health status. If a child is being bullied, investigate what anti-bullying policies and practices the school district abides by and encourage the family to explore these with the school administration even prior to making specific symptom-based recommendations. Aside from a specific bullying experience, other negative peer interactions can add significant stress to children's school experience and increase impairment. Here is an example of a statement we would add to a school letter specific to coping with peer stress and improving peer relationships, as demonstrated with our patient Alex, as he transitions back to school:

> To alleviate some of the negative social interactions Alex may experience at school, he would benefit from a schedule that allows him to interact with his preferred peer group to facilitate his social and emotional well-being. As much as possible, please integrate Alex into his preferred lunch, classes, and study groups with his close friends.

Information Sharing

Finally, the last part of our letter asks that the information be appropriately shared with *all* school staff who interact with the student. We have worked with many children and families who created a wonderful school plan, only to have it fall flat when the child tried to use it and was stopped by a school staff member who had no idea the child had somatic symptoms, let alone a plan to cope with them. For example, a child we worked with was appropriately taking his relaxation break by leaving the class and going to the quiet library, but his teacher didn't know this and as a result instituted a "missing person" alert to the entire school in an effort to find him. You can imagine the stress it caused that student to hear his name called out over the loudspeaker! In addition to making the request that all relevant staff be kept in the loop, we again provide education so that they understand why we make this request, which also provides an opportunity to help them take the perspective of the child in the situation.

Children with somatic symptoms generally dislike talking about their symptoms or special needs in front of teachers or peers in their classrooms; like many same-age peers, they are striving to look as *normal* as possible and are avoiding being different or standing out in any way. It is already difficult for them to be in the position of having a special plan to manage symptoms at all; layering on the stress of having to explain to a teacher why they have a plan or need to use it is simply too much for many of them to overcome. We have worked with many children who are reticent about using their skills for these reasons, even if it means that they suffer more from symptoms. In addition to the struggle of just looking different, it is embarrassing for children to ask a teacher for permission to cope with private and sometimes sensitive health issues surrounding symptoms. If children think they will be questioned by the teacher about what's wrong and potentially put on the spot to talk about their health in front of the whole class, it will be yet another deterrent to them asking for or receiving any kind of help. Finally, schools are actually putting themselves in a difficult situation if they are discussing children's symptoms in front of the class, as they are releasing protected health information. For all of these reasons, it is crucial to emphasize the importance of the school's discretion and supportive communication with students.

Something that is often overlooked when implementing these strategies across the school setting is ensuring that special occasions will also be covered, including substitute teachers or field trips. Strategies that have been successful for children to ensure that they are able to use accommodations in these special circumstances are for the parent to be informed about upcoming changes in teachers or trips to help the child plan, or for the child to have another point person available for them in school or on the field trip who is knowledgeable about their situation. It is sometimes difficult for schools to plan ahead for these occasions, in which case it is beneficial to have multiple members of the school staff who are involved in children's other educational activities aware of these accommodations.

In addition, we like to inform the school that children will be engaging in further treatment, so everyone has the correct expectation that this will be ongoing work and therefore continued school communication and support will be helpful and necessary. Here are the recommendations we make related to these topics for our patient Johnny:

> Please communicate the information in this letter to all of Johnny's teachers so they are aware of his medical concerns and these special accommodations. It adds additional stress for students when they have to explain their coping requests or medical situations to teachers, especially when they are in class or in front of other students. This communication will help teachers be sensitive to Johnny's needs and provide accommodations in their classrooms without the need for further explanation by Johnny.
>
> Johnny will need to attend future doctor's appointments for symptom management. It would be helpful if the school could support him should he need to miss school for these appointments.

We end the letter with the importance of the school working with the family to implement the plan and thank them for their assistance. Although you are providing these recommendations, we also want to support parents' ability to advocate for their children and know their rights in the school setting, as they are the experts on their own children and you are not going to be working with them forever. We have found that engaging parents in this process of communicating with the school is a way of training them for future school interactions, and they will be much more likely to do that successfully and independently having had this experience with you as the guide but them as the implementers. In addition to supporting parents' advocacy for children at school, it is helpful to encourage parents to implement plans at home to reward children for positive school performance despite their symptoms. School notes or short meetings with teachers on a daily or weekly basis can provide parents with information about how their child is coping during the school day. Finally, we like to express our appreciation for the extra time and effort involved in the school's collaboration:

> Johnny's family will be happy to work out the details of implementing this plan with you. Johnny is committed to being a good student with regular attendance despite his condition, and it is our hope that attending to his current school stressors, along with treating his symptoms and encouraging increased function, can help get him back on track physically, academically, and emotionally. Thank you in advance for your assistance in creating as supportive an environment as possible as Johnny copes with his condition. Ongoing communication between Johnny's school, family, and treatment team is vital to ensuring his success in these efforts, so I welcome contact with you [provide your own contact information directly in the letter].

In our practice, we have found that the information and accommodations we have covered in this letter template are effective in creating a supportive school environment for children with somatic symptoms. Again, not all children require each of these accommodations, and a plan should be developed that makes sense for each child's individual needs. Children and their parents benefit from being actively involved as you create this letter with them; they often have very good ideas for what will help the child the most in school and they appreciate knowing they have the backing of their therapist to implement these supports in school so that it will be a safe and productive environment for the child.

SCHOOL RESOURCES

In the final section of this chapter, we address what resources exist within the school setting itself that can be helpful for children coping with somatic symptoms, as well as providing standardized testing and college recommendations. It is helpful to be aware of these resources so you can educate families about the options that are out there for additional help, but it is up to the children and families to advocate for these services.

In the United States, formal educational accommodations are required by law for children with any kind of impairing disability to ensure there is no discrimination in education by publicly funded schools. Many times, the school letter sent by the mental health provider in combination with the family's advocacy will lead to the school or the family calling a meeting to formalize the recommendations and be in accordance with the law. This typically results in the creation of either a Section 504 plan, which *accommodates the environment* to make the curriculum more accessible for a child who has a medical condition or specific learning disability, or a more comprehensive Individualized Education Program (IEP), which *modifies the regular curriculum* to provide effective education to the child, accounting for medical, learning, or developmental challenges. The goal of both plans is to ensure that the child is effectively educated within the school setting, but they focus on different aspects of the changes that need to be made for that to happen. The 504 plan does that by changing aspects of the environment that will make the child more successful in school (e.g., allowing access to the bathroom, providing special seating, allowing for breaks), whereas the IEP does that by changing the content of the curriculum itself (e.g., instruction through a special education or resource classroom). In that sense, the 504 is a "lower level" plan in terms of the environmental accommodations, whereas the IEP is a "higher level" plan that requires much more involvement on the part of the school. More information can be found about these plans on the U.S. Department of Education website (*www.ed.gov*). Private schools do not have to adhere to these federal regulations because they are not publicly funded entities, but many follow a similar format, so it is still worth checking on the educational support services offered if a child is in a private school setting.

For children to qualify for either type of formal educational plan, the law requires that they must have a mental, physical, or learning impairment that substantially limits one or more major life activities (e.g., physical abilities such as hearing, seeing, or moving, emotional coping, communication abilities, social function). Thus, a medical, educational, or psychological diagnosis alone does not qualify children for special services in school; they need to have associated impairment as well. If they meet these qualifications, children must then be referred by parents, teachers, or school staff for evaluation; note that health care providers are *not* on this list of people who can refer a child for formal educational services. This is yet another reason to include parents in school communication efforts and educate them about ways they can further advocate for their child in the school setting, as they will have to be the ones to ask for these services. The school then conducts the evaluation, which can include a combination of formal observation of the child, administering standardized tests or assessments, conducting interviews with the parent, teacher, and/or child, and review of medical information provided by the family. The information is synthesized and a determination of eligibility is conducted, typically through a meeting involving parents, teachers, and the child (if appropriate) in which a formal plan is developed, including provisions about who will implement each aspect of the plan. A 504 plan typically provides accommodations for students who remain in regular classrooms, whereas an IEP provides special education services to address a health condition (in a category called "Other Health Impairment" or OHI) and learning or developmental needs (e.g., autism, learning disability) either through provision of supplementary services within regular education classrooms or by pulling students out for some or all classes in special education classrooms.

In our experience, a 504 plan is the most common and appropriate plan for children with somatic symptoms; an IEP is less common for children with somatic symptoms alone and more common for children who also have other learning or developmental diagnoses who need a specially designed curriculum. If children are highly impaired and require significant modifications to testing or attendance based on their somatic symptom disorder, then an IEP is typically considered under the OHI category. A positive aspect of children going through this formal evaluation process is that it creates an opportunity for teachers, parents, school staff, and children to work together to improve the educational setting in a proactive manner. For both plans, the school conducts a yearly review to readdress accommodations or modifications and makes any necessary changes as children progress throughout their education, including transferring between schools (i.e., elementary to middle, middle to high school).

Finally, there are a few other accommodation ideas that can be helpful to know about, especially for older adolescents who are preparing for the future by taking standardized tests and planning to go to college. For national standardized tests, there are forms available online that the family can complete to request accommodations for alterations to the testing environment for medical and psychological reasons. These can include spreading testing across several days, allowing for breaks, conducting testing in a private room, and having water and/or snacks available. Families need a letter documenting the child's medical condition, similar to what is done in the school template, with formal requests for the specific accommodations. In our practice, we provide these letters to the families and then they provide them to the testing body.

When students are preparing to go to college and need to think about accommodations for symptoms in that setting, the office of student disabilities is their best resource. Colleges are actually very supportive of students with medical concerns and offer a variety of creative ideas for assistance, including priority registration to get classes at advantageous times, living in dorms that are in the center of campus, having access to tutoring services, having professors provide class notes, and receiving testing accommodations so that students can take tests in private rooms proctored by tutors with allowance for breaks. Student health centers on campus are also good resources. It is helpful for students and families to communicate with the health center ahead of time so that they have information at the ready regarding a possible symptom episode to better facilitate care should the student require it. College counseling centers are also excellent resources for adolescents who need to continue to receive psychological support on campus. Although there are lots of reasons that adolescents and families are worried about the transition to college, it can be a very positive shift in the educational environment in terms of symptom management. When students are able to have more flexibility in classes, feel more independent in their educational choices, and are more motivated to engage in fields that feel more closely tied to their future goals, our experience is that even children who were quite significantly disabled by symptoms in high school succeed.

CHAPTER SUMMARY AND TAKE-AWAY POINTS

- Children with somatic symptoms experience associated school impairment at a low, medium, or high level. Assess these areas of difficulty and help children improve their functioning in the school setting.

- Communicating with the school through a letter is an effective way to educate the school about the child's condition while asking for tailored supports that will help the child improve function in that setting. Closely involve the family in this process to help them become advocates for the child.

- Schools have a number of resources to support children with medical, emotional, and learning challenges, such as the creation of a 504 plan or an IEP. Families can pursue these additional supports through the school as necessary.

CHAPTER 11

Health Care Colleagues

Collaborating with health care colleagues is critical to the success of psychological treatment for children with somatic symptoms in order to ensure that they are on the right track in *all* aspects of their care. In fact, it would not be possible to do this work without involving children's medical providers. If a child started having stomachaches one morning and began CBT for that problem later the same day, the first question should be "Have you seen your doctor?" It would be highly ineffective and potentially dangerous to engage in CBT for the stomach flu! Working alongside health care colleagues gives therapists, children, and families the assurance that it is safe to engage in a functional approach to symptom management. It ensures that all other appropriate aspects of treatment are carried out to give children the best chance of success in overcoming their condition (e.g., medication, nutrition, physical therapy).

Just as we rely on this collaboration and see it as complementary to the care we provide, health care colleagues are equally grateful for our role in the treatment of children with somatic symptoms. When thinking about medical collaboration, at first you may think about the importance of what you learn about the medical and physical aspects of the child's condition from health care colleagues, but keep in mind they are just as eager to learn from you about the way in which we talk about symptoms, the psychological factors that play a role in children's symptom presentations, and how they can support the use of coping tools we teach to children. Effectively treating children with somatic symptoms is truly a team effort.

For effective communication, return to the themes reviewed in the first section of the book regarding the medical field's understanding—and *mis*understanding—of somatic symptoms, as these themes come up when collaborating with health care providers. Typically, these challenges are *not* related to providers' desire to help or lack of medical ability; rather, they generally come from a lack of knowledge or understanding about somatic symptoms or a feeling of frustration with the failure of usual care. Unfortunately, this a common occurrence in the field of somatic symptoms, which is not well understood from the medical perspective.

Health care professionals who practice within a biopsychosocial model have a more integrated view of somatic symptoms. Thus, they will be more likely to truly collaborate with mental health providers versus placing a referral and discharging the patient from their care (i.e., "This is not medical, so see a mental health provider instead."). For example, a study of physicians working with patients who have functional neurological disorders demonstrated a strong belief that a biopsychosocial approach is most effective in diagnosis and treatment (de Schipper, Vermeulen, Eeckhout, & Foncke, 2014). While understanding somatic symptoms from a biopsychosocial model is important conceptually, there is variability in how effectively providers employ that framework in patient care. Research among neurologists and psychiatrists demonstrated that while they all agreed that psychological factors play a role in conversion disorder *and* saw it as their responsibility to inform patients of this, they did not routinely assess for or discuss those factors as part of the diagnosis, especially if the patient was not receptive (Kanaan, Armstrong & Wessely, 2011). Physicians understand the importance of providing an adequate, integrated explanation of a somatic symptom diagnosis but often feel incapable of doing so (Olde Hartman, Hassink-Franke, Lucassen, van Spaendonck, & van Weel, 2009). This tells us that even when physicians are biopsychosocially minded, they may lack the skill or ability to effectively relate the role of psychosocial factors in somatic symptoms.

Likely related to these challenges of understanding and treating somatic symptoms, physicians have high levels of frustration, uncertainty, helplessness, and discomfort when working in this patient population (Dalton, Drossman, Hathaway, & Bangdiwala, 2004). Some of this stress may be due to a lack of knowledge of effective treatment options for somatic symptoms. For instance, among primary care physicians treating adults with panic disorder, all of them believed medication effectively relieved panic symptoms, but only one-third knew that CBT is an effective treatment (Teng, Chaison, Bailey, Hamilton & Dunn, 2008).

A way to address these challenges is to teach physicians to talk about psychological factors with patients and offer CBT as another effective treatment avenue along with medical recommendations. A positive development is that training in the biopsychosocial model and communication about somatic symptoms is gaining attention in medical education. A short communication training program for physicians was found to be effective in improving their ability to explain somatic symptoms, reassure patients effectively, and avoid unnecessary diagnostic testing, all of which were found to increase their interviewing and information-giving skills (Weiland et al., 2015). This study demonstrates that while physicians understand the psychosocial correlates of somatic symptoms, many need our help in communicating about symptoms to children and families, which can be doubly helpful in alleviating their own frustration as well as providing efficacious treatment to children and families through CBT. Although studies such as this one have primarily been conducted among physicians, we can assume that providers in other medical disciplines (e.g., physical therapy, nursing) encounter similar challenges in understanding and treating somatic symptoms. Keep these ideas in mind as you interact with your health care colleagues, and if you encounter some who seem frustrated or dismissive, remember that their distress is understandable: as care providers they very much want to help but may not have all of the tools to do so. The key to a successful collaboration is recognition that in this line of work, no individual provider has all of the tools, and it takes a team to effectively treat children with somatic symptoms.

While this book is for mental health providers, it can also be an educational tool for medical providers, especially with regard to understanding somatic symptoms within a biopsychosocial context and explaining the role of CBT. We can empower our health care colleagues with this information. In our experience, when medical providers advocate for the role of CBT in children's care, families are more amenable to follow through with treatment. In addition, mental health collaboration relieves frustration on the part of health care providers by giving them additional treatment options. Adopting a biopsychosocial framework and effective communication gives much-needed relief for both medical providers and families when they see that non-medical interventions are useful for somatic symptoms.

In this chapter, we address the factors that are pertinent in working with our health care colleagues in the treatment of children with somatic symptoms. First, we address the logistical aspects of collaboration, including discussion of how teams work in different settings and how to communicate about somatic symptoms. Then we focus on the experience of collaborating on a patient's care after receiving a referral and how to facilitate that communication with families and medical teams. Finally, we cover when to make a referral either to another provider (e.g., a psychiatrist) or to a higher level of care, such as a day or inpatient treatment program.

HELPING COLLEAGUES COMMUNICATE ABOUT SOMATIC SYMPTOMS AND CBT

Collaboration with health care colleagues in the care of children with somatic symptoms begins before we have even met the child. Before we receive the mental health referral, typically, a medical provider has made that recommendation to the child and family. However, medical providers often have difficulty communicating with children and families about somatic symptoms and their treatment, so sometimes the first form of contact we have with health care colleagues is consultation around how to effectively explain the role of psychological factors in somatic symptoms, and how to refer families for CBT in the first place. The most frequently asked question we get from our health care colleagues is "What can I do when I try to refer a family to you and all they tell me is that they're not crazy?" We reinterpret this question as "How can I talk to my patients and families more effectively about the different aspects of treatment that are effective for somatic symptoms?" There is significant variability in how psychological information is taught and integrated into practice in health care disciplines. We have worked with colleagues who have quite a bit of training and experience in this area and others who have very little; however, despite the formal education they have received, many providers still feel unsure of how to approach a discussion of the role of psychological intervention for treatment of somatic symptoms with a patient and family in clinical encounters. For all of these reasons, when colleagues ask us for help in communicating with patients, we like to get a brief understanding of what they know already about psychological treatment for somatic symptoms (e.g., background, area of specialty training), specifically listening for how much of a biopsychosocial approach they incorporate into their medical and clinical thinking. Then, knowing how much to emphasize that based on their response, we focus on modeling the subtlety of language necessary to help them communicate with their patients about somatic symptoms and the role of psychological intervention. Here is an example for providers we often use with patients and families:

> "Seeing a psychologist is part of the treatment for somatic symptoms. As we've discussed, these symptoms are real, although we know that they are not caused by something dangerous happening in your brain, your stomach, or your heart, and the way to help them get better is to help your body get back in balance again and learn to do activities in a functional way. Your body does not work without your mind, and your mind does not work without your body; there is a strong connection between the two, which can make symptoms really hard to deal with, but you can also learn how to use this mind–body connection to make the symptoms easier to deal with. We want you to have the best life you can, and learning how deal with the symptoms is the first step to getting better. That is where the mental health provider fits in. Therapists help you understand the connection between the brain and body and teach you tools to calm your body down, distract your brain, and manage your thoughts so that symptoms do not keep you from doing what you want to do. This treatment is called CBT or cognitive-behavioral therapy, and there are many studies that show that it is extremely helpful for children dealing with somatic symptoms, just like you. I will keep seeing you as you are working with the therapist, and we'll work together as a team to make sure that we are giving you all of the treatments we know about that can help you get back to your life."

In the best-case scenario, providers can easily integrate this explanation into their existing biopsychosocial framework, feeling more confident in the language needed to describe CBT and the mind–body connection.

However, there are still medical providers who do not share the biopsychosocial approach—who see somatic symptoms as not real or legitimate, feel these patients are taking up the time a "truly sick" child could have, and send them to a mental health provider because they are frustrated with their overuse of health care services or because they really do think it is all in their heads! Other times, providers are biopsychosocially minded, but they just do not have a good understanding of what somatic symptoms are or what to do about them. This does not happen because they are bad medical providers; it happens because one cannot learn everything about everything. For example, if a medical student decides to focus on epilepsy, she might learn a lot about how to diagnose and explain epileptic seizures, but not learn a lot about how to talk about nonepileptic seizures, even if she learns that this is the term for certain types of neurological symptoms that are not epilepsy. In these scenarios, helping providers see the role of biopsychosocial factors in illness—*all* illness—and building their somatic symptom vocabulary are two ways that you can help them be more productive in their conversations, something that will be more satisfying for them as well as for patients and their families.

For example, we worked with a psychologically minded physician who felt that she was appropriately representing the importance of CBT to her patients; however, every referral we received stated, "CBT recommended to address the role of stress in symptom presentation." While it was wonderful that she was speaking to her patients about the role of stress in their symptom presentations and offering evidence-based treatment options to address that, we could not help but think that our colleague was missing a big part of the benefit of engaging in CBT for somatic symptoms: the benefit to biological and social factors. We suggested that she instead considered saying, "You will benefit from CBT to cope with your symptoms, integrate medical recommendations into your daily routine, get the right kind of help from the people around you, and understand the impact that stress may have on your body."

In our experience, from the perspective of the family, when children and families feel as though they hear the message "Nothing is wrong with you" or "It's all in your head" in their medical encounters, they do not feel validated, and if they do follow up on the psychology referral (we imagine many might not), the buy-in to treatment is always more challenging. We understand that many providers may not intend to send this message; however, sometimes the art of practicing medicine gets lost in the hustle of managed care, productivity requirements, and billable hours. In terms of communicating effectively about somatic symptoms, mental health providers have it easier because longer sessions allow for time to delve more deeply into symptom impairment and coping factors, in contrast to a specialty provider who is double booked and has to assess symptoms and provide a differential diagnosis within a shorter period of time, with less information. On the other hand, sometimes our health care colleagues give the perfect description of CBT, and the child and family are just not able to hear it. Many people do not think they need (or want) to see a therapist for a medical problem and feel frustrated with the medical provider when it is suggested they consider this, even when done with *exactly* the right words and within a biopsychosocial framework. In either scenario, we reassure providers that they can only focus on what *they* can do to effectively explain the role of psychological factors and CBT for treatment of somatic symptoms, and when children and families are ready to hear the message, they will.

We encourage our colleagues to be mindful of four factors when considering whether a mental health referral will aid in the child's treatment: (1) the degree of impairment a child is experiencing, including missing school or doing poorly in school, (2) a significant decline in activity level, such as physical or social function, (3) changes in sleep, or (4) changes in mood, such as an increase in anxiety, behavioral changes, or a decrease in positive mood. While we do not often have direct control over when a mental health referral is made for a child with somatic symptoms, it is most effective to do so early on in the child's medical treatment, so that the biopsychosocial approach is represented from the beginning. Even if children are still undergoing medication trials or have an additional test or procedure to do, we believe it is beneficial to engage them in psychological care, as our treatment will still be focused on coping with symptoms regardless of the origin. Further, delaying psychological referral until the medical workup is complete sends a (likely unintentional) biomedical message of "Well, we've confirmed there's nothing physically wrong with you—now we'll have to check out your mind." We would venture to guess that it would be more difficult to have that conversation with a child and family than it would be to suggest mental health treatment as a complement to their medical care as it's happening in real time. In an outpatient health care setting, this may mean that the child sees the medical provider and/or specialist for a visit, initial treatment recommendations are made, and a mental health referral is placed at that point, or the child comes back for a medical/specialty follow-up, and if he or she is still struggling, a mental health referral is made at that time. In inpatient or outpatient multi- or interdisciplinary settings, a mental health evaluation is often built into part of the initial visit, which is an ideal way to ensure that psychosocial factors are equally valued and assessed for from the beginning of treatment.

THE LOGISTICS OF COLLABORATION

Once a referral has been received, practically, communication happens through many channels: secure e-mail, electronic medical record communications (e.g., copying a provider on a note within an institution), phone calls/voicemail exchanges. In a busy world of patient care, sometimes the most challenging aspect of collaboration is actually getting in touch with someone; be persistent, it is important to make these connections. In some institutions, mental health notes are protected, so be aware of confidentiality policies when sharing information.

In addition, discuss the goal of treatment collaboration with the child and family, see if there are any other providers they would like to include in the communication network, and, as necessary, get written consent. Ensure that the family understands they are active members in the child's treatment—it is *not* the goal for the mental health provider to be the go-between for the family and medical providers. Inform the family that they will still need to reach out to those providers directly if they have any questions regarding those treatments or symptoms those providers are managing, and that the goal of collaboration is to inform providers about CBT and receive or give any pertinent updates about other aspects of treatment.

In terms of the health care colleagues with whom collaboration is most frequent, first is the primary care provider, who may be a pediatrician, nurse practitioner, physician assistant, family medicine practitioner, or adolescent medicine specialist. This is the first-line provider for most children with somatic symptoms. Skilled primary care providers are often able to effectively treat children and refer them for psychological intervention without specialty care. For mental health providers in hospital settings or in multidisciplinary outpatient clinics (meaning providers from different disciplines seeing patients individually), collaboration is most likely to occur with pediatric medical specialists or subspecialists (e.g., gastroenterology, neurology, cardiology). Within a larger health care team or in interdisciplinary care (meaning providers from different disciplines coordinating patient care in real time), collaboration may be with providers from a wide variety of disciplines, including, but not limited to, nursing, physical therapy, occupational therapy, child life, speech therapy, recreation therapy, nutrition, acupuncture, massage therapy, music therapy, pet therapy, and art therapy. In any setting, it is helpful to exchange information about diagnosis, evaluation, prognosis, medications, restrictions, and treatment. In working with physical or occupational therapy colleagues, it is useful to know the child's level of physical function (e.g., limitations, how far they can walk in the community, exercise program, response to performing physical tasks in session) and ability to perform activities of daily living (e.g., dressing, feeding, bathing).

The frequency of communication varies between disciplines. Medical providers in outpatient settings typically see children every 2 to 3 months, whereas physical and occupational therapists see children on a weekly basis, similar to the mental health model. It is productive to communicate with medical providers immediately prior to a child's medical visit so they have the most current update on progress and can reinforce treatment goals in their visit. Based on the typical frequency of medical visits, that may mean only once every 2 or 3 months. For providers who see children more frequently on an outpatient basis, such as physical therapy, more frequent communication is appropriate.

Although communication happens in multiple manners and styles with various providers in different treatment settings, the goal of collaboration remains the same—to provide a consistent message to the family and stay connected with one another about children's progress in treatment. When providers know about one another's treatment, they can reinforce those elements of treatment in the context of their own care, creating a unified, integrated approach to care.

COLLABORATING ON CARE

Most commonly, the first point of contact with health care colleagues is when they refer one of their patients for mental health treatment. Referral requests are highly variable: they may directly reference somatic symptoms ("assess for psychological factors related to abdominal pain") or might make reference to both medical and psychological factors ("assess for anxiety, child having headaches"), or there may be no mention of somatic symptoms, although the child has them ("assess for depression/mood").

From this point, review the information from the referring provider prior to the initial assessment to determine if further communication is needed before meeting the child and family. If you are familiar with the referring provider's practice and have access to the most recent note in the medical record or it is attached with the referral, you may have all the information you need to move forward. For example, we have developed referral relationships with several pediatric specialists, so all that we need to see is a referral such as "chronic headache, dizziness, and syncope" and we know exactly what to do. However, if you are not familiar with the referring provider, or if it seems the symptom presentation is more nuanced than usual, those are good reasons to communicate directly with the provider. That would also allow the opportunity to gain more information on what the provider has spoken about with the family regarding the symptoms as well as any additional medical information that may be helpful (e.g., if a diagnosis been given, what workup has been completed, what has been ruled out, etc.).

Once the assessment is completed, it is helpful to communicate with referring providers whether or not you spoke with them before seeing the child. In an outpatient setting, we most commonly do this by sending the provider the "Referring Provider Letter Template" (in the Appendix) and/or a copy of our visit documentation.

Providers have told us that the most important information for them to receive is a summary of the presenting biopsychosocial concerns, the treatment plan, and the projected length of treatment—they even benefit from simply knowing that the child successfully made it into our office! This communication also provides a chance to share any new information that was reported about symptom presentation that could be medically pertinent, as well as to discuss the frequency of communication that you both prefer. If you are working in an inpatient setting, this contact may occur through a review of one another's notes in the electronic medical record, during rounds, or at a care conference. Since children who are treated in an inpatient setting have more impairing symptoms that necessitate a higher level of care, it is particularly beneficial for all team members to communicate well and frequently in order to be on the same page regarding treatment.

A note on the changing landscape of mental health referrals as the biopsychosocial model gains ground: our medical colleagues have shared that it is challenging for them when they communicate to the family the importance of CBT in treating somatic symptoms and the child indeed follows up with a mental health provider, sometimes after a fair amount of convincing, only to have the mental health provider send the child back to the medical provider with a note saying "No anxiety or depression, no need for treatment." Somatic symptoms can and should be treated with CBT principles—they work and children get relief from their symptoms, regardless of whether they meet criteria for a mental health diagnosis like anxiety or depression. Hopefully, this book can bridge the gap between the medical and mental health worlds so that children who stand to benefit from CBT interventions have the opportunity to engage in them.

The ongoing communication about a child's care after the initial assessment is extremely variable, based on practice setting as well as preferences of the providers. In outpatient care, some of our health care colleagues want and need to be kept in the loop on a more frequent basis (i.e., every session to every few sessions), whereas others effectively discharge the child from their care once the somatic symptom diagnosis is made and do not want to be kept in the loop. This is a tough situation, as it involves differences in health care delivery within hospitals and medical practices, understanding of the treatment of somatic symptoms, and each provider's approach to care. If we got to choose, we would always want children with somatic symptoms to have at least one follow-up appointment with the medical specialist after initiation of CBT to address any questions related to the diagnosis of somatic symptoms and the treatment plan prior to being discharged from medical care. We suggest having a conversation with the referring or other treating providers if there are concerns regarding the child's ability to receive follow-up medical care.

In addition to the importance of the medical provider receiving updates about the progress of the child receiving CBT, it is equally essential to provide information regarding potential stressors or acute situations that may trigger symptoms and result in calls to the provider with medical questions. For example, we worked with a child with nonepileptic seizures who was also being followed by a psychiatrist who had prescribed medication to address anxiety. During finals, the child had a symptom flare (i.e., increased frequency of and impairment from somatic symptoms) that prompted an urgent call from the family to the psychiatrist with a concern that the anxiety medication was not working. In this case, it was crucial that we had been in close communication with the psychiatrist regarding this child, as the psychiatrist knew the other factors leading to the flare (i.e., school stress) and as a result was able to guide the family through the acute stressor rather than make unnecessary and reactive medication changes. Perhaps most important, this was an opportunity for the child and family to hear a consistent message about the treatment approach from both providers.

If you are working with a child who is in clear need of medical follow-up, as is the case for our case example patients Alex and Ashley, it is recommended that you discuss who will have what responsibility for which aspects of the child's care with the referring provider. For example, the neurologist who initially diagnosed Alex with a conversion disorder may be thinking, "Well, it's not a neurological disorder, so he'll be in great hands with the psychologist!" But the psychologist might be thinking, "How will I get a wheelchair for this child, and who will tell me when he can walk longer distances?" Similarly for Ashley, although we would feel confident teaching her to cope with her existing cardiac symptoms, if she had a new onset complaint of numbness and tingling in her extremities, we would rely on her medical provider to make an assessment of whether or not that is consistent with her underlying somatic symptom condition or a new concern deserving of further medical attention. In both of these situations, it is easy to see the benefit of having a medical provider working with you to best care for the child, one who understands that treatment for somatic symptoms cannot be solely psychological intervention without medical support.

In order to establish a collaborative working relationship with a medical provider or team, consider asking the following questions:

1. How often would communication be helpful?
   a. For the medical specialist?
   b. For the primary care provider?
   c. For other therapists (e.g., physical therapist, occupational therapist)?
   d. For you?

2. Will communication be problem or summary based (e.g., getting in touch only when there is a question or a regular update based on time or progress)?
   a. What is the most helpful information to be shared?
   b. What is the best method of communication?

3. If the child continues to have impairing symptoms that affect physical safety and/or require medical support (e.g., a wheelchair), who is responsible for that?

4. Who will sign permission for homebound instruction or medical excuses for missing school (typically, an MD signature is required)?

5. What should the family expect in terms of follow-up care from the medical provider?
   a. Frequency of visits (e.g., as needed or on a regular basis)?
   b. Any more procedures/diagnostic workup to be done?

6. What are the medical interventions that would be helpful to support in CBT?
   a. Adherence to medication, exercise, hydration?

7. When is the child cleared medically (when can he or she go back to school, drive, etc.) and how will this decision be made?
   a. Fewer symptoms?
   b. Less impairment?
   c. Time since last symptom flare?

Establishing the working relationship up front allows you and the medical provider to offer more coordinated care to the child and family and reduces frustration in the event that a challenging question or problem arises by helping providers know to whom to direct families.

As with the three levels of school impairment presented in the previous chapter, children can also be thought of as having three levels of collaborative need: low, moderate, and high. Consider each of those levels in the context of our three patients who we have described throughout the book.

For Johnny, a child with a relatively straightforward somatic symptom presentation, our treatment required an overall low level of medical collaboration. We sent an initial letter to the referring physician (a gastroenterologist) via electronic medical record summarizing the current concerns and impairment, the diagnosis and clinical impressions, and a description of treatment that was provided to the family in the initial assessment session. The physician communicated back and indicated Johnny's family needed medical follow-up in 3 months or as needed or if symptoms worsened, and that she would continue a low dose of his medication in the meantime. Since treatment progressed as expected for Johnny and his symptoms and impairment improved, Johnny's physician discontinued the medication at the follow-up visit. We touched base with his physician again when Johnny was discharged from our care by copying her on our final note, which included Johnny's ongoing coping plan to manage stress and pain. If you are working within a system that does not have an electronic medical record, we would recommend sending a discharge summary in the form of a letter to the provider that made the referral. This should follow a similar template to the referral letter (i.e., symptoms/impairment at discharge), with the addition of a *brief* summary of coping skills and interventional strategies taught during treatment. This way, the referring provider is aware of the outcome and disposition of the patient (in this case, with good results and no indication for follow-up care) and now has some concrete treatment information so he or she can potentially ask the patient about the use of coping skills at a future visit, if one should happen. In total, there were two points of contact with the referring provider for our example of a child with a low level of medical collaboration need: referral and discharge.

Alex is an example of a child with a moderate level of medical collaborative need for successful treatment because he had a more significant presentation of somatic symptoms. Alex continued to struggle with motor symptoms after beginning CBT, as is typical for children with conversion disorder, and our communication with his treating physicians was more complicated because everyone was not on the same page at the beginning of treatment. Alex's neurologist felt it would be counterproductive to provide a wheelchair, as she was understandably concerned that it would reinforce illness behaviors rather than healthy behaviors. We definitely saw this side of the argument; using a wheelchair does reinforce impairment rather than function. However, Alex wasn't walking *at all* at first, which meant he was not engaging in many activities outside the home that he needed to do for improved function, and Alex's parents could not carry him around to get him back into the world. Most importantly, we considered that having a wheelchair would enable him to attend school (with accommodations), which was a critical step toward increased function in our initial stages of treatment.

Our next step was contacting Alex's primary care provider, with the agreement of Alex's neurologist, who had not planned to be further involved in his care. This physician was happy to work with us, but he had not cared for many children with conversion disorder and was eager to learn more about it. After relaying a summary of diagnosis and treatment, we also provided assurance that we would carefully monitor wheelchair use to ensure it *increased* engagement in the community (e.g., school) to be consistent with our treatment goal of improving function. The pediatrician was in agreement with the plan and wrote a 1-month prescription for a wheelchair. He asked to stay involved in Alex's care, communicating every few sessions so he could most effectively support the family.

We also worked closely with Alex's physical therapist to know *how* he should use the wheelchair and make progress in his practice of walking. It is valuable to collaborate with physical therapy colleagues to know how to support children's function in our treatment, as well as to share information about coping tools that children could use in other therapy sessions. Imagine you are having the child walk down the hall to your office and you do not know what the physical therapist has recommended in terms of gait or muscle cues or posture changes—wouldn't that feel like a lost opportunity to assess the child's progress and increase function? And imagine that child is having a hard time with an exercise in physical therapy and the physical therapist doesn't know what coping skills to recommend—isn't that missing a chance to practice a coping tool in a difficult moment? This is the power of the team approach: even if you are not working in an interdisciplinary setting, you can still promote one another's treatment, which can enhance your own care. Most importantly, a united front is presented to the family, which helps them also focus on returning the child to functioning, confident that the whole team supports this approach, and avoids opportunities for team splitting or mixed messages.

Finally, throughout this collaboration, we also had conversations with his mother about who to call when Alex's symptoms were causing impairment. We decided that she would call the school contact person (his guidance counselor) to address school issues before calling us, with assurances that we were glad to help but wanted to help her feel empowered to address issues in the context in which they were happening. She also called Alex's pediatrician with health concerns, although our shared mantra was "unless he has a fever or needs to go to the emergency department for a new concern, he needs to go to school." And in fact, he did have a brief bout of fever during treatment that necessitated a call to the pediatrician and luckily required only an easy over-the-counter treatment. Through this coordinated approach, Alex's mother felt she had a better understanding of who to call when and did not feel she needed to defer to us to do the coordination, which made his treatment go much more smoothly for all parties.

Finally, for a child with a more complicated somatic symptom presentation, like our patient Ashley, a high level of medical collaboration is required. In this case, you may communicate frequently and may even need to consider whether a higher level of care is indicated depending on how treatment progresses. First we discussed her complicated case with her cardiologist. He planned to see her every 1 to 2 months, was interested in hearing any major points of intervention he could reinforce, and asked us to integrate improving adherence to hydration and exercise recommendations as part of treatment. He supported our treatment approach and agreed that although she may initially feel more symptoms from moving, this was in fact the most important thing for her to do. We asked about any barriers to physical function, and he assured us that Ashley did not need any activity restrictions beyond sitting down when she felt dizzy.

Next, we contacted Ashley's primary care provider, a pediatrician who had known her for many years, who was able to provide additional background that helped us put Ashley's current symptoms into a larger context, including a family history of significant health anxiety in her mother, as well as difficulty Ashley had with managing stress in late middle school prior to the current symptom onset. In turn, we shared our assessment and treatment plan with her, and she expressed gratitude for knowing how Ashley's treatment would look going forward so she could check in with her and support her progress. The conversation with both providers was invaluable, as all providers were able to give basically the same recommendation with support from the others. Had either doctor ordered that one extra test, the family would have had a more difficult time buying into the overall biopsychosocial treatment approach to somatic symptoms. Good team communication improves care from this angle as well.

After assessment, in the initial stages of treatment, Ashley still experienced significant impairment, so our communication with her cardiologist and primary care provider occurred after every session at first. This connection was crucial for us in knowing how to progress her functional plan as well as to keep her physicians in the loop regarding her response to initial treatment efforts. She saw her physicians regularly during this time as well. They supported our efforts to further increase her function, and our close communication enabled them to positively support the role of CBT in her care, which helped mitigate her initial distrust of working with a mental health provider. In addition to our communication with Ashley's primary medical providers, during her treatment we also discovered that the family was seeking out second and third opinions. We communicated with the family about this, telling them that our treatment would not change based on the cause of Ashley's symptoms, so that even if the new opinions found a rare disease that had otherwise been missed, she still needed help coping with feeling dizzy.

After this productive but slow start to treatment, Ashley had a setback as we entered level two intervention. She contracted a cold, a simple viral illness, but based on her poor physical condition, it set her back significantly so that her symptoms increased and she began to decline instead of progress in function (e.g., was unable to walk due to dizziness, did not get out of bed some days). We consulted with the pediatrician on whether she needed a higher level of care to get back on track, such as a hospital admission to stabilize symptoms and improve function, but the family elected to treat her at home. During this time, we got into an "every other" pattern for sessions in her CBT intervention; one time we would be on track learning the skills, the next time it would be crisis management for the latest symptom flare, next time back on track, and so forth. After about a month of this, Ashley and her family were concerned that CBT wasn't working for them and we were, too, until we stood back and realized that in six sessions, we'd only delivered 50% of the treatment we had planned because of all of the distractions. The lack of treatment success was in fact because we hadn't been delivering the treatment!

While we knew that Ashley was having symptom exacerbations after her viral illness, we also reflected that in some unintentional way, the symptoms were reinforcing an avoidance cycle with regard to learning new strategies, because the family was very scared about her increasing function, and the symptom setback was getting them out of facing a lot of fears. This is something we remind ourselves of in challenging patient situations, which can be very difficult in terms of managing the family's anxiety or distress around crises; setting a treatment agenda and sticking to it is an important part of the treatment process, including explaining that rationale to the family.

Fortunately, Ashley and her mom were able to hear this rationale and stay the course in treatment. We stayed with level one interventions while she followed her pediatrician's recommendations for home care, and soon her symptoms returned to their baseline level. We were then able to progress through the rest of treatment. Ashley's function improved with her more consistent use of coping skills, especially as she transitioned into level three treatment, and she was able to go back to school for half days.

The most challenging functional barrier for Ashley to overcome was driving, and for this decision we deferred to the cardiologist. It is our recommendation that medical providers take responsibility for driving recommendations. You can help them track frequency of and impairment from symptoms as well as the teenager's awareness of triggering events in treatment, so the patient and family can present this information for further discussion with the physician. There are no well-established criteria for driving with somatic symptoms. This is less pertinent for chronic pain and GI symptoms than it is for neurological (e.g., nonepileptic seizures, gait disturbances, conversion disorder) and cardiac presentations (e.g., syncopal episodes). In Ashley's case, her cardiologist recommended that she refrain from driving until she had a period where her symptoms were stable and didn't result in any blackout episodes, and after that recommended that she drive short distances with supervision.

For children at any level of impairment and collaborative need, as you gain more experience in treating children with somatic symptoms, you will quickly become the expert, confidently providing symptom information and a cohesive treatment plan for diagnoses that feel confusing for medical and mental health providers. They will look to you for guidance when you may have intended to call *them* for the guidance!

We encourage you to adopt this role as you feel comfortable; everyone has something to learn from others when it comes to communicating about care. As with the advice we offer to parents to be structured but flexible, you will provide this type of support for health care collaborators too. When medical providers cannot "fix" their patients and find themselves feeling frustrated or ineffective, you can help them realize that none of you have to fix it; better yet, take a flexible approach of normalizing the up-and-down nature of recovery and reiterate the importance for the whole team of staying the course.

MAKING REFERRALS

So far in this chapter, we have primarily focused on how to facilitate effective collaboration with health care colleagues when they refer a child with somatic symptoms to you for treatment. While this is the more common scenario, it can also happen that you need to *make* a referral for a child with whom you are working. In this section, we review the common scenarios we encounter when making a referral, including frequent referral resources as well as knowing when other treatment modalities would be effective in the care of the child with whom you are working. We discuss the most common referrals that we make, including to other mental health providers, psychiatry providers, primary care providers, and for additional testing. In general, when making a referral, include information about what diagnostic terminologies have been shared with the family, the family's understanding of the symptoms, what interventions were most helpful in your work with the child, and what the family was told about the role of the referring provider.

You might make a referral when you believe it is time to consider a different level of care entirely. Despite our best efforts, sometimes children require a higher level of intervention than is effectively provided in an outpatient setting. In our practice, when children do not attend school consistently or are unable to carry out the interventions taught to them in the outpatient setting, it is typically time to refer to a higher level of care. If the barrier is comorbid mood disorders (e.g., severe anxiety or depression affecting ability to use coping skills), then consider referral to a psychiatric day treatment program or inpatient program if there are safety concerns, with the assumption the child will return to outpatient care once he or she is stabilized. If the barrier is symptom acuity (e.g., too disabled to attend sessions or carry out recommended coping strategies at home), an inpatient or day treatment program that targets functional restoration can be an appropriate and helpful next step to increase the structure, dose, and intensity of care (e.g., chronic pain programs).

Another referral that therapists make is to other mental health providers, when children step down (or up) from one treatment level to another or require intervention for a comorbid mood disorder. For instance, an inpatient psychologist or mental health provider may focus on mood stabilization and behavioral activation and then transfer care for longer-term work to an outpatient provider upon discharge. Depending on the facility and the reason for the stay, the child might be discharged still having symptoms (e.g., after an acute medical hospitalization for an additional workup or procedures) or stable but not fully recovered (e.g., after a course of day treatment or inpatient rehabilitation). If you are the referring provider, it is important to communicate with the next mental health provider. If you are working in an acute, inpatient, rehabilitation, partial hospitalization, or day treatment program, you have access to a rich setting for seeing the child in different environments with different expectations. These observations are valuable to share with the outpatient provider, as it is helpful for him or her to know how the child functioned in a highly structured setting. Also, the outpatient provider will likely be appreciative of what you have been able to do in treatment in the acute setting and will be able to advance that work in the outpatient setting. For comorbid psychological concerns, you may consider transferring treatment or working simultaneously on mood as well as somatic symptoms.

Referrals for evaluations are sometimes warranted in the course of children's care, either to medical providers or psychologists. As mentioned in the case example with Ashley, children should be referred to primary care providers for acute medical concerns (e.g., viral illness) or attentional concerns, such as evaluation and treatment for ADHD. At times, children also benefit from referral for psychological or neuropsychological testing if there are concerns regarding behavior, memory, attention, or learning beyond the challenges related to somatic symptoms.

Finally, there is no perfect guideline on when to refer a child to see a psychiatry provider, including a physician or nurse practitioner, to discuss pharmacological treatment. Some children with somatic symptoms are referred for mental health intervention from psychiatrists, as it is relatively rare for psychiatrists to provide CBT in the scope of their practice, but most commonly, the children we see have not already seen a psychiatrist or nurse practitioner. Our rule of thumb for considering the addition of medication to treatment is that if the child is using the strategies consistently with minimal success, it is appropriate to consider a referral. For some children, their level of physiological arousal is just too high to be able to make good use of behavioral or cognitive strategies without psychopharmacological intervention—in such cases, using diaphragmatic breathing can be like trying to put out a house fire with a squirt gun.

Although there are some empirical investigations of the use of selective serotonin reuptake inhibitors in the management of psychogenic nonepileptic seizures, conversion disorders, and vasovagal syncope in adults, there are no randomized controlled trials in the pediatric population. Anecdotally, psychopharmacological intervention for children with somatic symptoms can be useful in treating co-occurring anxiety or depression that may hinder their ability to use cognitive-behavioral strategies targeted at improving function. With regard to FGIDs, a multisite randomized controlled trial found that amitriptyline was no more effective than placebo in treating GI pain (Saps et al., 2009). Overall, there is minimal information on the treatment of somatic symptoms from a psychopharmacological perspective. Medication is not the only line of treatment that should be recommended for children with somatic symptoms, and it is fair to say that the treatment for which we have the most evidence of success in children with somatic symptoms is CBT.

CHAPTER SUMMARY AND TAKE-AWAY NOTES

- Open communication with health care colleagues about treatment is a necessary part of working with children with somatic symptoms in order to achieve a team-based, collaborative approach to care, while empowering families to continue their direct communication with medical providers as well.

- We conceptualize three levels of collaboration—low, moderate, and high—based on children's level of impairment related to symptoms. The level of collaboration impacts the frequency and content of communication for effective treatment. Providers can learn about one another's approach to support and coordinate treatment to enhance overall care.

- Make a referral for another level of care or to another provider when a child would benefit from additional medical support, psychiatric evaluation or treatment, or further mental health support or testing.

CHAPTER 12

Summary, Challenges, and Successes

As you finish this book, we hope that you have found these chapters helpful in understanding, assessing, educating, treating, and finally collaborating on the care of children with somatic symptoms. We have both dedicated our practice and professional careers to working with children in this population and find it to be incredibly rewarding work. We are always eager to add more providers to our group of colleagues in the world of somatic symptoms. Our goal in writing this book was to provide you with the techniques and tools we use on a daily basis, so that you could pick up this book and feel successful and competent in providing this treatment. Children with somatic symptoms are everywhere, and they significantly benefit from psychological intervention. We are excited at the prospect of this information aiding in the treatment of children and families who are in need of your services. We want to leave you with just a few thoughts on the challenges and successes of working in the world of somatic symptoms.

While there are many successes in delivering treatment in this patient population, there are also a number of challenges, as there are in any population of children and families seeking mental health services. For children with somatic symptoms, the major way in which the challenges present is typically medical, such as children becoming more disabled, having additional symptoms, or seeking more medical work-up and treatment, which often results in families and providers becoming discombobulated regarding what the problems are and exactly "who's on first" to address them. There are several factors to think about when working with these types of challenging cases.

First, once the organic medical piece has been ruled out or accounted for, the next step is to figure out the purpose of the symptoms or health-care-seeking behavior. Is it anxiety driven? On the part of the family or the child? Families who seek additional help or treatment in those circumstance may be engaging in a process that is akin to an avoidance strategy—as long as providers are busy seeking solutions or researching treatments or referring to other providers, the pressure to get better is lifted from the child and the family. Assess buy-in to treatment in these scenarios, standing behind evidence-based treatment, and not making too many reactive changes to the plan. Otherwise, their idea that your treatment will fail will become a self-fulfilling prophecy, because you will not have delivered it in the manner or context in which you would typically do. We go by the rule that the harder or more challenging the situation, the less we change the treatment and, in fact, the more dogmatically we follow it unless there is clear indication to change course (e.g., new medical or psychological diagnosis).

Second, consider how burdened with work you are feeling in these challenging situations. Are you working harder than the child on creating change? What is that reflective of in your process or in the child's process? Making sure you have a close network of colleagues, both mental health providers as well as our allied health partners, is critical to ensure that *you* have an outlet to seek consultation on difficult cases as well as to manage your own emotional stress that can come with tolerating a child and family's significant distress. We believe this is a large part of our job as clinicians working with these families, to tolerate distress. Remember that our job is not to fix it—we are setting out to help children and families fix *themselves* with the right education and tools—our job is to sit in the same room with someone who might be in pain, or dizzy, or unable to walk, and interact with them as if they are a person who can get better, while modeling calm coping in the face of distress. Keep in mind it is a difficult job to work with children who are struggling with symptoms and be able to encourage them to keep going. In any other situation, we would be racing out to find a physician if a child we were working with had a medical problem in the course of a CBT session! Instead, we sit with children through these experiences, modeling how to cope with them. One of the most challenging things we are asked to do as human beings is *not* respond to another's distress as we are innately wired to do, and it is important for you to recognize the normal distress associated with going against that natural desire and to get support when it feels overwhelming.

In addition to the challenges of working with children with somatic symptoms and their families, there are many successes, such as the efficacy of this approach to treatment, which we cite whenever given the opportunity—whether it be with families or children or colleagues or our own family members who are curious about our professional lives. This means we talk about how CBT is an *evidence-based treatment* for somatic symptoms. Sometimes people who are unfamiliar with psychological interventions, especially as they pertain to treating medical problems, might not know that these are interventions that are studied and tested with scientific rigor, in the same way that medical interventions are evaluated. This lack of knowledge can perpetuate the myth that psychological intervention is somehow less scientific or less justified as a treatment. From a solid evidence base, we can say with confidence that CBT is helpful for coping with mood, stress, and somatic symptoms. A study that we often remind ourselves of found that parents of children with chronic pain actually felt that psychological treatment was not only acceptable, but potentially *one of the most effective therapies* for their children (Claar & Scharff, 2007). This is also important to remember, because as much as we are prepared to justify what we do, there are many children and families out there who are open to and eager for the type of intervention we have to offer. By and large, our experience is that most families we encounter are looking for different treatment options for their children, are aware of CBT, and are willing to try it.

Another way to successfully talk about this work to others is to frame CBT as coping skills training, which helps demystify it and ensure that people understand what the treatment actually is, versus falling back on preconceived notions of psychological treatment. When appropriate, share a story of a time that these skills were helpful for you or your colleagues. For example, when making a CBT referral for children with somatic symptoms, a physician colleague we worked with got into the practice of sharing his own experience of learning progressive muscle relaxation and how it helped him fall back to sleep after he got paged in the middle of the night. This was such a simple story to share, but so powerful because he modeled how coping skills training was something so normal and helpful that even a physician would do it! We both have shared stories about times when we used the same coping skills we are teaching to children, even highlighting the times the skills did not work perfectly, such as using diaphragmatic breathing and cognitive reframing to calm down, guided imagery to manage pain, and pleasant activities to manage stress. Or, you could always consider sharing stories about other children (anonymously, of course) who have gone through treatment and learned to manage their somatic symptoms, and what they have found helpful. Children learn best through examples, as many adults do as well, and personalized stories go a long way in making children feel hopeful about the positive impact coping skills could have on their lives, too.

Perhaps our favorite reason for working with children with somatic symptoms is to witness their feats of success in the face of great distress. We get to see firsthand the effects of hope and resilience that children have a knack for embodying. There is such joy to be experienced when a child walks unassisted for the first time, makes it through a whole day of school without having a stomachache even once, or sends you a letter years later to let you know that he graduated from high school and is heading off to college to pursue a dream he previously thought was impossible. Our wish for you is that you also feel the happiness that comes with being a part of this journey with children and families, and take the time to celebrate the big and small accomplishments along the way.

And finally, we have to acknowledge the treatment successes of the many children and families with whom we have worked, who have shared so many positive messages with us about how we have given them the tools to understand and recover from their symptoms. We have heard from children about the value they felt in being heard, listened to, understood, worked with, and supported through the ups and downs that somatic symptoms bring to children's and family's lives. We have heard from their parents about how they felt guided, like they had a partner in this journey, and the confidence they took from our modeling of how to support their children. The most important message to give to a child with somatic symptoms is "These symptoms are real, they come from normal body processes that just aren't working normally, they are not your fault, and there are really helpful coping skills you can learn to manage them." Ultimately, through this approach and treatment, we can get children back on their feet and into their lives.

Reproducible Materials

The materials presented in the Appendix are designed to be both educational and interactive. Children and families benefit from concrete description of concepts during treatment sessions, as well as having something to reference when they go home. These handouts and worksheets illustrate the concepts described in the sections on assessment, education, intervention, and collaboration, and are presented in the order in which they are referenced in the book. This list also serves as a guide for the order in which treatment is delivered. It is suitable to print these materials for each child you work with and keep them in a file folder to use as you progress through treatment, or provide them to children in their own coping skills binder that they bring to each session.

THE FIGHT–OR–FLIGHT RESPONSE

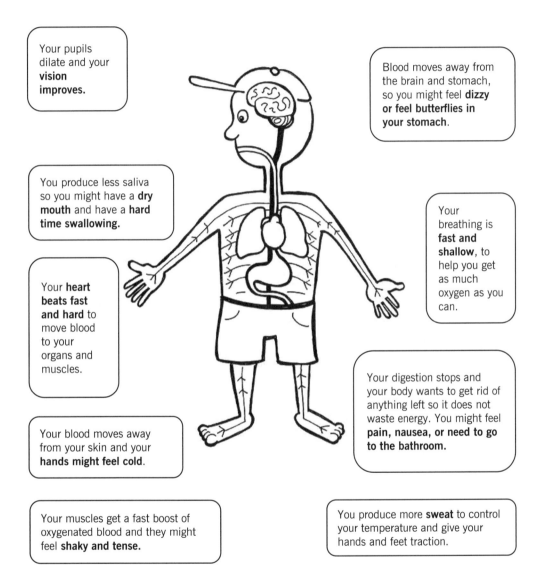

Your short-term memory changes so you can pay attention to danger, which means it is **hard to concentrate** on other things.

Epinephrine triggers a release of blood sugar which gives you a **rush of energy.**

Your pupils dilate and your **vision improves.**

Blood moves away from the brain and stomach, so you might feel **dizzy or feel butterflies in your stomach**.

You produce less saliva so you might have a **dry mouth** and have a **hard time swallowing.**

Your breathing is **fast and shallow**, to help you get as much oxygen as you can.

Your **heart beats fast and hard** to move blood to your organs and muscles.

Your digestion stops and your body wants to get rid of anything left so it does not waste energy. You might feel **pain, nausea, or need to go to the bathroom.**

Your blood moves away from your skin and your **hands might feel cold**.

Your muscles get a fast boost of oxygenated blood and they might feel **shaky and tense.**

You produce more **sweat** to control your temperature and give your hands and feet traction.

THE REST-AND-DIGEST RESPONSE

Your short-term memory functions normally and you can use your thinking and problem solving skills again as your **concentration improves.**

Blood sugar stabilizes and is stored for future activity, and **the body is able to be at rest.**

Your pupils constrict and your **vision is back to normal**.

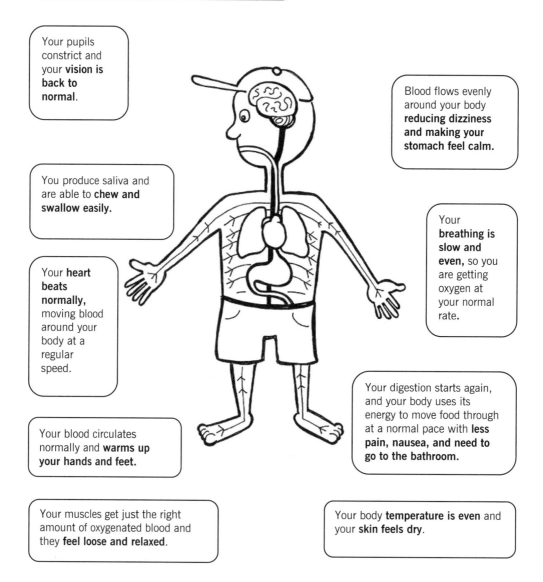

Blood flows evenly around your body **reducing dizziness and making your stomach feel calm.**

You produce saliva and are able to **chew and swallow easily.**

Your **breathing is slow and even,** so you are getting oxygen at your normal rate.

Your **heart beats normally,** moving blood around your body at a regular speed.

Your digestion starts again, and your body uses its energy to move food through at a normal pace with **less pain, nausea, and need to go to the bathroom.**

Your blood circulates normally and **warms up your hands and feet.**

Your muscles get just the right amount of oxygenated blood and they **feel loose and relaxed.**

Your body **temperature is even** and your **skin feels dry**.

LEARNING TO DRIVE THE "AUTO"NOMIC NERVOUS SYSTEM

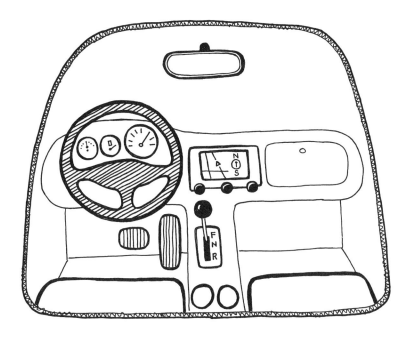

To understand how your body works and how that affects your symptoms, imagine your body is like a car and you're the driver. The autonomic nervous system is like the engine of your body, and just like a car, there are two important functions of the engine, accelerating and braking.

Your sympathetic nervous system, which controls the fight-or-flight response, is like hitting the gas pedal. Epinephrine (also known as adrenaline) is released to make your body go fast, use your energy, and respond to the situation. But if you go too fast for too long, this can make symptoms worse. What do you notice in your body when you're driving at top speed?

Your parasympathetic nervous system, which controls the rest-and-digest response, is like hitting the brakes. Acetylcholine and other chemicals are released to make your body slow down, save your energy, and help you recover. If you allow your body to slow back down to a normal speed, this can also make symptoms better. What do you notice in your body when you're going slowly?

The speedometer tells us how fast the engine is going. Since humans do not have speedometers, we use signs in our body like heart rate, breathing, muscle tension, and sweating to tell us if we are going at a low, relaxed speed, at a fast, stressed speed, or somewhere in the middle. The goal is to learn how to be a good driver, taking control of our "auto" and using the right balance of gas and brakes to help our body go at a moderate speed and feel the best it can.

THE GATE CONTROL THEORY OF PAIN

When pain signals arrive at the brain, they have to pass through something like a gate that can open and close.

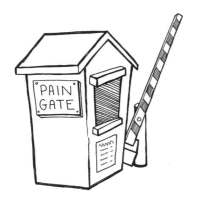

When the gate is open, all of the pain signals are allowed to come through, and your brain experiences the full amount of pain that is being communicated. You actually want the gate to be open to feel pain and protect yourself in case of acute injury (like touching a hot stove). However, for chronic pain, it's not helpful to have the gate open.

Gate openers: paying attention to pain, the fight-or-flight response, feeling nervous or upset, stressful situations.

If the gate is halfway open, the signals can still get in, so the pain will be more than if the gate was closed, but less than if the gate was all the way open. Pain signals still get into the brain, but in a slower fashion, lessening the pain experience.

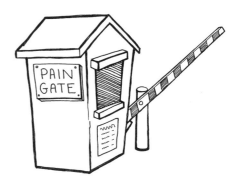

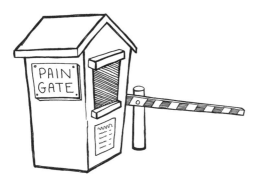

When the gate is closed, pain signals are not able to carry their message to your brain, and you do not feel any pain, even if the signals are there. You want the gate to be closed if you have chronic pain.

Gate closers: distraction from pain, the rest-and-digest response, feeling calm and happy, the right support from family and friends.

BIOPSYCHOSOCIAL ASSESSMENT TOOL

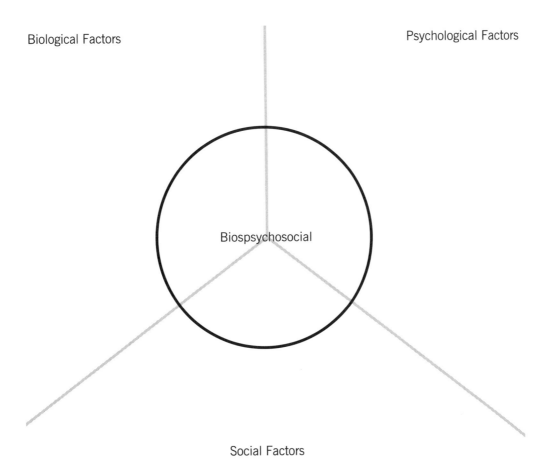

Biological Factors

Psychological Factors

Biospsychosocial

Social Factors

CARDIAC SYMPTOMS FACT SHEET

Terminology: neurocardiogenic syncope (NCS), neurally mediated syncope, vasovagal syncope, vasodepressor syncope, neurally mediated hypotension, syncope, passing out, fainting, psychogenic syncope, presyncope, dizziness, shortness of breath, dysautonomia, postural orthostatic tachycardia syndrome (POTS), orthostatic intolerance, noncardiac chest pain

WHAT ARE CARDIAC SYMPTOMS?

Syncope is the most common cardiac symptom and happens in response to something stressful, like pain, emotion, or a quick change in position. There is a release of epinephrine (also called adrenaline), followed by an increase and then slowing of the heart rate, which drops blood pressure and limits oxygenated blood flow to the brain. Children then feel dizzy and may have blurry vision, weakness, sweating, or nausea, or may pass out. Psychogenic syncope means fainting without changes in heart rate or blood pressure. POTS is related to poor regulation of the autonomic nervous system and happens when the heart rate increases rapidly and causes dizziness when going from sitting to standing. Somatic symptoms are biological in nature and are *real*. They are not voluntary or produced on purpose. They are a physical way that children experience stress and are more likely to occur in situations where the body is physically or emotionally activated, like in times of excitement, worry, or high activity.

Symptoms and disease are often thought of together, but in reality they are separate. Symptoms are a person's own experience of changes in the body, and disease is a detectable problem in the body. A person may have a disease with no symptoms, but somatic symptoms are the opposite: symptoms with no current damage, injury, or infection in the body. Somatic symptoms are the result of a triggering of the stress response and a change in the way normal body processes work. In addition to being seen by a medical provider to make sure they receive any necessary evaluations or treatments, children with these types of symptoms are often referred to a mental health provider to help them manage their symptoms, be less affected by symptoms, and be able to return to their normal activities.

HOW ARE THESE SYMPTOMS MANAGED?

Cognitive-behavioral therapy (CBT) is an evidence-based treatment that helps children and adolescents improve their coping and management of somatic symptoms by focusing on the connections between their thoughts, feelings, body responses, and actions. CBT teaches children how to engage in positive and realistic thinking patterns, as well as use relaxation, healthy habits, and participation in pleasant activities as coping skills. The goal of CBT is to change the way children think, feel, and act on their somatic symptoms, allowing them to do more of the things they enjoy, even if they cannot always control or predict when their symptoms will occur. CBT is structured and skill-based. It is something the child actively learns, does, and practices outside of session. Through CBT, children will learn:

- How to understand symptoms physically, emotionally, behaviorally, and socially
- How to identify thoughts, feelings, and behavior patterns that affect symptoms
- How to choose the best coping skills for their symptoms

Parents have an important role in encouraging their children as they use their skills outside of session. It is also important to collaborate with the school and health care providers. Together, they can use this approach to help children learn the skills they need to be successful and build a network to support children in returning to their normal activities.

GASTROINTESTINAL SYMPTOMS FACT SHEET

Terminology: functional gastrointestinal disorders (FGIDs), disorders of brain–gut interaction, functional abdominal pain (FAP), functional bowel disorder (FBD), irritable bowel syndrome (IBS), gastroparesis, belly pain, rumination, functional nausea, functional vomiting, abdominal migraine

WHAT ARE GASTROINTESTINAL SYMPTOMS?

Gastrointestinal (GI) symptoms, like abdominal pain, nausea, and diarrhea, all share the feature of ongoing or frequent symptoms resulting from problems in the way the brain and the gut communicate with each other, instead of structural abnormality or disease. Somatic symptoms are biological in nature and are *real.* They are not voluntary or produced on purpose. They are a physical way that children experience stress and are more likely to occur in situations where the body is physically or emotionally activated, like in times of excitement, worry, or high activity.

Symptoms and disease are often thought of together, but in reality they are separate. Symptoms are a person's own experience of changes in their body, and disease is a detectable problem in the body. A person may have a disease with no symptoms, but somatic symptoms are the opposite: symptoms with no current damage, injury, or infection in the body. Somatic symptoms are the result of a triggering of the stress response and a change in the way normal body processes work. In addition to being seen by a medical provider to ensure that they receive any necessary evaluations or treatments, children with these types of symptoms are often referred to a mental health provider to help them manage their symptoms, be less affected by symptoms, and be able to return to their normal activities.

HOW ARE THESE SYMPTOMS MANAGED?

Cognitive-behavioral therapy (CBT) is an evidence-based treatment that helps children and adolescents improve their coping and management of somatic symptoms by focusing on the connections between their thoughts, feelings, body responses, and actions. CBT teaches children how to engage in positive and realistic thinking patterns, as well as use relaxation, healthy habits, and participation in pleasant activities as coping skills. The goal of CBT is to change the way children think, feel, and act on their somatic symptoms, allowing them to do more of the things they enjoy, even if they cannot always control or predict when their symptoms will occur. CBT is structured and skill-based. It is something the child actively learns, does, and practices outside of session. Through CBT, children will learn:

- How to understand symptoms physically, emotionally, behaviorally, and socially
- How to identify thoughts, feelings, and behavior patterns that affect symptoms
- How to choose the best coping skills for their symptoms

Parents have an important role in encouraging their children as they use their skills outside of session. It is also important to collaborate with the school and health care providers. Together, they can use this approach to help children learn the skills they need to be successful and build a network to support children in returning to their normal activities.

NEUROLOGICAL SYMPTOMS FACT SHEET

Terminology: conversion disorder, functional neurological symptom disorder, psychogenic non-epileptic seizures (PNES), nonepileptic seizures, pseudoseizures, functional movement disorder, functional gait disorder, functional gait imbalance, psychogenic movements, spells, numbness, tingling, paresthesia, psychogenic blindness

WHAT ARE NEUROLOGICAL SYMPTOMS?

Functional neurological symptoms, like spells, muscle weakness, or tremors, are motor move-ment or sensation problems that are not due to injury or disease in the brain, but rather are due to problems in the way the nervous system communicates with the body. Somatic symptoms are biological in nature and are *real*. They are not voluntary or produced on purpose. They are a physical way that children experience stress and are more likely to occur in situations where the body is physically or emotionally activated, like in times of excitement, worry, or high activity.

Symptoms and disease are often thought of together, but in reality they are separate. Symp-toms are a person's own experience of changes in the body, and disease is a detectable prob-lem in the body. A person may have a disease with no symptoms, but somatic symptoms are the opposite: symptoms with no current damage, injury, or infection in the body. For example, children with nonepileptic seizures have shaking episodes that resemble epileptic seizures but are not associated with abnormal brain electrical activity. Children with a functional gait disor-der have difficulty walking or leg paralysis that is not associated with an identified brain injury. Somatic symptoms are the result of a triggering of the stress response and a change in the way normal body processes work. In addition to being seen by a medical provider to ensure that they receive any necessary evaluations or treatments, children with these types of symptoms are often referred to a mental health provider to help them manage with their symptoms, be less affected by symptoms, and be able to return to their normal activities.

HOW ARE THESE SYMPTOMS MANAGED?

Cognitive-behavioral therapy (CBT) is an evidence-based treatment that helps children and ado-lescents improve their coping and management of somatic symptoms by focusing on the connec-tions between their thoughts, feelings, body responses, and actions. CBT teaches children how to engage in positive and realistic thinking patterns, as well as use relaxation, healthy habits, and participation in pleasant activities as coping skills. The goal of CBT is to change the way children think, feel, and act on their somatic symptoms, allowing them to do more of the things they enjoy, even if they cannot always control or predict when their symptoms will occur. CBT is structured and skill-based. It is something the child actively learns, does, and practices outside of session. Through CBT, children will learn:

- How to understand symptoms physically, emotionally, behaviorally, and socially
- How to identify thoughts, feelings, and behavior patterns that affect symptoms
- How to choose the best coping skills for their symptoms

Parents have an important role in encouraging their children as they use their skills outside of session. It is also important to collaborate with the school and health care providers. Together, they can use this approach to help children learn the skills they need to be successful and build a network to support children in returning to their normal activities.

Terminology: amplified musculoskeletal pain syndrome (AMPS), widespread chronic pain, fibromyalgia, complex regional pain syndrome (CRPS), reflexive sympathetic dystrophy (RSD), chronic migraine, chronic headache, functional pain disorder, chronic pain syndrome, primary pain disorder

WHAT ARE PAIN SYMPTOMS?

A chronic pain syndrome is characterized by recurrent or chronic pain that has persisted for 3 or more months in the absence of identifiable disease or lasting longer than what would be expected after recovery from injury. Chronic pain is caused by problems in the activity of the central nervous system. Somatic symptoms are biological in nature and are *real.* They are not voluntary or produced on purpose. They are a physical way that individuals experience stress and are more likely to occur in situations where the body is physically or emotionally activated, like in times of excitement, worry, or high activity.

Symptoms and disease are often thought of together, but in reality they are separate. Symptoms are a person's own experience of changes in their body and disease is a detectable problem in the body. A person may have a disease with no symptoms, but somatic symptoms are the opposite: symptoms with no current damage, injury, or infection in the body. Somatic symptoms are the result of a triggering of the stress response and a change in the way normal body processes work. In addition to being seen by a medical provider to ensure that they receive any necessary evaluations or treatments, children with these types of symptoms are often referred to a mental health provider to help them cope with their symptoms, reduce symptom-related impairment, and improve their function.

HOW ARE THESE SYMPTOMS MANAGED?

Cognitive-behavioral therapy (CBT) is an evidence-based treatment that helps children and adolescents improve their coping and management of somatic symptoms by focusing on the connections between their thoughts, feelings, body responses, and actions. CBT teaches children how to engage in positive and realistic thinking patterns, as well as use relaxation, healthy habits, and participation in pleasant activities as coping skills. The goal of CBT is to change the way children think, feel, and act on their somatic symptoms, allowing them to do more of the things they enjoy, even if they cannot always control or predict when their symptoms will occur. CBT is structured and skill-based. It is something the child actively learns, does, and practices outside of session. Through CBT, children will learn:

- How to understand symptoms physically, emotionally, behaviorally, and socially
- How to identify thoughts, feelings, and behavior patterns that affect symptoms
- How to choose the best coping skills for their symptoms

Parents have an important role in encouraging their children as they use their skills outside of session. It is also important to collaborate with the school and healthcare providers. Together, they can use this approach to help children learn the skills they need to be successful and build a network to support children in returning to their normal activities.

HEALTHY HABITS

Drinking	Eating
No caffeine, 64 ounces of fluids per day (or as directed) **My goals:**	Eat regular meals, including a well-balanced diet of protein, vegetables, dairy, grains, and fruits (or as directed) **My goals:**
Sleeping 12 years and under, 9–12 hours; 13 years and older, 8–10 hours **My goals:**	**Moving** 60 minutes per day (or as directed) **My goals:**

SYMPTOM TRACKING

Date	Description of symptoms (+/−)	How long did symptoms last?	What was I doing?	What was I thinking about?	What was I feeling?

DAILY SCHEDULE TEMPLATE

Time	Activity	Did I do it?
6 A.M.		
7 A.M.		
8 A.M.		
9 A.M.		
10 A.M.		
11 A.M.		
12 P.M.		
1 P.M.		
2 P.M.		
3 P.M.		
4 P.M.		
5 P.M.		
6 P.M.		
7 P.M.		
8 P.M.		
9 P.M.		
10 P.M.		

Wake times, mealtimes, and bedtimes should be consistent: do not change them by more than about an hour from day to day. Give yourself a reward after finishing tasks on your schedule, such as taking a short break to play a game, spend time with a pet, go outside, or watch a show you enjoy.

FEELINGS IDENTIFICATION

Feeling: Situation(s): Body Responses:	Feeling: Situation(s): Body Responses:
Feeling: Situation(s): Body Responses:	Feeling: Situation(s): Body Responses:

THE ROADMAP

Feelings

Thoughts

Actions

Body Responses

DISTRACTING AND PLEASANT ACTIVITIES

It is important to do things you enjoy every day. Even little things can make a *big* difference in how you are feeling. Put an X by the activities you would like to do more often.

- ☐ Watch a movie or TV show
- ☐ Listen to music
- ☐ Look out the window
- ☐ Laugh
- ☐ Learn a new joke
- ☐ Listen to others
- ☐ Read a magazine
- ☐ Learn a new recipe
- ☐ Think about my good qualities
- ☐ Go ice skating
- ☐ Play basketball
- ☐ Join a sports team
- ☐ Find a relaxing scent
- ☐ View some art
- ☐ Doodle
- ☐ Think about people I love
- ☐ Stretch
- ☐ Put on scented lotion
- ☐ Take care of a plant
- ☐ Think about things I'd like to buy
- ☐ Make a list of things I'd like to do
- ☐ Learn about a foreign country
- ☐ Look at photos
- ☐ Teach my pet a new trick
- ☐ Paint my nails
- ☐ Think about how I've improved
- ☐ Say "I love you" to someone important
- ☐ Say thank you
- ☐ Get a back rub
- ☐ Sing a song
- ☐ Write 10 things I'm thankful for
- ☐ Talk to someone about my feelings
- ☐ Imagine myself at the beach
- ☐ Sew
- ☐ Make a gift for someone
- ☐ Make decorations for my room
- ☐ Make a collage
- ☐ Design a T-shirt
- ☐ Make a list of goals
- ☐ Face paint
- ☐ Go online

- ☐ Make a necklace
- ☐ Wash the car
- ☐ Mow the lawn
- ☐ Play catch with a ball
- ☐ Do jumping jacks
- ☐ Color
- ☐ Write in a journal
- ☐ Plan a party
- ☐ Write a story
- ☐ Draw
- ☐ Do arts and crafts
- ☐ Daydream
- ☐ Plan what I'll do when I grow up
- ☐ Meditate
- ☐ Play an instrument
- ☐ Play a game
- ☐ Read/write song lyrics
- ☐ Knit/crochet
- ☐ Join a soccer league
- ☐ Shovel snow
- ☐ Lift hand weights
- ☐ Learn a magic trick
- ☐ Text/call a friend
- ☐ Visit friends' profiles on social media
- ☐ Read a book
- ☐ Act
- ☐ Be alone
- ☐ Write a supportive letter to myself
- ☐ Try a new hobby/sport
- ☐ Use a cold/warm compress
- ☐ Use Play-Doh or clay
- ☐ Do a crossword or Sudoku puzzle
- ☐ Practice yoga or take a class
- ☐ Learn something new
- ☐ Make some music
- ☐ Walk around a museum or zoo
- ☐ Think about happy times with friends
- ☐ Turn off electronics
- ☐ Fly a kite
- ☐ Watch the stars
- ☐ Offer to help someone

(continued)

DISTRACTING AND PLEASANT ACTIVITIES

- ☐ Dance or imagine myself dancing
- ☐ Think about something I did well
- ☐ Invite someone to sit and talk
- ☐ Run through the sprinkler
- ☐ Take a walk
- ☐ Play on a softball team
- ☐ Train for a running race
- ☐ Be with other people
- ☐ Think about what makes me special
- ☐ Imagine the future
- ☐ Look up new words
- ☐ Do a jigsaw puzzle
- ☐ Go rollerblading
- ☐ Put on temporary tattoos
- ☐ Take the stairs instead of an elevator
- ☐ Join a swim team
- ☐ Play an active video game
- ☐ Keep a gratitude journal
- ☐ Light a candle/aromatherapy
- ☐ Make a homemade gift
- ☐ Play cards/solitaire
- ☐ Try skiing
- ☐ Spend time with a pet
- ☐ Give myself a facial
- ☐ Squeeze a stress ball
- ☐ Take a bike ride
- ☐ Swing on a swing
- ☐ Go mountain biking
- ☐ Paddle a canoe or kayak
- ☐ Row a boat
- ☐ Complete a random act of kindness
- ☐ Cook or bake
- ☐ Learn a card game
- ☐ Read/write poetry
- ☐ Walk around the mall
- ☐ Call a relative
- ☐ Play tennis
- ☐ Go swimming
- ☐ Watch the clouds
- ☐ Sit in nature
- ☐ Think about happy times with my family
- ☐ Solve a riddle
- ☐ Walk around the block
- ☐ Walk a dog
- ☐ Play volleyball
- ☐ Go sledding
- ☐ Rake the leaves

- ☐ Plant a garden
- ☐ Work out to exercise videos
- ☐ Try karate
- ☐ Take a dance class
- ☐ Play Frisbee
- ☐ Jump rope
- ☐ Chew my favorite gum
- ☐ Clean/organize my room
- ☐ Use colored pens
- ☐ Paint
- ☐ Sketch
- ☐ Go for a scenic drive
- ☐ Go to the park
- ☐ Hike/take a nature walk
- ☐ Join a new club
- ☐ Invent something
- ☐ Take a bubble bath or shower
- ☐ Volunteer
- ☐ Look up tutorials online
- ☐ Do a word search
- ☐ Do a logic puzzle
- ☐ Create or build something
- ☐ Make a playlist
- ☐ Pop bubble wrap
- ☐ Solve a maze
- ☐ Make a video
- ☐ Go to the library
- ☐ Hula hoop
- ☐ Send an encouraging e-mail
- ☐ Learn a new language
- ☐ Play I Spy
- ☐ Go on a scavenger hunt
- ☐ Be silly
- ☐ Build a blanket fort
- ☐ Climb a tree
- ☐ Play outside
- ☐ Watch cute animal videos
- ☐ Play a board game
- ☐ Rearrange my room
- ☐ Plan my dream vacation
- ☐ Blow bubbles
- ☐ Build with Legos
- ☐ Go fishing
- ☐ Video chat with a friend
- ☐ Jump on a trampoline
- ☐ Open a lemonade stand
- ☐ Add my own idea: _____

MINDFULNESS AND THE FIVE SENSES

Much of the stress and tension people experience on a daily basis comes from what is taken in through the senses—what people see, hear, smell, taste, and touch. You can also use the five senses to create a calm atmosphere, reduce stress, and enhance relaxation. This is a strategy called mindfulness, which is a way of placing all of your attention and focus in the moment on something nice and relaxing by just noticing and letting yourself experience it.

See: Looking at calm, slow-moving, or peaceful scenes improves relaxation, mood, and symptoms. You can look out the window at slow-moving clouds, trees, flowers, or water. Inside, look at photographs with nature scenes, loved ones, or happy times. It is also relaxing to look at bubbles floating, a lava lamp, rain falling, or fish swimming in a tank.

Hear: Listening to certain sounds, such as music or nature sounds, provides calm and relaxation. In fact, pleasing music lowers heart rate and blood pressure and calms brain activity. Slower music works better than faster music, but pick music you enjoy. You can also listen to nature sounds like raindrops, wind, rivers, waves, or birds, either by opening the window or with a sound machine, app, or recording.

Smell: Certain scents enhance mood and relaxation, which can help with symptoms. These scents include lavender, vanilla, rose, jasmine, and fruit. To be relaxing, it needs to be a scent that you like! Surround yourself with pleasing scents by using oils, candles, potpourri, or lotions.

Taste: Some tastes also increase relaxation. Having your favorite food can be comforting, soothing, and improve mood. Warm milk or caffeine-free teas can relax your body. When using the sense of taste to help relax, be careful not to feed your emotions or overdo it. Use this one in moderation.

Touch: Physical touch and massage can be healing and lower stress hormones in your body. Massage and heat can reduce somatic symptoms by loosening stiff joints and muscles, and by bringing more blood flow and oxygen to areas of the body that might uncomfortable or tense. This can be done by a professional or at home. You can also take a warm bath or shower or use a hot water bottle or heating pad. It also feels good to get a hug, wear soft comfortable fabrics, roll or squeeze a stress ball in your hand, or pet an animal with soft fur.

A shorter version of mindfulness of the five senses can be used in times of acute stress or symptom flares. We call this "5-4-3-2-1," and you count down five different things you can see in a favorite color, if you would like, such as blue things, four different textures or surfaces you can feel, three different sounds you can hear, two different scents you can smell, and one flavor you can taste or imagine tasting. This is a nice strategy to use when you do not have access to the usual things you find calming to your senses.

DIAPHRAGMATIC BREATHING

Under conditions of stress, either physical or emotional, the body takes short breaths through the upper chest. This kind of shallow breathing disrupts the balance of oxygen and carbon dioxide and increases the heart rate, which makes the body feel *more* stressed as part of the fight-or-flight response.

Diaphragmatic breathing, or belly breathing, reduces stress by lowering heart rate and increasing relaxation. This kind of breathing uses the diaphragm muscle, which is a dome-shaped muscle located under the ribs and above the stomach. Instead of moving the chest, diaphragmatic breathing moves the stomach because the lungs are taking in more air. When inhaling, the diaphragm muscle pushes the stomach *out*; when exhaling, the diaphragm moves back to resting position and the stomach goes back *in*. There is little or no upper chest movement. Diaphragmatic breathing is the process of taking deep breaths that provide a good balance of oxygen and carbon dioxide for the body and slow the heart rate, turning on the relaxation response.

GETTING STARTED: FIND YOUR DIAPHRAGM

Place one hand on your stomach at the bottom of your sternum and just above your belly button. Sniff quickly as if you have a runny nose to feel the diaphragm muscle move or jump under your fingers. Keep your hand on your stomach while you slowly breathe in and feel your stomach move out against your hand, then breathe out and feel your stomach moving back in. That is what breathing through your diaphragm feels like!

- Inhaling makes the diaphragm push down to inflate the lungs and the stomach moves out.
- Exhaling makes the diaphragm go back up to a resting position and the stomach moves in.

DIAPHRAGMATIC BREATHING TECHNIQUE

- Lie down or sit comfortably in a chair. When practicing this breathing technique, keep your upper chest and neck muscles as loose and relaxed as possible.
- Place one hand on your upper chest by your collarbone, and the other just below your rib cage at the bottom of your sternum. This will allow you to feel your diaphragm move as you breathe and make sure that your upper chest stays still. You can also try putting something light, like a stuffed animal, on your stomach as a visual reminder.
- Breathe in slowly through your nose so that your stomach moves out against your hand. The hand on your chest should remain as still as possible.
- Slowly breathe out, letting your stomach fall back in as you exhale through your mouth. Keep the hand on your upper chest as still as possible.

KEEP PRACTICING!

Breathe in a cycle; the ideal time for a relaxed breath in and out is 10 seconds altogether—5 seconds in and 5 seconds out—for a total of six breaths per minute. Breathe in slowly and comfortably until your lungs feel like they are full but not bursting, then just hold your breath until it has been 5 seconds, then slowly let your air out and just pause until it has been 5 seconds before you slowly inhale again. Practicing this breathing technique for 10 minutes twice a day will strengthen the diaphragm muscle, train your relaxation response to turn on, and leave you with a nice relaxed feeling. Remember, you have to breathe anyway, so you can practice this strategy anytime, anywhere!

ACTIVE PROGRESSIVE MUSCLE RELAXATION

This exercise loosens up your body from your toes to your head by first tensing each muscle group and then relaxing it. Do each exercise three times, holding for 5 seconds and then relaxing for 5 seconds. As you practice, pace it with deep breathing. As you inhale, tense the muscles, and as you exhale, relax the muscles.

Get started: Get in a relaxed position, either sitting comfortably in a chair or lying down on your bed. Keep your arms at your sides and either put your feet flat on the floor if you are sitting or keep your legs straight if you are lying down. Let your body sink into the chair or bed and close your eyes. Take three deep breaths through your stomach and let your body begin to relax.

Toes: Starting with your toes, curl them up and hold for 5 seconds, then relax. Curl them up again; relax. Tense them one more time; now relax and wiggle them around.

Legs: Lift your legs straight out in front of you, either off the floor or the bed, and hold them up for 5 seconds. Slowly lower them down and feel your leg muscles relax. Lift them again and hold; slowly lower them down. Lift your legs one more time and hold them up, then lower them down again and feel the muscles relax. Your feet and legs are nice and relaxed.

Stomach: Take three deep, relaxing breaths in slowly through your stomach. Tighten the muscles in your stomach and hold; relax and let your stomach muscles move out. Tighten again; then relax. For the last time, breathe in while you tighten in your stomach muscles and hold your breath in, then slowly relax and breathe out. Feel the relaxation in your stomach muscles.

Back: Lift your arms up and stretch them over the top of your head, reaching as far as you can for 5 seconds, then relax and bring them back down by your sides. Reach over your head again and hold, then relax them down by your side. Once more, reach as far as you can over your head, stretching even more this time, and then bring your arms back down feeling loose and relaxed.

Shoulders: Shrug your shoulders up to touch your ears and hold; relax and let your shoulders fall down. Scrunch them up again to your ears; then relax. Once more scrunch them up and feel the tightness, then let your shoulders fall down, even farther than they were before.

Hands: With both hands, make a fist and squeeze as hard as you can for 5 seconds, using your forearm and bicep muscles, too. Relax your hands. Squeeze again, then relax. The last time, squeeze, then relax and wiggle your fingers, letting your hands and arms be loose and relaxed.

Jaw: Slowly and gently clench your teeth together so you feel the tightness in your jaw for 5 seconds. Relax your jaw by opening your mouth, like a yawn. Clench your teeth again; then relax by opening your jaw. Once more clench your teeth, and relax.

Eyes: Close your eyes tightly; hold for 5 seconds, then relax. Squeeze your eyes closed again; hold, then relax. The last time, squeeze and relax.

Forehead: Lifting up your eyebrows, hold for 5 seconds, and relax. Pull your eyebrows up again, hold, then relax. The last time, pull up your eyebrows and wrinkle your forehead, then relax.

End up relaxed: Stay sitting or lying down quietly with your eyes closed. Notice how loose, warm, and relaxed your body feels from your toes all the way up to your head. If there is any leftover tension, go back and loosen that spot. Enjoy the feeling of relaxation.

PASSIVE PROGRESSIVE MUSCLE RELAXATION

This exercise should take about 4–5 minutes.

Find a comfortable position. Lie on your back or sit in a chair with your back supported. Place your hands at your sides. Close your eyes and begin to relax. Take long, slow, deep breaths. Your stomach gets bigger as you breathe in and smaller as you breathe out. Begin to notice how comfortable your body feels. Notice the rhythm of your breathing as you relax. As you exhale, release any tension, any stress from any part of your body. Your body and your mind relax and let go with each breath. Let go of any pain, sadness, or worry with each breath out.

Slowly take a deep breath in . . . pause for a moment . . . and then exhale slowly. Now imagine a shimmering ray of light starting right above your head. You can imagine it to be any color that makes you feel relaxed. Maybe it is blue, or green, or pink, or silver. The light enters at the top of your head and travels over your scalp, relaxing any areas that feel tight. The light moves slowly across your forehead and face, bringing feelings of relaxation to each place that it touches. The light relaxes your eyes, your cheeks, your jaw, and your mouth. In its path it leaves feelings of warmth and calm.

Now imagine the light moving slowly down your neck and into your shoulders, softening them. The light travels slowly across your shoulders, down your right arm and into your hand and fingers, releasing tension and bringing feelings of warmth, then traveling back up your arm and to your left shoulder, bringing feelings of warmth to your left arm, hand, and fingers. You may notice your arms and hands feeling heavy. Take a deep breath in . . . pause for a moment . . . and out . . . feeling relaxation in your body, and letting go of any negative thoughts or feelings.

Feel the shimmering light move down your back, one vertebra at time, releasing tension and pain as it goes. Allow the light to circle around to the front of your body, breathing relaxation and warmth into your chest. Take a deep breath in . . . pause . . . and let the air out . . . releasing any tension. Now imagine breathing the shimmering light into your stomach, filling your body with calm feelings, and breathing out pain or discomfort. Notice how calm and relaxed your head, neck, shoulders, back, and stomach feel.

Let the shimmering light move into your lower body, through your hips and legs, going down your right leg, past your knee, into your calf, and into your foot, pushing stress out of your body as it moves and leaving warmth behind. The light moves slowly back up your leg, and over to your left leg, through your thigh muscle, swirling around your knee, through your calf muscle and out through your toes. Take a deep breath in . . . pause . . . and exhale slowly.

Now the shimmering light has moved through your whole body, relaxing and warming everything along its path, and pushing out pain, tension, or negative feelings. Scan your body to see if there are any areas that still feel tight, and breathe deeply, pulling the light into this area, and letting it relax. Take as much time as you need. Your body feels relaxed and heavy. When you are ready, you can open your eyes and come back, bringing feelings of relaxation and calm with you.

IMAGERY

A fun way to relax is by imagining a calming picture in your mind. It could be a place, real or imaginary, or a picture of something you like. Thinking of a calming place or picture in your mind actually makes your body feel less stressed and more relaxed. Here's how to get started:

- Pick a quiet place and time, so no one will disturb you.
- Get in a comfortable position, either sitting or lying down.
- Close your eyes and imagine your picture.
- Using all of your senses, imagine your picture in lots of detail:
  - Seeing: what are the colors, shapes, and look of things?
  - Hearing: what sounds do you hear?
  - Smell: what do you smell?
  - Taste: what do you taste?
  - Feel: how does your body feel and what emotions do you feel?
- Really imagine yourself in your picture, like you are actually there.
- As you think of your picture, notice how calm and relaxed your body is.

Here is an example: Imagine being on a tropical beach by the ocean.

- Picture yourself on the beach with lots of details—maybe it's a beach you have been to before or one you've seen in a picture or just imagine in your mind.
  - See the blue water, the yellow sun, green palm trees, and brown sand.
  - Hear the sound of the waves, seagulls, and boats passing by.
  - Smell the sunscreen and saltwater.
  - Taste the salty air and a cool refreshing glass of water.
  - Feel the warm sun, cool ocean breeze, and relaxed feeling in your body.
- Imagine this picture in such detail that you actually *feel* like you are there at the beach, and notice how your body feels calm and relaxed.

Remember, you can pick any picture that is special and calming for YOU! It is a good idea to practice imagery every day. The more you practice, the easier it will be to imagine your picture and the quicker your body will feel calm and relaxed. Good times to practice are at night before you go to bed, if you find your mind thinking too much, or anytime you feel stressed.

COPING SKILLS TOOLKIT

Distracting Tools	**Relaxing Tools**
Pleasant, fun, active, calming activities	Imagery, diaphragmatic breathing, muscle relaxation
My favorite tools:	**My favorite tools:**
Living Tools	**Thinking Tools**
Sleep, exercise, hydration, healthy foods, daily schedule	Reframing, problem solving, goal setting
My favorite tools:	**My favorite tools:**

WHAT AFFECTS SOMATIC SYMPTOMS?

SITUATION

If you are busy doing something that holds your attention, is distracting, or fun, symptoms will be less noticeable and bothersome than if you are bored and doing something uninteresting.

- **Goal:** Distraction, completing daily activities, and having fun

FEELINGS

If you are feeling sad, unhappy, frustrated, or worried, symptoms will be worse than if you are feeling happy, relaxed, or calm.

- **Goal:** Calm and neutral emotions

DEGREE OF CONCERN ABOUT SYMPTOMS

If you feel the somatic symptoms mean that something scary is happening in your body, you will feel the symptoms more intensely. The more confident you are about what somatic symptoms are, the better you will be able to manage them.

- **Goal:** Remember that symptoms are real but not dangerous

AMOUNT OF CONTROL OVER SYMPTOMS

If you feel out of control when symptoms happen or like they will take over your whole day, chances are symptoms will negatively affect you. Remembering the strategies you have to manage symptoms if they happen will ensure that you are in charge, not the symptoms.

- **Goal:** Even if you do not have control over when symptoms happen, you do have control over how to cope with them.

Learning how to have positive and realistic thought patterns allows your mind and body to focus on more helpful situations, manage your feelings and the amount of concern you have about your symptoms, and give you a sense of control over your symptoms, all of which improve the symptom experience and allow you to place more focus on function.

THINKING, FEELING, AND DOING

Thoughts affect how you feel emotionally, what body responses you have, and what actions you take. It is important to pay attention to your thoughts and figure out whether they are helping you or making situations harder. Let's look at a few pictures that can help you understand how thoughts affect feelings and actions.

This child won a trophy. What is she thinking? How does she feel?

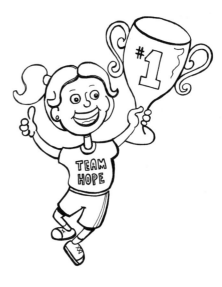

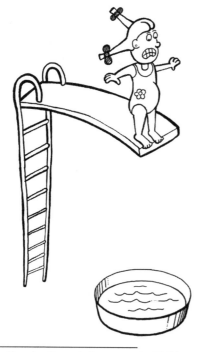

This child is standing on a diving board. What is she thinking? How does she feel? What are her body responses?

(continued)

From *Treating Somatic Symptoms in Children and Adolescents* by Sara E. Williams and Nicole E. Zahka. Copyright © 2017 The Guilford Press. Permission to photocopy this handout is granted to purchasers of this book for personal use or use with individual clients (see copyright page for details). Purchasers can download enlarged versions of this material (see the box at the end of the table of contents).

THINKING, FEELING, AND DOING

This picture shows two children in the same situation, but they have very different thoughts about it. How do their thoughts lead to different feelings, body responses, and actions?

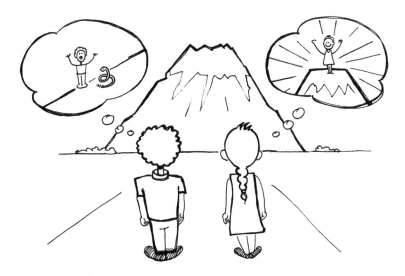

Two people can have different feelings, body responses, and actions in the same situation, all because of how they think about it. Here is an example of one person in a situation who could be having two very different thoughts—one positive and one negative.

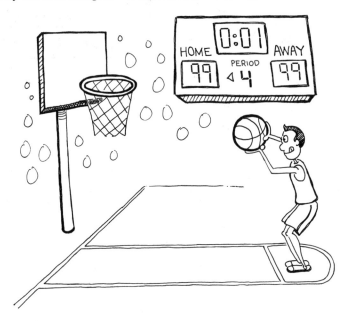

How would those thoughts affect his feelings, body responses, and actions differently? If you were any of these characters, how would you choose to think and why?

245

INFORMATION PROCESSING

When information comes into your brain, you have to think about it to know how to react to it. How you process information can be related to previous experiences, how you are feeling, and what you are paying attention to. Brains are designed to pay more attention to danger than to safety, something called an "attention bias," which is supposed to protect you against danger, like checking for cars before you cross the street. But sometimes this negative attention bias isn't helpful, like when you pay attention to how bad your symptoms might be in a situation. In fact, you're more likely to notice things that prove your negative thoughts *right* and end up missing the things that are good or could help you.

Here is a child who has a lot of information coming into his brain about going to school. There are a few examples of what he is thinking about in the bubbles and a few blank bubbles for you to add your own examples.

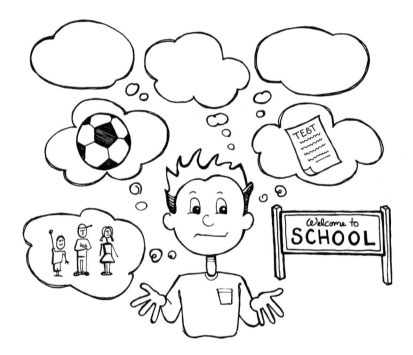

If he has a negative attention bias to processing information about school, how would he think about taking a test? Or playing sports in gym class? Or meeting other kids? What about the things you wrote in the bubbles? How would these things make him feel emotionally and in his body?

Is there another way to process the same information about school in a more positive way? If he had those thoughts, how would his feelings and body responses be different?

What can you take away about how you can process information in any situation?

COGNITIVE DISTORTIONS

Cognitive distortions are exaggerated thought patterns that reinforce negative thoughts. They are like *thinking traps* that people get stuck in, and *unhelpful thinking styles*, because they do not help you get to your goals!

All-or-Nothing Thinking: When you see things as all good or bad, in black and white, without seeing the middle ground or the shades of gray.
- If I don't get an A on the test, I'll fail the class.

Mental Filter: When you pay attention only to negative evidence and dwell on it.
- I didn't make the shot and we lost the game.

Jumping to Conclusions: There are two ways to jump to conclusions.
  Mind Reading: When you guess what others are thinking about you or your situation.
  - My teacher thinks I'm faking being sick.

  Fortune Telling: When you try to predict the future or outcome of a situation.
  - I'm going to get a stomachache at the recital and have to run to the bathroom.

Emotional Reasoning: When you make decisions based on how you feel; "I feel it; therefore, it is true."
- I feel anxious; therefore, it's a bad situation and it means I should avoid it.

Labeling: When you give yourself or other people a label.
- I'm the sick kid.

Overgeneralizing: When you assume a pattern based on one event and draw broad conclusions.
- I always give the wrong answer in history class, so I'm just bad at history.

Disqualifying the Positive: When you ignore the good things that happen.
- Today was just OK (not counting hanging with friends, fun at lunch, good grade, etc.).

Catastrophizing: When you exaggerate or magnify the importance of things, like your mistake or someone else's success.
- Missing today's practice means I'm never going to get to play on the team.

Minimizing: The opposite of catastrophizing, when you shrink your successes.
- It doesn't count as a good day just because I stayed at school; I still felt dizzy all day.

"Should" Statements: When you try to motivate yourself with words like "should," "shouldn't," "must," or "ought"; this causes guilt. When you use these statements to describe others, you may feel frustrated with them.
- I should be able to walk around the mall with my friends.
- My friends should be more supportive of my symptoms.

Personalization: When you feel responsible for something that was not your fault.
- It's my fault my teacher looks frustrated because I asked for extra help to get caught up.

THOUGHT RECORD

Date	Situation What happened?	Thoughts What was I thinking about?	Body Responses What was going on in my body?	Feelings What was I feeling?	Actions What did I do?

REFRAMING THOUGHTS

Situation: _____

Thoughts

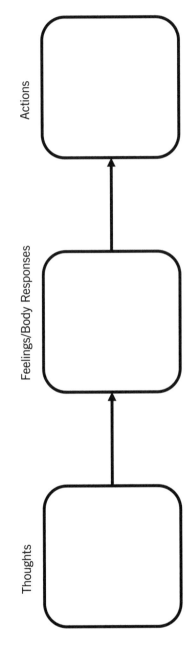

Feelings/Body Responses

Actions

Are these thoughts true? Are they helpful? Are there any other ways to think that might lead to different feelings/body responses and actions?

NEW Thoughts

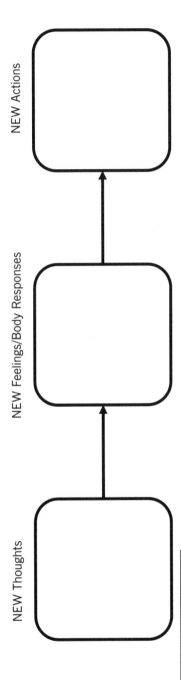

NEW Feelings/Body Responses

NEW Actions

WAYS TO CHALLENGE THOUGHTS

What evidence goes against this thought?

What would I say to someone else in my shoes?

What new knowledge do I have that could help in this situation?

What would happen if I kept thinking this way?

What would really be so bad about that?

Am I able to read minds?

What happened the last time?

Is there anything good that could happen?

How likely is that to happen?

Has that ever happened before?

So what if it does happen?

Do I really know this to be true?

Am I focusing on one detail or mistake rather than the whole picture?

Is this thought helpful?

Are there times when this was not true?

Is there a middle ground?

Can I predict the future?

Am I thinking too far ahead?

Am I missing any positives?

Is there something I'm not giving myself credit for?

Is this thought true?

Is there another way to think about it?

Do I have control over this?

Is there anything I can change about the situation?

PROBLEM SOLVING

Step 1: Identify the problem—What is the problem or thing you would like to change?
- Pick one problem.

Step 2: Set the goal—What would you like to have happen?
- Write the goal in achievable terms.

Step 3: Brainstorm solutions—How are you going to get it done?
- 4–6 ideas; be creative, no judgment.

	Rating

Step 4: Evaluate solutions—Is this a good idea?
- Rate solutions on a scale from 1 (not so great) to 10 (will probably work). Think about benefits/drawbacks.

Step 5: Choose your best solution and try it out—Did it work?
- Be patient, it might not work right away.

Step 6: If needed, go back to the list and try again—What's your second choice?
- Pick another solution to try

COPING PLAN

Strategy	What it helps	When to use it	How long to use it
Healthy habits			
Schedule			
Breathing			
Muscle relaxation			
Imagery			
Distracting activities			
Reframing			
Problem solving			
Goal setting			
Other			

TAKE A BREAK

The phrase "Take a BREAK!" helps children remember their coping skills, including the importance of:

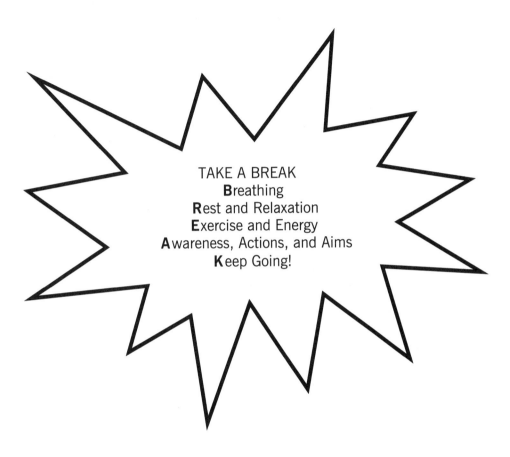

TAKE A BREAK
Breathing
Rest and Relaxation
Exercise and Energy
Awareness, Actions, and Aims
Keep Going!

B: diaphragmatic breathing
R: good sleep and use of relaxation skills
E: healthy habits including exercise, good eating, and hydration
A: awareness of thoughts and feelings, distracting activities, and goals
K: the importance of continuing to use skills for symptoms and challenges

PROVIDING SUPPORT TO CHILDREN WITH SOMATIC SYMPTOMS

It can be hard to find the right balance between supporting children with somatic symptoms *and* encouraging them to participate in their activities and use positive coping skills. These tips provide guidance on how to help children with somatic symptoms cope with challenges and improve function. These are helpful for parents, extended family, coaches, teachers, babysitters, and friends to follow.

- **Encourage normal activity:** Stick to a regular routine every day and during somatic symptom episodes, both at school and at play. If a reduction in activity is necessary, provide no special treatment.

- **Tolerate distress:** Demonstrate to the child you can handle his or her distress by showing minimal worry or concern and remaining calm. Somatic symptoms can be scary and can seem worse if adults look worried.

- **Balance attention to symptoms:** Do not ask about symptoms, as attention to symptoms only makes them worse. Encourage the child to place attention on something else, such as an active or distracting coping strategy.

- **Promote positive coping:** Reinforce the child's use of a new skill or positive coping strategy by specifically praising the effort, not the outcome. Pay attention to what the child *can* do, rather than what he or she *cannot*.

- **Respond flexibly:** Above all, adopt a flexible approach. Try to look at the circumstances, identify the problem, and help the child choose from their toolkit of coping strategies. There isn't just one answer. Keep the overall focus on function.

GENERAL SCHOOL LETTER TEMPLATE

(Insert individual information for words in ALL CAPS.)

Dear Administration:

This letter is to confirm that GRADE student NAME is receiving cognitive-behavioral therapy (CBT) in the Psychology Clinic. Specifically, NAME is receiving treatment for CONDITION, which is a chronic medical condition characterized by SYMPTOMS caused by a dysregulation in the nervous system/CAUSE. The symptoms are real, but are not dangerous in the sense that they are not caused by acute illness, injury, or disease. These challenging problems have interfered with NAME's ability to attend a regular school day and keep up with HIS/HER work this academic year. Thank you for all you have done to support HIM/HER in school. As a child psychologist/ therapist specializing in somatic symptoms, I am working with NAME, HIS/HER family, and HIS/HER medical team to help manage HIS/HER symptoms and increase HIS/HER ability to function.

Somatic symptoms have both physical and psychosocial components. Physically, it's difficult for children with somatic symptoms to remain in school for a full day. Sitting in hard-back chairs increases stiffness and musculoskeletal pain, dizziness and problems with walking are magnified in crowded hallways and stairwells, and limited bathroom breaks make stomach symptoms hard to manage. Waking up early in the morning and the demand on concentration are additional physical challenges. Like any medical condition, somatic symptoms are made worse by emotional and social stress, so it is typical for symptoms to increase on school days when a child encounters worry or frustration with academic work, has to cope with intense symptoms in a public setting, or has difficult peer interactions. The recommendations include a variety of strategies aimed at improving school attendance and performance as well as managing stressful situations that may exacerbate the cycle of symptoms and disability. Please keep in mind that while stress and symptoms are closely related, this does *not* mean that the symptoms are made up or that psychosocial challenges alone cause the symptoms.

Somatic symptom intensity fluctuates. Children often ignore or distract themselves from symptoms by functioning in positive activities and then experience more symptoms during times of stress, leading to varying levels of observable symptoms and distress. In a school setting, this can result in NAME appearing to be quite "well" at times and in significant distress at other times, which can be misleading and cause confusion about the nature of symptoms, particularly when NAME appears well during fun activities and distressed during difficult times. However, when this presentation leads to NAME or HIS/HER family being questioned about how "real" the condition is, it only adds stress and frustration for HIM/HER. Eliminating questions about the validity of HIS/HER condition is the most helpful approach for promoting HIS/HER ability to positively manage symptoms.

We strongly encourage children like NAME with this condition to engage in as much normal functioning as possible, including attending school. This condition is not associated with any specific time line in terms of recovery, which varies greatly by individual. It would be helpful for NAME to have a *flexible* school plan that meets HIS/HER educational needs while HE/SHE engages in treatment by allowing the following accommodations:

(continued)

GENERAL SCHOOL LETTER TEMPLATE

1. From a physical standpoint, NAME would benefit from additional time to transfer between classes and not be counted as tardy, not only so HE/SHE can pace HIS/HER physical exertion but also so HE/SHE has a chance to use the restroom if needed. Please provide a second set of books for NAME to keep at home to minimize the weight of the backpack HE/SHE carries to and from school. Please allow HIM/HER to use the elevator on days when HE/SHE's unable to use the stairs in a safe and timely manner.

2. If NAME has periods of substantially increased work to either make up or complete, it would be useful to modify the assignments in the short term so that HE/SHE is at less risk of falling behind in the long term. Having less work to make up will limit the stress that accompanies and worsens chronic conditions, making it easier for HIM/HER to stay engaged in HIS/HER classes. Having teachers grade work that has been completed instead of giving zeros for missing assignments would also help HIM/HER keep up HIS/HER usual level of performance.

3. NAME is being taught to use breaks and relaxation strategies to cope with symptoms right there in the school setting rather than being sent home. Please allow NAME to spend 5–10 minutes in the bathroom, nurse's office, or another quiet place as needed to cope with symptom flares. HE/SHE should also be allowed to stand up, stretch, and move around in the classroom as needed to manage discomfort that comes with sitting for long periods of time; a seat in the back of the classroom would help HIM/HER to do this without feeling out of place or being disruptive to the class.

4. Please allow NAME to carry a water bottle in school. Dehydration is a trigger for symptoms and the length of the school day does not allow for adequate hydration to achieve HIS/HER daily fluid intake goal. It would be helpful if NAME could have a permanent pass to allow for bathroom breaks, which will be more frequent.

5. Please communicate the information in this letter to all of NAME's teachers so they are aware of HIS/HER medical concerns and these special accommodations. It adds additional stress for students when they have to explain their coping requests or medical situations to teachers, especially when they are in class or in front of other students. This communication will help teachers be sensitive to NAME's needs and provide accommodations in their classrooms without the need for further explanation by NAME.

6. NAME will need to attend future doctor's appointments for symptom management. It would be helpful if the school could support HIM/HER should HE/SHE need to miss school for these appointments.

NAME's family will be happy to work out the details of implementing this plan with you. NAME is committed to being a good student with regular attendance despite HIS/HER condition, and it is my hope that attending to HIS/HER current school stressors, along with treating HIS/HER symptoms and encouraging increased function, can help get HIM/HER back on track physically, academically, and emotionally. Thank you in advance for your assistance in creating as supportive an environment as possible as NAME copes with HIS/HER condition. Ongoing communication between NAME's school, family, and treatment team is vital to ensuring HIS/HER success in these efforts, so I welcome contact with you.

Sincerely,

SCHOOL SUBJECT TRACKING FORM

Subject:	Mon.	Tues.	Wed.	Thurs.	Fri.
Turns in homework					
Is prepared for class					
Gets right to work					
Follows directions					
Gives good effort					
Stays on task					
Total					

Parent signature: _____

Teacher signature: _____

SPECIFIC SCHOOL SYMPTOM PLAN TEMPLATE

(Insert individual information for words in ALL CAPS.)

Dear Administration,

Thank you for your ongoing communication in regards to GRADE student NAME, who as you know has CONDITION, which is a medical condition characterized by SYMPTOMS caused by a dysregulation in the nervous system/CAUSE. The symptoms are real, but are not dangerous in the sense that they are not caused by acute illness, injury, or disease. If NAME has episodes of SOMATIC SYMPTOMS in the school setting, we recommend the following plan for how school staff should interact with HIM/HER to promote a focus on function, which is the way NAME is being taught to cope with symptoms in treatment:

1. When discussing NAME's school plan or symptoms, focus on ways that NAME can positively cope with symptoms and engage in school as normally as possible, rather than focus on ways that HE/SHE is sick or disabled. Help HIM/HER to problem-solve which coping skills to use if worried about or focusing on symptoms in a functional way, which is what HE/SHE is being taught to do in treatment.

2. Provide and stick to a structured, consistent routine on a daily basis, *especially* during times of increased symptoms. If NAME has an episode, have HIM/HER return to HIS/HER regular schedule as soon as possible. Provide rewards for engagement in a normal routine.

3. Please allow NAME to visit the nurse's office as needed for medication that has been prescribed by the doctor. After taking the medicine, HE/SHE may either take a short break to cope with symptoms or return to class. We do not recommend that HE/SHE call home or expect to go home when experiencing typical symptoms at school. Under extreme conditions, or in the face of unusual symptoms, such as fever, the school nurse should use discretion with this guideline.

4. Encourage NAME to manage HIS/HER symptoms independently. Do not rush in or overly comfort HIM/HER. While it's natural to want to help, this response can increase stimulation when HE/SHE needs to calm down and focus, which HE/SHE can best accomplish on HIS/HER own.

5. Do not ask NAME about physical health or symptoms. Even when school staff mean well by checking on how HE/SHE is feeling, this increases attention to symptoms, which makes them worse. Instead, make positive comments about how NAME is functioning or say, "Good to see you" in instead of "How are you?"

6. Overall, please allow NAME to engage in meaningful activities in school that do not center around symptom management, such as helping a teacher in the classroom before school or during lunch. This allows NAME to feel positive about HIS/HER effect in school and gives HIM/HER something to look forward to doing in the school setting.

Thank you again for your assistance in creating a supportive and productive learning environment for NAME. Please continue to stay in touch as this plan is implemented in school.

Sincerely,

REFERRING PROVIDER LETTER TEMPLATE

(Insert individual information in blanks and for words in ALL CAPS.)

Dear Referring Provider,

Recently, I met with NAME and FAMILY in response to your referral for assessment and treatment of SOMATIC SYMPTOMS. During the biopsychosocial assessment, NAME and FAMILY reported concerns in the following areas: _____. Symptoms are affecting NAME's quality of life and are causing impairment in functioning. NAME and FAMILY did/did not report mood concerns, including _____. NAME meets diagnostic criteria for the following: DIAGNOSIS.

    During the consultation, a summary of cognitive-behavioral therapy (CBT) intervention was provided to the family, including description of treatment efficacy, course, and content. Skills relevant to coping with somatic symptoms include understanding and use of healthy habits, a daily schedule, hydration, sleep, diet, and exercise, relaxation and diaphragmatic breathing, the role of distracting and pleasant activities, and cognitive techniques (e.g., reframing, problem solving). Active treatment is likely to last approximately 8 to 16 weekly to biweekly sessions. NAME may require additional treatment as needed for maintenance of skills.

    NAME and FAMILY appear to be willing and able to adhere to treatment recommendations and were scheduled for follow up on DATE. Questions and concerns were addressed during this consultation.

Thank you for referring NAME for treatment of SOMATIC SYMPTOMS. I will contact you to discuss frequency of communication necessary for effective collaborative care. Please contact me should you have any questions or concerns.

Sincerely,

References

American Psychiatric Association. (2013). *Diagnostic and statistical manual of mental disorders* (5th ed.). Arlington, VA: Author.

Anthony, K. K., & Schanberg, L. E. (2005). Pediatric pain syndromes and management of pain in children and adolescents with rheumatic disease. *Pediatric Clinics of North America, 52,* 611–639.

Aronowitz, R. A. (2001). When do symptoms become a disease? *Annals of Internal Medicine, 134,* 803–808.

Bagayogo, I. P., Interian, A., & Escobar, J. (2013). Transcultural aspects of somatic symptoms in the context of depressive disorders. *Advances in Psychosomatic Medicine, 33,* 64–74.

Bakvis, P., Spinhoven, P., & Roelofs, K. (2009). Basal cortisol is positively correlated to threat vigilance in patients with psychogenic nonepileptic seizures. *Epilepsy and Behavior, 16*(3), 558–560.

Bandura, A. (1986). *Social foundations of thought and action: A social cognitive theory.* Englewood Cliffs, NJ: Prentice-Hall.

Bao, C. H., Liu, P., Liu, H. R., Wu, L. Y., Jin, X. M., Wang, S. Y., et al. (2016). Differences in regional homogeneity between patients with Crohn's disease with and without abdominal pain revealed by resting-state functional magnetic resonance imaging. *Pain, 157*(5), 1037–1044.

Bass, C., & Halligan, P. (2014). Factitious disorders and malingering: Challenges for clinical assessment and management. *Lancet, 383*(9926), 1422–1432.

Bauer, A. M., Quas, J. A., & Boyce, W. T. (2002). Associations between physiological reactivity and children's behavior: Advantages of a multisystem approach. *Journal of Developmental and Behavioral Pediatrics, 23*(2), 102–113.

Beck, A. T., Rush, A. J., Shaw, B. F., & Emery, G. (1979). *Cognitive therapy of depression.* New York: Guilford Press.

Beck, J. E. (2008). A developmental perspective on functional somatic symptoms. *Journal of Pediatric Psychology, 33*(5), 547–562.

Belmaker, E., Espinoza, R., & Pogrund, R. (1985). Use of medical services by adolescents with non-specific somatic symptoms. *International Journal of Adolescent Medicine and Health, 1,* 150–156.

Black, D. N., Seritan, A. L., Taber, K. H., & Hurley, R. A. (2004). Conversion hysteria: Lessons from functional imaging. *Journal of Neuropsychiatry and Clinical Neurosciences, 16*(3), 245–251.

Blount, R. L., Davis, N., Powers, S. W., & Roberts, M. C. (1991). The influence of environmental factors and coping style on children's coping and distress. *Clinical Psychology Review, 11*(1), 93–116.

Blount, R. L., Simons, L. E., Devine, K. A., Jaaniste, T., Cohen, L. L., Chambers, C. T., et al. (2008). Evidence-based assessment of coping and stress in pediatric psychology. *Journal of Pediatric Psychology, 33*(9), 1021–1045.

Boyce, W. T., Quas, J., Alkon, A., Smider, N. A., Essex, M. J., & Kupfer, D. J. (2001). Autonomic reactivity and psychopathology in middle childhood. *British Journal of Psychiatry, 179*(2), 144–150.

Bronfenbrenner, U. (1979). *The ecology of human development: Experiments by nature and design.* Cambridge, MA: Harvard University Press.

Byars, K. C., Brown, R. T., Campbell, R. M., & Hobbs, S. A. (2000). Psychological adjustment and coping in a population of children with recurrent syncope. *Journal of Developmental and Behavioral Pediatrics, 21*(3), 189–197.

Campo, J. V. (2012). Annual research review: Functional somatic symptoms and associated anxiety and depression—developmental psychopathology in pediatric practice. *Journal of Child Psychology and Psychiatry, 53*(5), 575–592.

Campo, J. V., & Fritsch, S. L. (1994). Somatization in children and adolescents. *Journal of the American Academy of Child and Adolescent Psychiatry, 33*, 1223–1235.

Carson, A. J., Ringbauer, B., Stone, J., McKenzie, L., Warlow, C., & Sharpe, M. (2000). Do medically unexplained symptoms matter?: A prospective cohort study of 300 new referrals to neurology outpatient clinics. *Journal of Neurology, Neurosurgery, and Psychiatry, 68*, 207–210.

Chan, E., Piira, T., & Betts, G. (2005). The school functioning of children with chronic and recurrent pain. *Pediatric Pain Letter, 7*(2–3), 11–16.

Claar, R. L., & Scharff, L. (2007). Parent and child perceptions of chronic pain treatments. *Children's Health Care, 36*, 285–301.

Coghill, R. C., Sang, C. N., Maisog, J. M., & Iadarola, M. J. (1999). Pain intensity processing within the human brain: A bilateral, distributed mechanism. *Journal of Neurophysiology, 82*(4), 1934–1943.

Compas, B. E., Connor-Smith, J. K., Saltzman, H., Thomsen, A. H., & Wadsworth, M. E. (2001). Coping with stress during childhood and adolescence: Problems, progress, and potential in theory and research. *Psychological Bulletin, 127*(1), 87.

Creed, F. (2009). Medically unexplained symptoms—blurring the line between "mental" and "physical" in somatoform disorders. *Journal of Psychosomatic Research, 67*(3), 185–187.

Dalton, C. B., Drossman, D. A., Hathaway, J. M., & Bangdiwala, S. I. (2004). Perceptions of physicians and patients with organic and functional gastrointestinal diagnoses. *Clinical Gastroenterology and Hepatology, 2*, 121–126.

de Schipper, L. J., Vermeulen, M., Eeckhout, A. M., & Foncke, E. M. (2014). Diagnosis and management of functional neurological symptoms: The Dutch experience. *Clinical Neurology and Neurosurgery, 122*, 106–112.

Deary, V., Chalder, T., & Sharpe, M. (2007). The cognitive behavioural model of medically unexplained symptoms: A theoretical and empirical review. *Clinical Psychology Review, 27*(7), 781–797.

Dengler-Crish, C. M., Horst, S. N., & Walker, L. S. (2011). Somatic complaints in childhood functional abdominal pain are associated with functional gastrointestinal disorders in adolescence and adulthood. *Journal of Pediatric Gastroenterology and Nutrition, 52*(2), 162–165.

Diers, M., Koeppe, C., Yilmaz, P., Thieme, K., Markela-Lerenc, J., Schiltenwolf, M., et al. (2008). Pain ratings and somatosensory evoked responses to repetitive intramuscular and intracutaneous stimulation in fibromyalgia syndrome. *Journal of Clinical Neurophysiology, 25*(3), 153–160.

Drossman, D. A. (1998). Gastrointestinal illness and the biopsychosocial model. *Psychosomatic Medicine, 60*, 258–267.

Drossman, D. A. (2016). Functional gastrointestinal disorders: History, pathophysiology, clinical features, and Rome IV. *Gastroenterology, 150*(6), 1262–1279.

Due, P., Holstein, B. E., Lynch, J., Diderichsen, F., Gabhain, S., Scheidt, P., et al. (2005). Bullying and symptoms among school-aged children: International comparative cross sectional study in 28 countries. *European Journal of Public Health, 15*(2), 128–132.

Eccleston, C., Palermo, T. M., Williams, A., Lewandowski, A., & Morley, S. (2009). Psychological therapies for the management of chronic and recurrent pain in children and adolescents. *Cochrane Database of Systematic Reviews, 2*(2).

Eisenberg, L. (1977). Disease and illness: Distinctions between professional and popular ideas of sickness. *Culture, Medicine and Psychiatry, 1,* 9–23.

Eminson, D. M. (2007). Medically unexplained symptoms in children and adolescents. *Clinical Psychology Review, 27*(7), 855–871.

Eminson, M., Benjamin, S., Shortall, A., Woods, T., & Faragher, B. (1996). Physical symptoms and illness attitudes in adolescents: An epidemiological study. *Journal of Child Psychology and Psychiatry, 37*(5), 519–528.

Engel, G. (1977). The need for a new medical model: A challenge for biomedicine. *Science, 196,* 129–136.

Escobar, J., & Gureje, O. (2007). Influence of cultural and social factors on the epidemiology of idiopathic somatic complaints and syndromes. *Psychosomatic Medicine, 69*(9), 841–845.

Folkman, S., & Lazarus, R. S. (1985). If it changes it must be a process: Study of emotion and coping during three stages of a college examination. *Journal of Personality and Social Psychology, 48*(1), 150–170.

Friedrich, W. N., & Schafer, L. C. (1995). Somatic symptoms in sexually abused children. *Journal of Pediatric Psychology, 20*(5), 661–670.

Fritz, G. K., Fritsch, S., & Hagino, O. (1997). Somatoform disorders in children and adolescents: A review of the past 10 years. *Journal of the American Academy of Child and Adolescent Psychiatry, 36*(10), 1329–1338.

Garralda, M. E. (1999). Practitioner review: Assessment and management of somatisation in childhood and adolescence: A practical perspective. *Journal of Child Psychology and Psychiatry, 40*(8), 1159–1167.

Gatchel, R. J., Peng, Y. B., Peters, M. L., Fuchs, P. N., & Turk, D. C. (2007). The biopsychosocial approach to chronic pain: Scientific advances and future directions. *Psychological Bulletin, 133,* 581–624.

Grubb, B. P., Gerard, G., Wolfe, D. A., Samoil, D., Davenport, C. W., Homan, R. W., et al. (1992). Syncope and seizures of psychogenic origin: Identification with head-upright tilt table testing. *Clinical Cardiology, 15*(11), 839–842.

Grubb, B. P., & Karabin, B. (2008). Postural tachycardia syndrome: Perspectives for patients. *Circulation, 118*(3), e61–e62.

Gunnar, M. R., Bruce, J., & Hickman, S. E. (2001). Salivary cortisol response to stress in children. *Advances in Psychosomatic Medicine, 22,* 52–60.

Hatcher, J. W., Powers, L. L., & Richtsmeier, A. (1993). Parental anxiety and response to symptoms of minor illness in infants. *Journal of Pediatric Psychology, 18,* 397–408.

Hofmann, S. G., Asnaani, A., Vonk, I. J., Sawyer, A. T., & Fang, A. (2012). The efficacy of cognitive behavioral therapy: A review of meta-analyses. *Cognitive Therapy and Research, 36*(5), 427–440.

Hubbard, C. S., Becerra, L., Heinz, N., Ludwick, A., Rasooly, T., Wu, R., et al. (2016). Abdominal pain, the adolescent and altered brain structure and function. *PLoS One, 11*(5), e0156545.

Husain, K., Browne, T., & Chalder, T. (2007). A review of psychological models and interventions for medically unexplained somatic symptoms in children. *Child and Adolescent Mental Health, 12*(1), 2–7.

Jessop, D. J., & Stein, R. (1985). Uncertainty and its relation to the psychological and social correlates of chronic illness in children. *Social Science and Medicine, 20,* 993–999.

Kanaan, R. A., Armstrong, D., & Wessely, S. C. (2011). Neurologists' understanding and management of conversion disorder. *Journal of Neurology, Neurosurgery, and Psychiatry, 82*(9), 961–966.

Kanner, A. D., Feldman, S. S., Weinberger, D. A., & Ford, M. E. (1987). Uplifts, hassles, and adaptational outcomes in adolescents. *Journal of Early Adolescence, 7*(4), 371–394.

Kaplan, R. M., Ganiats, T. G., & Frosch, D. L. (2004). Diagnostic and treatment decisions in US healthcare. *Journal of Health Psychology, 9,* 29–40.

Kashikar-Zuck, S., Flowers, S. R., Claar, R. L., Guite, J. W., Logan, D. E., Lynch-Jordan, A. M., et al. (2011). Clinical utility and validity of the Functional Disability Inventory in a multicenter sample of youth with chronic pain. *Pain, 152*(7), 1600–1607.

Kendall, P. C., & Pimentel, S. S. (2003). On the physiological symptom constellation in youth with generalized anxiety disorder (GAD). *Journal of Anxiety Disorders, 17*(2), 211–221.

Keller, N. R., & Robertson, D. (2006). Familial orthostatic tachycardia. *Current Opinion in Cardiology, 21*(3), 173–179.

Kiecolt-Glaser, J. K., McGuire, L., Robles, T. F., & Glaser, R. (2002). Psychoneuroimmunology: Psychological influences on immune function and health. *Journal of Consulting and Clinical Psychology, 70*(3), 537–547.

Korsch, B. M., Gozzi, E. K., & Francis, V. (1968). Gaps in doctor–patient communication: 1. Doctor-patient interaction and patient satisfaction. *Pediatrics, 42*(5), 855–871.

Kozlowska, K., English, M., & Savage, B. (2013). Connecting body and mind: The first interview with somatising patients and their families. *Clinical Child Psychology and Psychiatry, 18*(2), 224–245.

Kozlowska, K., Palmer, D. M., Brown, K. J., Scher, S., Chudleigh, C., Davies, F., et al. (2015). Conversion disorder in children and adolescents: A disorder of cognitive control. *Journal of Neuropsychology, 9*(1), 87–108.

Kozlowska, K., Scher, S., & Williams, L. M. (2011). Patterns of emotional–cognitive functioning in pediatric conversion patients: Implications for the conceptualization of conversion disorders. *Psychosomatic Medicine, 73*(9), 775–788.

Kroenke, K., & Mangelsdorff, A. (1989). Common symptoms in ambulatory care: Incidence, evaluation, therapy, and outcome. *American Journal of Medicine, 86,* 262–266.

LaFrance, W. C., Reuber, M., & Goldstein, L. H. (2013). Management of psychogenic nonepileptic seizures. *Epilepsia, 54*(Suppl. 1), 53–67.

Lazarus, R. S., & Folkman, S. (1984). *Stress, appraisal, and coping.* New York: Springer.

Legrain, V., Van Damme, S., Eccleston, C., Davis, K. D., Seminowicz, D. A., & Crombez, G. (2009). A neurocognitive model of attention to pain: Behavioral and neuroimaging evidence. *Pain, 144*(3), 230–232.

Levant, R. F. (2005). Psychological approaches to the management of health and disease: Health care for the whole person. In N. A. Cummings, W. T. O'Donohue, & E. V. Naylor (Eds.), *Psychological approaches to chronic disease management* (pp. 37–48). Reno, NV: Context Press.

Levy, R. L., Whitehead, W. E., Walker, L. S., Von Korff, M., Feld, A. D., Garner, M., et al. (2004). Increased somatic complaints and health-care utilization in children: Effects of parent IBS status and parent response to gastrointestinal symptoms. *American Journal of Gastroenterology, 99*(12), 2442–2451.

Logan, D. E., Simons, L. E., Stein, M. J., & Chastain, L. (2008). School impairment in adolescents with chronic pain. *Journal of Pain, 9*(5), 407–416.

Lynch-Jordan, A. M., Sil, S., Peugh, J., Cunningham, N., Kashikar-Zuck, S., & Goldschneider, K. (2014). Differential changes in functional disability and pain intensity over the course of psychological treatment for children with chronic pain. *Pain, 155*(10), 1955–1961.

Mayer, E. A., Naliboff, B. D., Chang, L., & Coutinho, S. V. (2001). Stress and irritable bowel syndrome. *American Journal of Physiology; Gastrointestinal and Liver Physiology, 280,* G519–G524.

McCracken, L. M., & Gauntlett-Gilbert, J. (2011). Role of psychological flexibility in parents of adolescents with chronic pain: Development of a measure and preliminary correlation analyses. *Pain, 152*(4), 780–785.

McGrady, A. (1996). Good news–bad press: Applied psychophysiology in cardiovascular disorders. *Biofeedback and Self-Regulation, 21*(4), 335–346.

McGrath, P. J. (1995). Annotation: Aspects of pain in children and adolescents. *Journal of Child Psychology and Psychiatry, 36*(5), 717–730.

Melzack, R., & Wall, P. D. (1967). Pain mechanisms: A new theory. *Survey of Anesthesiology, 11*(2), 89–90.

Merskey, H., & Bogduk, N. (1994). *Classification of chronic pain: IASP Task Force on Taxonomy.* Seattle, WA: International Association for the Study of Pain Press.

Minuchin, S., Baker, L., Rosman, B. L., Liebman, R., Milman, L., & Todd, T. C. (1975). A conceptual model of psychosomatic illness in children: Family organization and family therapy. *Archives of General Psychiatry, 32*(8), 1031–1038.

Olde Hartman, T. C., Hassink-Franke, L. J., Lucassen, P. L., van Spaendonck, K. P., & van Weel, C. (2009). Explanation and relations: How do general practitioners deal with patients with persistent medically unexplained symptoms: A focus group study. *BMC Family Practice, 10*(1), 68.

Paruthi, S., Brooks, L. J., D'Ambrosio, C., Hall, W. A., Kotagal, S., Lloyd, R. M., et al. (2016). Recommended amount of sleep for pediatric populations: A consensus statement of the American Academy of Sleep Medicine. *Journal of Clinical Sleep Medicine, 12*(6), 785–786.

Plioplys, S., Doss, J., Siddarth, P., Bursch, B., Falcone, T., Forgey, M., et al. (2014). A multisite controlled study of risk factors in pediatric psychogenic nonepileptic seizures. *Epilepsia, 55*(11), 1739–1747.

Puzanovova, M., Arbogast, P. G., Smith, C. A., Anderson, J., Diedrich, A., & Walker, L. S. (2009). Autonomic activity and somatic symptoms in response to success vs. failure on a cognitive task: A comparison of chronic abdominal pain patients and well children. *Journal of Psychosomatic Research, 67*(3), 235–243.

Rafanelli, C., Gostoli, S., Roncuzzi, R., & Sassone, B. (2013). Psychological correlates of vasovagal versus medically unexplained syncope. *General Hospital Psychiatry, 35*(3), 246–252.

Raj, S. R. (2013). Postural tachycardia syndrome (POTS). *Circulation, 127*(23), 2336–2342.

Rangel, L., Garralda, M. E., Levin, M., & Roberts, H. (2000). The course of severe chronic fatigue syndrome in childhood. *Journal of the Royal Society of Medicine, 93*(3), 129–134.

Reid, G. J., Gilbert, C. A., & McGrath, P. J. (1998). The pain coping questionnaire: Preliminary validation. *Pain, 76*(1), 83–96.

Reynolds, C., & Kamphaus, R. (2015). *Behavior Assessment System for Children, Third Edition (BASC-3).* Bloomington, MN: Pearson.

Rouster, A. S., Karpinski, A. C., Silver, D., Monagas, J., & Hyman, P. E. (2016). Functional gastrointestinal disorders dominate pediatric gastroenterology outpatient practice. *Journal of Pediatric Gastroenterology and Nutrition, 62*(6), 847–851.

Sapolsky, R. M. (2004). *Why zebras don't get ulcers* (3rd ed.). New York: Macmillan.

Saps, M., Youssef, N., Miranda, A., Nurko, S., Hyman, P., Cocjin, J., et al. (2009). Multicenter, randomized, placebo-controlled trial of amitriptyline in children with functional gastrointestinal disorders. *Gastroenterology, 137*(4), 1261–1269.

Sawchuk, T., & Buchhalter, J. (2015). Psychogenic nonepileptic seizures in children: Psychological presentation, treatment, and short-term outcomes. *Epilepsy and Behavior, 52*, 49–56.

Schechter, N. (2014). Functional pain: Time for a new name. *JAMA Pediatrics, 168*(8), 693–694.

Sharpe, M., & Carson, A. (2001). "Unexplained" somatic symptoms, functional syndromes, and somatization: Do we need a paradigm shift? *Annals of Internal Medicine, 134*, 926–930.

Shelby, G. D., Shirkey, K. C., Sherman, A. L., Beck, J. E., Haman, K., Shears, A. R., et al.. (2013). Functional abdominal pain in childhood and long-term vulnerability to anxiety disorders. *Pediatrics, 132*(3), 475–482.

Simons, L. E., Logan, D. E., Chastain, L., & Stein, M. (2010). The relation of social functioning to school impairment among adolescents with chronic pain. *Clinical Journal of Pain, 26*, 16–22.

Simons, L. E., Moulton, E. A., Linnman, C., Carpino, E., Becerra, L., & Borsook, D. (2014). The human amygdala and pain: Evidence from neuroimaging. *Human Brain Mapping, 35*(2), 527–538.

Skinner, B. F. (1953). *Science and human behavior.* New York: Simon & Schuster.

Sowder, E., Gevirtz, R., Shapiro, W., & Ebert, C. (2010). Restoration of vagal tone: A possible mechanism for functional abdominal pain. *Applied Psychophysiology and Biofeedback, 35*(3), 199–206.

Stewart, J. L., & Mishel, M. H. (2000). Uncertainty in childhood illness: A synthesis of the parent and child literature. *Scholarly Inquiry for Nursing Practice, 14,* 299–319.

Stone, A. L., & Walker, L. S. (2016). Adolescents' observations of parent pain behaviors: Preliminary measure validation and test of social learning theory in pediatric chronic pain. *Journal of Pediatric Psychology.* Online publication ahead of print.

Stone, J., Carson, A., & Sharpe, M. (2005). Functional symptoms and signs in neurology: Assessment and diagnosis. *Journal of Neurology, Neurosurgery, and Psychiatry, 76*(Suppl. 1), i2–12.

Strieper, M. J., Auld, D. O., Hulse, J. E., & Campbell, R. M. (1994). Evaluation of recurrent pediatric syncope: Role of tilt table testing. *Pediatrics, 93*(4), 660–662.

Susman, E. J., Dorn, L. D., & Schiefelbein, V. L. (2003). Puberty, sexuality, and health. In R. M. Lerner, M. A. Easterbrooks, & J. Mistry (Eds.), *The comprehensive handbook of psychology* (Vol. 6, pp. 293–324). New York: Wiley.

Tache, Y., Martinez, V., Million, M., & Rivier, J. (1999). Corticotropin-releasing factor and the brain–gut motor response to stress. *Canadian Journal of Gastroenterology, 13*(Suppl. A), 18A–25A.

Taylor, D. C., Szatmari, P., Boyle, M. H., & Offord, D. R. (1996). Somatization and the vocabulary of everyday bodily experiences and concerns: a community study of adolescents. *Journal of the American Academy of Child and Adolescent Psychiatry, 35*(4), 491–499.

Temple, J. L., Ziegler, A. M., Graczyk, A., Bendlin, A., Sion, T., & Vattana, K. (2014). Cardiovascular responses to caffeine by gender and pubertal stage. *Pediatrics, 134*(1), e112–e119.

Teng, E. J., Chaison, A. D., Bailey, S. D., Hamilton, J. D., & Dunn, N. J. (2008). When anxiety symptoms masquerade as medical symptoms: What medical specialists know about panic disorder and available psychological treatments. *Journal of Clinical Psychology in Medical Settings, 15*(4), 314–321.

Tobin, D. L., Holroyd, K. A., Reynolds, R., & Wigal, J. (1989). The hierarchical factor structure of the Coping Strategies Inventory. *Cognitive Therapy and Research, 13*(4), 343–361.

Tunaoglu, F. S., Olguntürk, R., Akcabay, S., Oguz, D., Gücüyener, K., & Demirsoy, S. (1995). Chest pain in children referred to a cardiology clinic. *Pediatric Cardiology, 16*(2), 69–72.

van Dijk, N., Quartieri, F., Blanc, J. J., Garcia-Civera, R., Brignole, M., Moya, A., et al. (2006). Effectiveness of physical counterpressure maneuvers in preventing vasovagal syncope: The Physical Counterpressure Manoeuvres Trial (PC-Trial). *Journal of the American College of Cardiology, 48*(8), 1652–1657.

van Geelen, S. M., Rydelius, P. A., & Hagquist, C. (2015). Somatic symptoms and psychological concerns in a general adolescent population: Exploring the relevance of DSM-5 somatic symptom disorder. *Journal of Psychosomatic Research, 79*(4), 251–258.

Van Slyke, D. A., & Walker, L. S. (2006). Mothers' responses to children's pain. *Clinical Journal of Pain, 22,* 387–391.

Varni, J. W., Seid, M., & Kurtin, P. S. (2001). PedsQL 4.0: Reliability and validity of the Pediatric Quality of Life Inventory Version 4.0 Generic Core Scales in healthy and patient populations. *Medical Care, 39*(8), 800–812.

Vervoort, T., Goubert, L., Eccleston, C., Bijttebier, P., & Crombez, G. (2006). Catastrophic thinking about pain is independently associated with pain severity, disability, and somatic complaints in school children and children with chronic pain. *Journal of Pediatric Psychology, 31*(7), 674–683.

Vitaliano, P. P., Russo, J., Carr, J. E., Maiuro, R. D., & Becker, J. (1985). The ways of coping checklist: Revision and psychometric properties. *Multivariate Behavioral Research, 20*(1), 3–26.

von Baeyer, C. L., Spagrud, L. J., McCormick, J. C., Choo, E., Neville, K., & Connelly, M. A. (2009). Three new datasets supporting use of the Numerical Rating Scale (NRS-11) for children's self-reports of pain intensity. *Pain, 143*(3), 223–227.

Vuilleumier, P. (2005). How brains beware: Neural mechanisms of emotional attention. *Trends in Cognitive Sciences, 9*(12), 585–594.

Wade, D. T., & Halligan, P. W. (2004). Do biomedical models of illness make for good healthcare systems? *British Journal of Medicine, 329*, 1398–1401.

Walker, E. A., Katon, W. J., Keegan, D., Gardner, G., & Sullivan, M. (1997a). Predictors of physician frustration in the care of patients with rheumatological complaints. *General Hospital Psychiatry, 19*, 315–323.

Walker, L. S., Beck, J. E., Garber, J., & Lambert, W. (2009). Children's Somatization Inventory: Psychometric properties of the revised form (CSI-24). *Journal of Pediatric Psychology, 34*(4), 430–440.

Walker, L. S., Dengler-Crish, C. M., Rippel, S., & Bruehl, S. (2010). Functional abdominal pain in childhood and adolescence increases risk for chronic pain in adulthood. *Pain, 150*(3), 568–572.

Walker, L. S., Garber, J., & Greene, J. (1993). Psychological correlates of recurrent abdominal pain: A comparison of pediatric patients with recurrent abdominal pain, organic illness, and psychiatric disorders. *Journal of Abnormal Psychology, 102*, 248–258.

Walker, L. S., Garber, J., Van Slyke, D. A., & Greene, J. W. (1995). Long-term health outcomes in patients with recurrent abdominal pain. *Journal of Pediatric Psychology, 20*, 233–245.

Walker, L. S., & Greene, J. W. (1989). Children with recurrent abdominal pain and their parents: More somatic complaints, anxiety, and depression than other patient families? *Journal of Pediatric Psychology, 14*, 231–243.

Walker, L. S., & Greene, J. (1991a). The Functional Disability Inventory: Measuring a neglected dimension of child health status. *Journal of Pediatric Psychology, 16*(1), 39–58.

Walker, L. S., & Greene, J. W. (1991b). Negative life events and symptom resolution in pediatric abdominal pain patients. *Journal of Pediatric Psychology, 16*(3), 341–360.

Walker, L. S., Smith, C. A., Garber, J., & Van Slyke, D. A. (1997b). Development and validation of the Pain Response Inventory for Children. *Psychological Assessment, 9*(4), 392–405.

Walker, L. S., Williams, S. E., Smith, C. A., Garber, J., Van Slyke, D. A., & Lipani, T. A. (2006). Parent attention versus distraction: Impact on symptom complaints by children and adolescents with and without chronic functional abdominal pain. *Pain, 122*, 43–52.

Walker, L. S., & Zeman, J. L. (1992). Parental response to child illness behavior. *Journal of Pediatric Psychology, 17*, 49–71.

Weiland, A., Blankenstein, A. H., Van Saase, J. L., Van der Molen, H. T., Jacobs, M. E., Abels, D. C., et al. (2015). Training medical specialists to communicate better with patients with medically unexplained physical symptoms (MUPS): A randomized, controlled trial. *PLoS One, 10*(9), e0138342.

Williams, S. E., Smith, C. A., Bruehl, S. P., Gigante, J., & Walker, L. S. (2009). Medical evaluation of children with chronic abdominal pain: Impact of diagnosis, physician practice orientation, and maternal trait anxiety on mothers' responses to the evaluation. *Pain, 146*(3), 283–292.

Woolf, C. J. (2011). Central sensitization: Implications for the diagnosis and treatment of pain. *Pain, 152*(3), S2–S15.

World Health Organization. (2015). *International statistical classification of diseases and related health problems* (10th rev.). Geneva, Switzerland: Author.

Zernikow, B., Wager, J., Hechler, T., Hasan, C., Rohr, U., Dobe, M., et al. (2012). Characteristics of highly impaired children with severe chronic pain: A 5-year retrospective study on 2249 pediatric pain patients. *BMC pediatrics, 12*(1), 1

Index